Author CONFERENCE ON EXPERIMENTAL MEDICINE AND SURGERY IN PRIMATES, 3rd, Lyon, 1972

Division of Im

GOLDSMITH E.I. & MOOR-JANKOWSKI J. (EDS.)
Medical Primatology 1972: Part III: Infectious Diseases, Oncology,
LOC: QY 60.P7/GOL 0001
~~0002551~~

AF795545

Selected papers from the Third Conference on Experimental Medicine and Surgery in Primates, Lyon, June 1972

Medical Primatology 1972

Part III

Infectious Diseases, Oncology, Pharmacology and Toxicology, Cardiovascular Studies

Edited by

EDWARD I. GOLDSMITH
Cornell University Medical College, New York, N.Y.

J. MOOR-JANKOWSKI
New York University School of Medicine, New York, N.Y.

In collaboration with

C. R. Austin
H. Balner
N. Barnicot
R. Cortesini
F. Deinhardt
N. Gengozian
G. A. Gresham
J. E. Hamner III
S. S. Kalter
R. Naquet
M. Panigel
F. T. Perkins
J. Ruffié
A. Schrier
M. Vastesaeger
G. Zbinden
E. Zuckerkandl

With 113 figures and 75 tables

S. Karger · Basel · München · Paris · London · New York · Sydney 1972

Medical Primatology 1970
XXII+997 p., 284 fig., 174 tab., 1971
ISBN 3-8055-1163-9

S. Karger · Basel · München · Paris · London · New York · Sydney
Arnold-Böcklin-Strasse 25, CH–4011 Basel (Switzerland)

All rights, including that of translation into other languages reserved. Photomechanic reproduction (photocopy, microcopy) of this volume or parts thereof without special permission of the publishers is prohibited.

© Copyright 1972 by S. Karger AG, Verlag für Medizin und Naturwissenschaften, Basel
Printed in Switzerland by Gassmann AG, Solothurn
ISBN 3-8055-1488-3

To Frank Glenn, MD

Professor of Surgery Emeritus, Cornell University Medical College, whose pioneering efforts on behalf of Medical Primatology have guided and encouraged the editors of these volumes

Contents

Part III

Infectious Diseases

Viral Oncology

Part I

General Primatology. Husbandry, Management, Breeding Choice of Species Conservation. Communication Media in Medical Primatology

Part II

Transplantation Immunology

Foreword

The three volumes of 'Medical Primatology 1972' consist of papers selected from communications presented at the Third Conference on Experimental Medicine and Surgery in Primates, held in Lyon, France, 21st–23rd June 1972. The program of the Conference was designed to gather new information to complement the former volume *Medical Primatology 1970*, which resulted from the Second Conference.

Papers chosen for the present volumes passed two selection procedures: (1) 246 abstracts were submitted of which 176 were accepted to be presented as papers at the Third Conference; (2) these complete papers were then evaluated for validity and relevance of the results presented. With the exception of review articles, only papers containing new information were accepted. The selection process led to some difficult decisions, as no time was available for resubmission of rejected papers. The chosen 120 papers were edited for style, correct simian taxonomy, bibliography, and appropriate cross references.

Despite the rigorous standards applied, we expect that shortcomings will still be found since little time was available for editing in order to obtain publication within seven months after the Conference. We hope, however, that *Medical Primatology 1972* will satisfy the objectives set at the First Conference in 1967, namely, to provide periodically an up-to-date and complete handbook and reference source covering the broad field of Medical Primatology.

Mr. THOMAS KARGER has continued to back up the new field of medical primatology despite the commercial risk involved. Miss DENISE GREDER and Mr. ROLF STEINEBRUNNER of the Karger firm, have assisted us at the Conference and during the following months of hard editorial labor. Miss

GETTA SKOTCHDOPOLE, Assistant Editor, attended most ably to the coordination of editorial efforts and to proof-reading. The Editors alone, being nonsimian primates, must accept the blame for inadequacies.

EDWARD I. GOLDSMITH, MD
Professor of Surgery
Cornell University Medical College, New York

J. MOOR-JANKOWSKI, MD
Research Professor
New York University School of Medicine, New York

Laboratory for Experimental Medicine and Surgery in Primates (LEMSIP) New York, November 1972

Organization Committee of the Third Conference on Experimental Medicine and Surgery in Primates 1972

WHO Delegates	W. I. B. BEVERIDGE, Geneva Z. FEJFAR, Geneva
National Delegates	
Belgium	Dr. ROBERT GORTZ University of Bruxelles Dr. J. MORTELMANS Institut de Médecine tropicale, Antwerp
Canada	Dr. SAMUEL SOLOMON Royal Victoria Hospital, Montreal
France	Dr. CHARLES MERIEUX Institut Merieux, Lyon Dr. ROBERT NAQUET Institut de Neuro-physiologie du CNRS, Marseille Dr. RENÉ TRIAU Fondation Merieux, Lyon
Germany	Dr. HANS-JÜRG KUHN Universität Frankfurt
Great Britain	Mr. K. R. HOBBS Medical Research Council, Carshalton Dr. F. T. PERKINS National Institute for Medical Research, London
Holland	Dr. HANS BALNER Radiobiological Institute TNO, Rijswijk
Israel	Dr. URI MARINOV National Council for Research and Development, Jerusalem

Italy	Dr. RAFFAELLO CORTESINI Università di Roma
Norway	Professor KARE BERG University of Oslo
Sweden	Professor ERNST BARANY Uppsala Universitet
Switzerland	Dr. HEINZ WEBER Sandoz AG, Basel Professor G. ZBINDEN Universität Zürich
United States	Dr. JULES S. CASS Veterans Administration, Washington, D.C. Dr. S. S. KALTER Southwest Foundation for Research and Education San Antonio, Texas Dr. C. H. KRATOCHVIL The Upjohn Company Kalamazoo
Scientific Secretary	Dr. J. RUFFIÉ Collège de France, Paris
Co-Chairmen	Dr. E. I. GOLDSMITH Cornell University Medical College, New York Dr. J. MOOR-JANKOWSKI New York University School of Medicine, New York

Sponsors and Benefactors of the Third Conference on Experimental Medicine and Surgery in Primates 1972

The Conference participants are greatly indebted to Dr. PIERRE DOROLLE, Deputy Director, World Health Organization, for the fruitful collaboration of WHO in the Conference.

The Conference was sponsored by the following international and national agencies:

International	European Society for the Study of Drug Toxicity International Association of Biologic Standardization
Belgium	Ministère de la Politique et Programmation Scientifique
Canada	McGill University, Montreal
France	Ministère de la Santé Publique et de la Sécurité Sociale Centre National de la Recherche Scientifique (CNRS) Institut National de la Santé et de la Recherche Médicale (INSERM) Université Paul Sabatier de Toulouse Université Claude Bernard de Lyon Fondation Merieux
Germany	German Pharmacological Society
Great Britain	The Royal College of Surgeons of England The Zoological Society of London
Holland	Netherlands Organization for Health Research
Israel	The Weizmann Institute

Italy	Italian Ministry of Health
Sweden	The Royal Swedish Academy of Sciences
Switzerland	Union of Swiss Societies of Experimental Biology
USA	New York University School of Medicine American Association for Laboratory Animal Science

The Conference Organization Committee is grateful to the governments and agencies which provided travel grants for their nationals to attend the Conference.

Our sincere thanks are due to Dr. CHARLES MERIEUX, the Merieux Foundation and the Merieux Institute. Their staff provided valuable scientific contributions to the Conference, assumed responsibility for the logistics, and offered warm hospitality to the participants, far beyond the usual role of hosts. The Merieux Foundation provided generously for the considerable expenditures of the local organization and helped many speakers to attend the Conference by defraying their expenses.

We wish to thank the following organizations, listed in alphabetical order, which contributed substantially to cover the expenses of the American participation in the Conference.

Major Contributors	*Baylor University* *Ciba-Geigy* *Generics Corporation of America* *Hoffmann-La Roche* *Schering Corporation* *The Upjohn Company*
Contributors	*Ortho Pharmaceutical Corporation* *Riker Laboratories, Inc.* *Sandoz Ltd. Basel* *Sherwood Medical Industries Inc.*

Infectious Diseases

Medical Primatology 1972. Proc. 3rd Conf. exp. Med. Surg. Primates, Lyon 1972, part III, pp. 2–12 (Karger, Basel 1972)

Diagnosis of Tuberculosis in Experimentally Infected Rhesus Monkeys *(Macaca mulatta)*

P. ACRED, PAMELA A. HUNTER, J. E. C. BYWATER and J. JAMES

Beecham Research Laboratories, Brockham Park, Betchworth, Surrey, Brittoncourt Tarm, Tyler Hill, Canterbury, Kent and Cooper-McDougal & Robertson Ltd., Berkhampstead, Herts

Introduction

Tuberculosis of nonhuman primates should no longer be considered a major hazard, either to the animals or the humans handling them, in view of the available diagnostic methods and therapy. However, despite available diagnostic methods there is still disagreement or rather lack of experimental assessment as to the value of the techniques. The principal methods used to diagnose tuberculosis are the intradermal tuberculin test and X-rays, with other methods, e.g. clinical appearance, body weight, erythrocyte sedimentation rate being of secondary importance. The allergic reaction to Koch's old tuberculin (KOT) in simians was first described in 1906 by BAERMAN and HALBERSTAEDTER, while the use of KOT for detection of tuberculosis in nonhuman primates was first reported by WHITE and FOX [1909]. This test which depended upon the temperature response of the monkeys to the s.c. administered tuberculin was time consuming and was not generally adopted. In 1938 SCHROEDER described his intrapalpebral technique for inoculating tuberculin purified protein derivate (PPD). Intradermal injection of 0.1 ml of a one-percent solution of PPD was given in the skin of the upper eye lid. A positive reaction consisting of oedema and erythema could be seen over a 72-hour post-inoculation period. Subsequent workers have established the value of the Schroeder technique [KENNARD and WILLNER, 1941; HABEL, 1947; BENSON *et al.*, 1955; HABERMANN and WILLIAMS, 1957; BYWATER *et al.*, 1962; STONES, 1969; HARTLEY, 1969].

Radiological examination, although of considerable value for detection of the advanced disease state, when animals may be anergic to tuberculin, is of limited value for detecting the early stages of the disease [SCHMIDT *et al.*, 1955; DOLOWY *et al.*, 1958; HIME, 1969]. Early diagnosis can also be confused by the presence of other pulmonary conditions, e.g. pneumonia, lung mites.

In monkeys, as in man, the erythrocyte sedimentation rate (ESR) increases during active tuberculosis, although this is not the only pathological condition giving rise to the response. FRANCIS [1956] reported that changes in the ESR proved a sensitive index of the effectiveness of various drugs against experimental tuberculosis in monkeys. Other diagnostic procedures which have been less frequently used were adequately reviewed by RUCH [1967].

This paper describes the procedures used to follow the course of a tubercular infection experimentally induced in rhesus monkeys, *Macaca mulatta*. The experiment was primarily set up to evaluate potentially useful antitubercular drugs, but as a consequence of the procedures used to follow the course of the infection, useful information relating to the diagnosis of tuberculosis in the rhesus monkey emerged.

Methods

The rhesus monkeys (weight 2.0–3.0 kg) used in the experiments were imported directly to the experimental quarters where they were quarantined for a period of six weeks. The animals were treated prophylactically on arrival for a period of three days with i.m. administered ampicillin at a dose of 50 mg/kg/day.

During the first week after arrival the thoraxes of the animals were X-rayed and tuberculin testing was carried out using the Schroeder intrapalpebral technique. Mammalian tuberculin PPD in a dose containing the equivalent of ten thousand IU old tuberculin (OT) was used for each monkey. Only those animals not responding to the tuberculin test and showing clear X-rays were used in the experiments.

Three experimental groups are considered:

(A) A group of 16 infected animals in which nine died by the end of the experiment (20 weeks post-infection).

(B) A group of seven infected animals treated daily i.m. with streptomycin sulphate 50 mg/kg; therapy being started 14 days post-infection.

(C) A group of three non-infected animals.

The monkeys were infected with *Mycobacterium tuberculosis* $H_{37}Rv$ by introducing a suspension of bacilli, prepared from an 18-day surface culture grown on Proskauer and Beck medium, directly into the main stem bronchus. This was achieved by placing the lightly anaesthetised animals (phencyclidine hydrochloride, 'Sernylan', Parke Davis and Co. 0.5–0.75 mg/kg) in a supine position and passing a tracheal tube down the trachea, the epiglotis being depressed by means of a modified canine vaginal speculum. The tube was passed to the bifurcation of the trachea and then into either the left or right main stem bronchus. The bacillary suspension containing 3×10^6 viable organisms/ml in a volume of 0.3 ml was injected into the bronchus, the mouth being held firmly closed for 30 sec to allow aspiration of the inoculum.

Diagnosis of the progress of the disease was determined by the following criteria:

(a) Body weight was recorded at weekly intervals throughout the 20-week period of the experiment.

(b) Clinical observations were carried out by daily visual and weekly physical examination of the monkeys.

(c) Hypersensitivity reactions to intradermal mammalian tuberculin PPD were determined at 14-day intervals throughout the 20 weeks of the experiment. Four dilutions of mammalian tuberculin PPD 2 mg/ml (equivalent in potency to 100,000 IU OT/ml) were used 10^{-1}, 10^{-2}, 10^{-3} and 10^{-4}. The four dilutions in volumes of 0.05 ml were injected intradermally into the shaved skin of the lower abdomen, which meant each monkey was injected with the equivalent of 500, 50, 5 and 0.5 IU OT. Hypersensitivity reactions were determined by measuring the increase in skin thickness at the site of the injection, the thickness being measured prior to and 72 h after injecting the PPD.

(d) ESR were determined by the Wintrobe method on the 1st and 2nd weeks of the test and thereafter at 14-day intervals to the 20th week.

(e) Radiology of the thorax was carried out at weekly intervals during the six weeks immediately following infection and then at 14-day intervals until the end of the test. The heavily sedated animals were strapped to a purpose-built table. Only dorsal/ventral aspect X-rays were taken. The tube/film distance was 36″, exposure $^1/_{20}$ sec., 50–55 kv, 40–60 mA, and a Schonander grid 75 lines/in was used. Lung inflation was not used as it was felt that in the more seriously affected animals inflation could further damage the lungs and affect the progress of the disease.

Results

Changes in body weight proved of no diagnostic consequence as it was only found when monkeys were in the final stages of the disease that any significant loss of body weight occurred. The monkeys in groups B and C, and those surviving in group A had a mean weight of 2.4 kg at the commencement of the experiment and the mean weight rose to 2.8 kg in the 20th week. The weights of the nine animals in group A dying as a consequence of the tubercular infection are shown in table I. The nine animals died between the 44th and 114th days post-infection with a mean time to death of 71 days.

Clinical observations were also of limited value, since it was only in the later stages of the disease that symptoms became obvious. Changes observed were loss of weight, anorexia, coughing in some animals, a distinctly grey pallor of the skin with wrinkling and dryness apparent, and associated with this was poor coat condition.

Table I. Body weights of rhesus monkeys *(Macaca mulatta)* infected experimentally with *Myocobacterium tuberculosis* $H_{37}Rv$

Group	Monkey	Weight, kg			Weeks from max. weight to death
		week 1	maximum	at death	
A	1	2.1	2.7	2.55	3
	2	2.8	3.2	1.9	5
	3	2.5	2.55	2.4	5
	4	1.9	1.9	1.5	7
	5	2.3	3.0	2.4	3
	6	2.1	2.5	1.95	3
	7	2.8	2.9	2.9	0
	8	2.3	2.55	2.15	4
	9	2.6	2.9	2.4	4
Mean		2.4	2.7	2.2	3.8

The three criteria proving of most use for continuously monitoring the disease were:

(1) Hypersensitivity reactions to intradermal mammalian tuberculin PPD.

(2) Changes in the chest X-ray.

(3) Changes in the ESR.

Responses to Purified Protein Derivative

The responses to the 10^{-1} dilution of PPD (a dose equivalent to 500 IU OT) are shown in figure 1. Sensitivity responses to the intradermal PPD were observed within two weeks of infecting the monkeys.

Measurement of skin thickness is obviously subject to individual variation making it difficult to interpret small changes in response to PPD. It was also regrettable that we were only able to use three animals in our non-infected controlled group. These animals were located in the experimental quarters at the point of maximum risk to airborne infection, namely near the air extraction system. Of these animals one responded to PPD (10^{-1} dilution) at weeks 6, 8, 10 and 12, the responses being 0.5, 0.2, 0.8 and 0.5 mm, respectively; thereafter the animal was negative to the end of the test. The second animal responded on two occasions at week 6 and week 16, the responses being 0.3 and 0.4 mm, respectively. The third animal showed responses from weeks 12, 14, 16 and 18, the responses being 0.9, 1.0, 6.3 and 1.2 mm, respectively, but

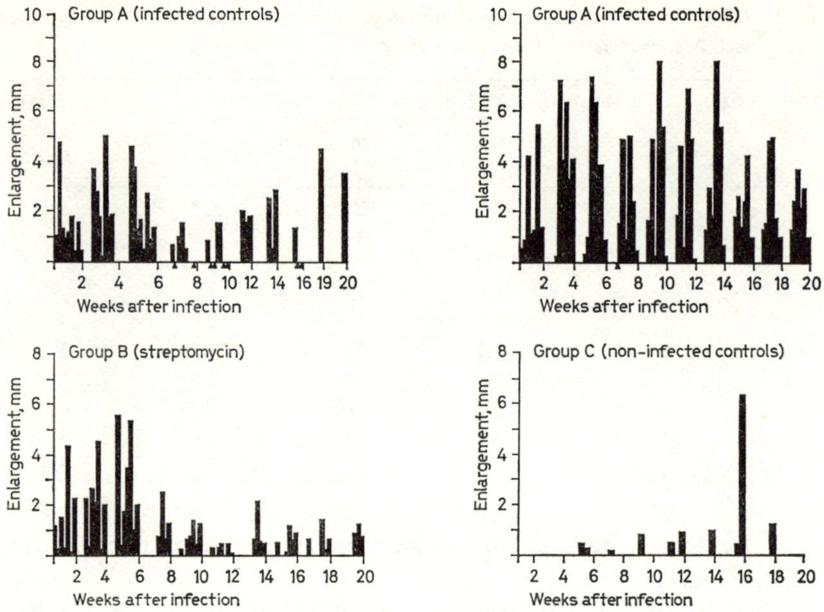

Fig. 1. Hypersensitivity responses in rhesus monkeys experimentally infected with *Mycobacterium tuberculosis* $H_{37}Rv$ to intradermal mammalian tuberculin PPD, containing the equivalent of 500 IU OT. ▲ = Monkey died.

there was no response on the 20th week of the test. Of these three animals only the third showed any evidence of tuberculosis and this was only seen on histopathological examination of the tracheobronchial lymphatics. The mean of the responses recorded in the two confirmed non-infected animals was 0.5 mm. If we take this as the potential error in our reading technique and regard any response above 0.5 mm as being of positive significance for diagnosis of tuberculosis, then in group A of 104 readings 84 were positive, the remaining 20 readings were made up of 10 zeros and a further 10 results with values of 0.5 or less. Of these 20 'negative' responses, 10 were obtained in animals immediately prior to death and could be interpreted as being due to the anergic condition of the animals. The remaining 10 responses occurred as single readings amongst strongly positive responses i.e. they were not found on successive occasions in the same monkey. In the streptomycin group, of 63 readings 39 positive readings were obtained during the early part of the experiment. Towards the end of the test three of seven animals gave repeated negative reactions which reflected the improved condition of the animals.

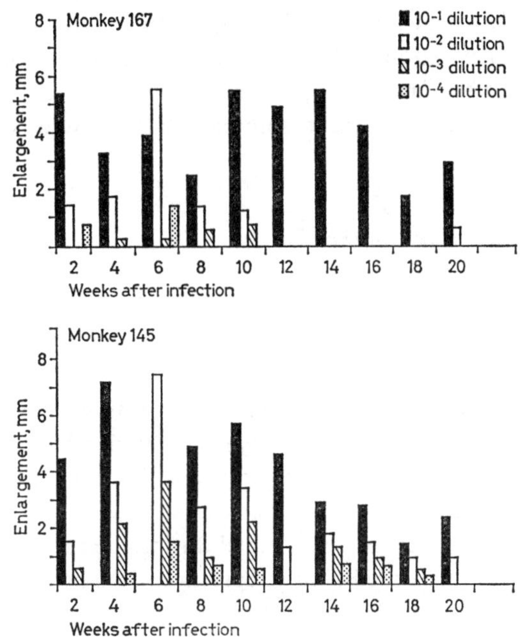

Fig. 2. Hypersensitivity responses in two rhesus monkeys, experimentally infected with *Mycobacterium tuberculosis* $H_{37}Rv$ to four dilutions of mammalian tuberculin PPD, containing the equivalent of 500, 50, 5 and 0.5 IU OT.

A gradation of responses to the four dilutions of PPD was observed, however the responses were not consistent. Examples of the responses seen in two of the monkeys are shown in figure 2. It can be seen that while monkey 167 showed a marked increase in skin thickness to the 10^{-1} dilution the animal rarely responded to the other dilutions of PPD. In contrast monkey 145 showed a graded response to the four dilutions. It was not possible to correlate the intensity of the reactions with the extent of the disease as seen in X-rays, or by retrospective correlation with the *post mortem* findings.

X-Rays

Radiological evidence of lung disease was observed within two weeks in all but one of the infected animals. In one animal the disease was not evident until the 4th week post-infection. All animals in the infected untreated group showed deterioration with increasing involvement either to death or necropsy. In one animal cavitation and pneumothorax was seen. The group receiving streptomycin, after an initial period during which the lung involvement increased, showed improvement from the 5th to 8th week until the end of the experiment.

Erythrocyte Sedimentation Rate

The ESR during the periods 0–1, 2–8, 10–20 weeks post-infection are shown in table II. The ESR responses were similar to those to PPD, viz. changes occurred from the 2nd week after infecting. During the two- to eight-week period marked increases in the sedimentation rates occurred in all of the infected animals, with peak increases occurring between the 2nd to 6th weeks post-infection. Following the peak period the ESR values in the infected control animals decreased but the sedimentation rates were always significantly greater than those obtained during the zero- to one-week period (see fig. 3). The group dosed with streptomycin showed a dramatic return to

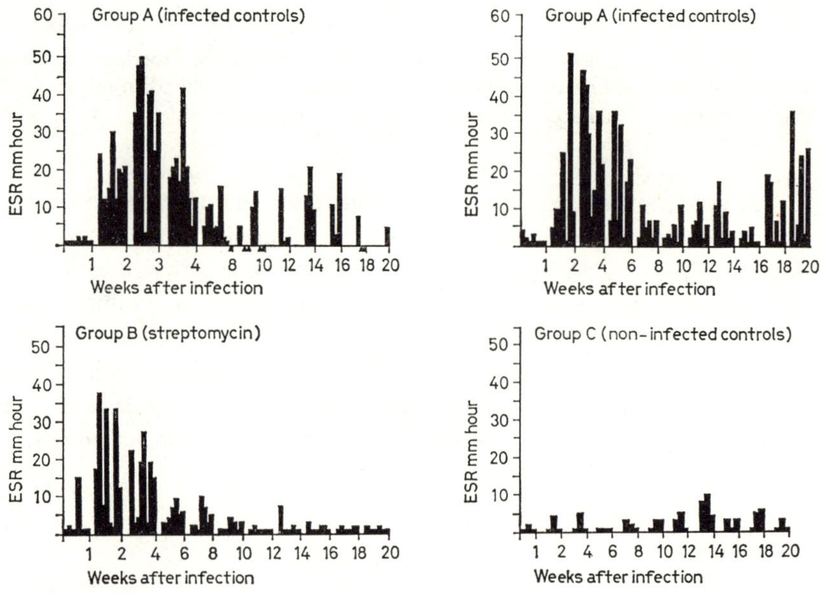

Fig. 3. ESR values in rhesus monkeys experimentally infected with *Mycobacterium tuberculosis* $H_{37}Rv$. ▲ = Monkey died.

Table II. Mean ESR values over a 20-week period in rhesus monkeys *(Macaca mulatta)* infected experimentally with *Mycobacterium tuberculosis* $H_{37}Rv$

Period weeks	Group A (infected control)	Group B (streptomycin)	Group C (non-infected control)
0–1	1.5	2.88	1.3
	(1–4)	(1–15)[1]	(1–2)
2–8	18.95	10.8	1.83
	(1–56)	(1–37)	(1–5)
10–20	7.66	1.9	3.2
	(1–21)	(1–4)	(1–10)
0–20	12.36	5.3	2.7

1 One animal in the group had an ESR value of 15, remaining animals 1 or 2.
Figures in parenthesis are the range of individual results.

normal ESR values. The three non-infected animals were showing increased ESR values towards the end of the experiment but only one animal, as already stated, was found to be obviously infected with tubercle.

Post mortem *and Histopathological Observations*

In all infected untreated monkeys caseation of lung tissue together with enlargement and caseation of the tracheobronchial lymph nodes was observed at *post mortem,* and was confirmed histopathologically. Acid fast bacilli were observed on microscopic examination of the lymph nodes and lung tissues. The liver of all the untreated infected animals showed varying degrees of congestion with round cells, and in one animal, foci of tuberculosis.

Post mortem examination of the animals dosed with streptomycin revealed moderately enlarged tracheobronchial lymph nodes with no evidence of caseation; there were many areas of scar tissue in the lungs, with very occasional areas of active tuberculosis. Histopathological examination of the lung tissues showed chronic inflammatory cells, large mononuclear cells and fibroblasts, but only in one animal were acid fast bacilli seen.

Apart from evidence of lung mite infection in one animal at *post mortem* the non-infected control animals showed no abnormalities. Histologically caseation of the tracheobronchial lymph nodes was seen in one of the non-infected control animals, but no acid fast bacilli were observed.

Discussion and Conclusions

The experiment described above was set up to evaluate potential antitubercular drugs and would have been designed somewhat differently if evaluation of the diagnostic techniques had been the objective. Nevertheless, useful information with respect to diagnosis emerged.

The hypersensitivity response to intradermally injected mammalian tuberculin proved a valuable diagnostic technique. The injections of PPD were made into the skin of the epigastric region for three reasons:

(1) It was impractical to make a comparison of the responses to various dilutions of the PPD by injecting intrapalpebrally.

(2) There were some indications that the abdominal site was more suitable [SCHMIDT, 1968; HARTLEY, 1969].

(3) By measuring skin thickness a quantifiable estimate of the hypersensitivity response was possible.

PPD was used and not OT, since it seemed more appropriate to use the purified reagent. There is a risk of non-specific responses with OT which is not seen with PPD; experimental confirmation of this factor was recently reported by CLARKE [1968].

The fortnightly measurements of skin thickening for the infected control animals showed no consistent pattern over the 20 weeks of the experiment. When the infected control monkeys, responses to intradermal injection of 500 IU PPD are analysed using the criteria that an animal is positively infected, if two of three consecutive fortnightly measurements of skin thickness show increases greater than 0.5 mm, then of 69 periods of three consecutive readings, 62 were positive for infection and seven indicated non-infected. The seven periods in which the response was 0.5 mm or less occurred in animals which were positive radiologically, and the ESR values were increased above normal. The animals were in all probability anergic. The non-infected group of three animals were correctly classified as two non-infected and one infected, which was confirmed at *post mortem*.

The WHO [1971] recommend a dose equivalent to 100 IU of OT for detection of tuberculosis. Others have used various doses ranging from 10,000 IU [HARTLEY, 1969; BYWATER *et al.*, 1962] to 1,000 IU [KENNARD and WILNER, 1941]. As a consequence of discussions held at the symposium 'Hazards of Handling Simians' [PERKINS and O'DONOGHUE, 1969], it was suggested a dose of tuberculin containing, 1,000–2,000 IU injected intrapalpebrally should be used for the diagnosis of tuberculosis. Our results indicate that a dose of tuberculin containing the equivalent of 500 IU is suitable for detection of the disease following inhalation of a large number of tubercle bacilli.

Radiology is undoubtedly of value for detection of the advanced disease but for the early detection of the disease there are certain limitations. Early uncalcified lesions are difficult to detect and are easily confused with other lung conditions. However, if good quality equipment and interpretation are available and if the results are taken in conjunction with other diagnostic criteria, radiology is of value.

The erythrocyte sedimentation rate proved a good index of the developing infection. In the first week of the experiment the majority of animals showed responses of 1 or 2, the mean ESR value for all animals being 1.92 (range 1–15). KING and GARGUS [1967] reported a mean ESR value of 1.3 $\pm$ 1.9 (range 0–13.0) for 109 observations in a group of female rhesus monkeys. Peak increases in ESR values occurred two to six weeks post-infection, after which time the values in the infected untreated animals remained significantly higher than normal. It would seem from these results that if ESR values are taken in conjunction with other diagnostic criteria, it is a useful index of tubercular infection.

This experiment indicates that hypersensitivity reactions to PPD, X-ray or ESR changes used alone are not 100% reliable for the diagnosis of a tubercular infection. However, we consider that, in view of the specificity of the hypersensitivity response to mammalian tuberculin, PPD (the risk of non-specific reactions to OT contraindicates its use) this test should be used, but always in conjunction with a second diagnostic test, either radiology or ESR.

References

BAERMANN, G. und HALBERSTAEDTER, L.: Experimentelle Hauttuberkulose bei Affen. Berl. klin. Wschr. *43:* 199 (1906).

BENSON, R. E.; FREMMING, B. D., and YOUNG, R. J.: A tuberculosis outbreak in a *Macaca mulatta* colony. Amer. Rev. Tuberc. *72:* 204 (1955).

BYWATER, J. E. C.; HARTLEY, E. G.; RUTTY, D. A., and ACKERLEY, E. T.: Observations in the intradermal palpebral tuberculin test and subsequent autopsy findings in monkeys. Vet. Rec. *74:* 1414 (1962).

CLARKE, G. L.: The relationship of hypersensitivity to shedding of *Mycobacterium tuberculosis* in experimentally infected *Macaca mulatta*. Amer. Rev. resp. Dis. *98:* 416–423 (1968).

DOLOWY, W. C.; FRANK, M. H.; COX, G. E., and HESSE, A. L.: Detection of pulmonary tuberculosis in laboratory monkeys be chest radiography. Amer. J. vet. Res. *19:* 225 (1958).

FRANCIS, J.: Natural and experimental tuberculosis in monkeys with observations on immunization and chemotherapy. J. comp. path. *66:* 128–135 (1956).

HABEL, K.: Tuberculosis in a laboratory monkey colony. Its spread and control. Amer. Rev. Tuberc. *55:* 77 (1947).

HABERMANN, R.T. and WILLIAMS, F.P., jr.: Diseases seen at necropsy of 708 *Macaca mulatta* (rhesus monkey) and *Macaca philippinensis* (cynomolgus monkey). Amer. J. vet. Res. *18:* 419 (1957).

HARTLEY, E.G.: Tuberculin testing in monkeys in PERKINS and O'DONOGHUE Hazards of handling simians. Lab. Animal Handbooks, vol. 4 (1969).

HIME, J.M.: Radiological examination of simian pulmonary tuberculosis in PERKINS and O'DONOGHUE Hazards of handling simians. Lab. Animal Handbooks, vol. 4 (1969).

KENNARD, M.A. and WILNER, M.B.: Tuberculosis and tuberculin tests in sub-human primates. Yale J. Biol. Med. *13:* 795 (1941).

KING, T.O. and GARGUS, J.L.: Normal blood values of the adult female monkey *(Macaca mulatta)*. Lab. Anim. Care *17:* 391–396 (1967).

PERKINS, F.T. and O'DONOGHUE, P.H. (ed.): Hazards of handling simians in Lab. Animal Handbooks, vol. 4 (1969).

RUCH, T.W.: Diseases of laboratory primates, pp. 199–253 (Saunders, Philadelphia 1967).

SCHMIDT, L.H.; HOFFMANN, R., and JOLLY, P.N.: Induced pulmonary tuberculosis in the rhesus monkey and its usefulness in evaluating chemotherapeutic agents. Chemo. Tuberc. Atlanta Georgia 226–231 (1955).

SCHMIDT, L.H.: Further on Koch's O.T. tuberculin *versus* P-P-D. for tuberculin testing. Lab. Primate Newsl., October 1968, p. 28.

SCHROEDER, C.R.: A diagnostic test for the recognition of tuberculosis in primates. A preliminary report. Zoologica, N.Y. *23:* 397 (1938).

STONES, P.B.: Incidence of tuberculosis in *Macaca mulatta* and *Cercopithecus aethiops* monkeys with special reference to the tuberculin test in PERKINS and O'DONOGHUE Hazards of handling simians. Lab. Animal Handbooks, vol. 4 (1969).

WHO: The health aspects of the supply and use of non-human primates for biomedical purposes. WHO Technical Report Series No. 470 (1971).

WHITE, C.Y. and FOX, H.: Results of tuberculin tests in monkeys at the Philadelphia Zoological Gardens. Arch. inter. Med. *4:* 517 (1909).

Authors' addresses: P. ACRED and PAMELA A. HUNTER, Beecham Research Laboratories, Brockham Park, *Betchworth, Surrey;* J.E.C. BYWATER, Brittoncourt Farm, Tyler Hill, *Canterbury, Kent;* J. JAMES, Cooper-McDougal & Robertson Ltd., *Berkhampstead, Herts* (UK). Requests for reprints should be sent to Mr. P. ACRED

Medical Primatology 1972. Proc. 3rd Conf. exp. Med. Surg. Primates, Lyon 1972, part III, pp. 13–21 (Karger, Basel 1972)

Experimental Malaria in Macaque Monkeys

The Effects of Splenectomy on Seroimmunological Phenomena[1]

P. AMBROISE-THOMAS, T. KIEN TRUONG, H. VERINE, ANDRÉE GOULLIER and C. DESCOURS

Laboratory of Parasitology and Tropical Medicine, Medical School of Grenoble University, La Tronche

Progressive appearance of acquired immunity to malaria is a long-recognized fact. The effect of this immunity is decrease of parasitemia, making reinfestation more difficult or limiting its consequences.

Various serological methods provide specific indication of the antiplasmodium serum antibodies and enable their evolution to be followed during attacks of malaria.

Are these antibodies responsible for the immunity or, on the contrary, are they merely evidence of infection? Arguments can be put forward for either theory. In order to separate the two phenomena (immunity and the presence of serum antibodies), we observed parasitemia and titration of anti-plasmodium antibodies in monkeys infected with *Plasmodium cynomolgi bastianellii*. Some of these animals had previously undergone splenectomy in order to prevent the appearance or the persistence of acquired immunity to malaria.

I. Material and Methods

Ten monkeys, nine *Macaca mulatta* and one *Macaca fascicularis* (S3 monkey) were used.

All animals were innoculated by i.v. injection of blood from previously-infected monkeys. After being citrated and treated with glycerin, the blood was preserved in liquid nitrogen for three to seven months [2]. Only the first inoculation of monkey S2 was carried

1 Work carried out with the financial aid of the World Health Organization.

out with fresh heparinized blood immediately after it was taken from another infected monkey. In all cases, the inoculate contained approximately 100 million plasmodia.

Five of the ten animals were splenectomized after general anesthesia with phencyclidine (Sernyvet®) 20 mg/ml, 0.3–0.4 ml i.m. according to weight [21]. During the operation care was taken to remove the entire spleen so as not to distort the experiment. Upon completion of the experiment, three of the five splenectomized monkeys were necropsied in order to verify the absence of accessory spleen.

Eight to ten days after splenectomy, infestation or reinfestation of the operated monkeys was carried out. Severity of the experimental malaria at times necessitated subcurative treatment (monkeys S2, S8 and S10) with i.m. injections of Chloroquine (3 mg/kg for three consecutive days). Parasitemia was determined in all animals every 24 or 48 h for the first ten days after inoculation. Later, these tests were repeated every five or ten days or at longer intervals for certain monkeys. Blood specimens were taken for the study of fluorescent antibodies in capillary tubes according to a method previously described [1].

The sera were studied at 1/20, 1/40 dilutions, etc., by the indirect immunofluorescence test with *Plasmodium cynomolgi bastianellii* antigen. Sera from all animals were studied simultaneously to provide controls even for slight variations of the fluorescent antibody titer.

II. Results

A. Non-Splenectomized Monkeys

(1) Inoculation produced experimental malaria in only two of the five non-splenectomized monkeys (S3 and S7), with negative serology at the onset of the experiment (fig. 1). Parasitemia appeared between the 6th and 10th day, and after attaining a maximum of 10–14% between the 12th and the 14th day, it decreased progressively and became negative between the 40th and 60th day. One of these monkeys had a slight parasitemic relapse from the 75th to the 85th day.

Development of fluorescent antibodies was parallel to that of parasitemia, but somewhat slower, confirming previous observations [2, 4, 10, 20, 23].

(2) Attempted infection failed in three nonsplenectomized monkeys, S4, S5 and S6 (fig. 2). All these animals had positive serology before inoculation, probably as a consequence of spontaneous malaria contracted before capture. Injection of infected blood provoked a rapid, but fleeting, rise in titer of the fluorescent antibodies. This corresponds to an anamnestic reaction provoked by the injection of parasitic blood.

Failure of infestation did not appear to be due to poor preservation of the inoculate. The same batch of frozen parasites was used for infection of monkeys S4, S5 and, three months later, S7.

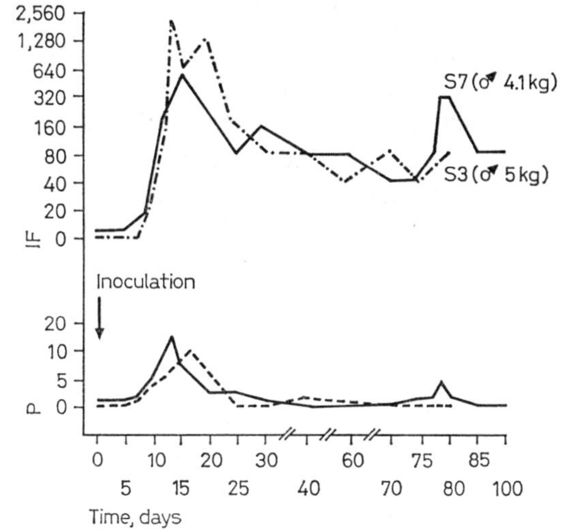

Fig. 1. Course of parasitemia and fluorescent antibodies during *Plasmodium cynomolgi bastianellii* infection in two unsplenectomized monkeys (S 3, *Macaca fascicularis* and S 7, *Macaca mulatta*). P = parasitemia; IF = immunofluorescence titres.

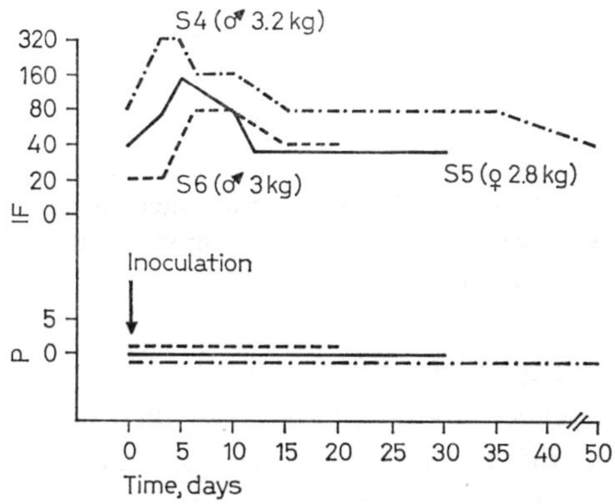

Fig. 2. Serology in three unsplenectomized *Macaca mulatta* resistant to experimental malaria. P = parasitemia; IF = immunofluorescence titres.

B. Splenectomized Monkeys

(1) Monkey S2 whose serology was positive at the outset proved resistant to the first infestation although it was infected with large number of organisms in blood freshly taken from another animal. Splenectomy was performed 64 days later and on the 72nd day a further attempt at infection provoked a bout of experimental malaria so intense as to require subcurative treatment. There was still 2% parasitemia on the 310th day, i.e. 238 days after the second inoculation (fig. 3).

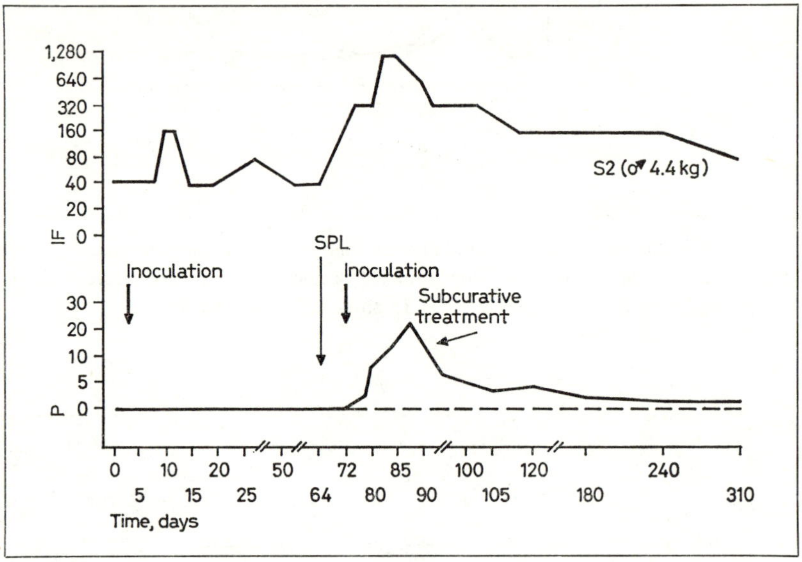

Fig. 3. Parasitemia and fluorescent antibody titres in one *Macaca mulatta* first resistant to experimental malaria, but developing intensive infection after splenectomy. SPL = splenectomy; P = parasitemia; IF = immunofluorescence titres.

(2) A similar experiment with monkey S1 resulted in repeated failures, and even after splenectomy the animal remained resistant (fig. 4).

(3) The other three monkeys (S8, S9 and S10) were first splenectomized and then infested eight days later. They rapidly developed intense malaria and, in two cases, subcurative treatment was necessary from the 12th to the 15th day (monkey S10) and from the 17th to the 20th day (monkey S8). Parasitemia persisted at least 150 (S9), 180 (S10) and 190 days (S8), which is

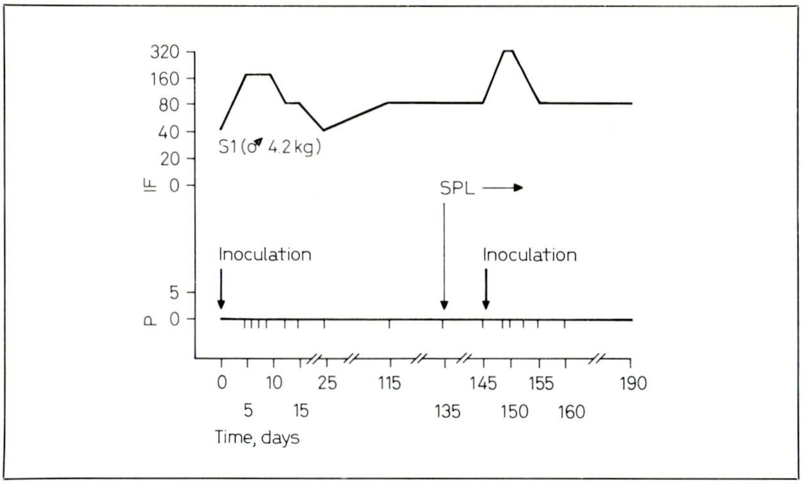

Fig. 4. Course of fluorescent antibodies in one monkey resistant to *Plasmodium cynomolgi bastianellii* infection before and after splenectomy. SPL = splenectomy; P = parasitemia; IF = immunofluorescence titres.

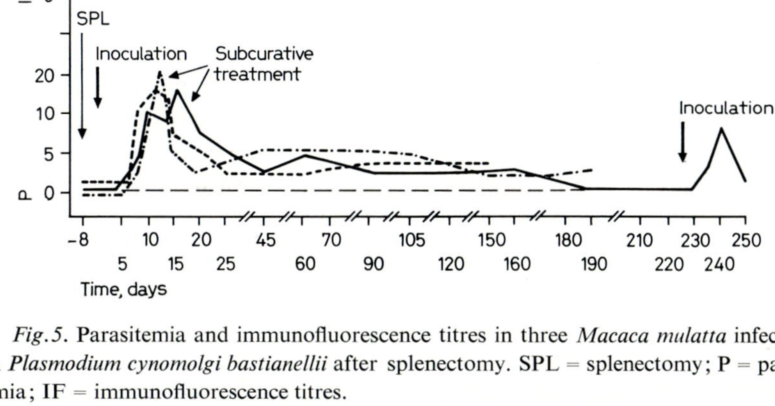

Fig. 5. Parasitemia and immunofluorescence titres in three *Macaca mulatta* infected with *Plasmodium cynomolgi bastianellii* after splenectomy. SPL = splenectomy; P = parasitemia; IF = immunofluorescence titres.

much longer than the normal duration of parasitism in non-splenectomized animals. Furthermore, on the 225th day, when no parasitemia was observed, monkey S 8 was successfully reinfected.

Serology was positive from the 5th to the 7th day after infestation in all splenectomized animals with persistent high titers.

III. Comments and Discussion

For a discussion of the possible protective role of serum antibodies, we shall consider two series of arguments taken from our own experiments or from the work of others.

A. Are Serum Antibodies Evidence of Infection?

(1) It is evident that antibodies develop or remain positive – sometimes with high titers – in infected animals in whom splenectomy has practically annulated antimalarial immunity. This lowered immunosuppressive action is shown in two ways: (a) *susceptibility* to a plasmodium against which the animals have an acquired immunity (this phenomenon is not constant, as shown by the case of monkey S 1) or natural immunity (splenectomized chimpanzees become receptive to *Plasmodium malariae*) [3, 11, 13–15, 17, 19]; (b) *severity and length of evolution of experimental malaria* in which the tendency to spontaneous cure disappears or, in any case, is greatly slowed down.

At the same time as immunity is lowered in this way by splenectomy, serum antibodies are produced to titers at least as high as in the control animals.

(2) Titers of serum antibodies rise in proportion to the extent of parasitemia. Malarial relapse is not preceded by a lowering of antibody titer (monkey S 7) but, on the contrary, is followed by an increase of serum antibodies. However, this aspect of the problem is questionable and does not resolve the relationship of serum antibodies to protection from disease. It is, in fact, possible that persistence or reappearance of parasites in the blood stream may be due to the development of 'antigenic variants' which escape the action of pre-existing specific antibodies [5, 22].

(3) Finally, antimalarial immunity is generally a specific phenomenon which is only effective against one species or even against a certain strain of plasmodia. On the other hand, numerous serologic cross-reactions are known to occur among all plasmodia of primates [2, 9, 19].

B. Are Serum Antibodies Protectors?

(1) It is striking to note that a monkey which appears unaffected by malaria almost always has positive serology prior to infestation presumably as a result of malaria contracted before capture.

These observations in experimental animals coincide with our observations in human studies during unsuccessful attempts at therapeutic infection (malariotherapy for general paralysis or for Buerger's disease) in former malaria sufferers [16].

(2) Schizontocidal treatment alone leaves a certain amount of acquired immunity and the serology decreases but remains positive.

However, complete course of treatment (with gametocidal medicaments) removes both immunizing protection and, sooner or later, the serum antibodies [2, 19, 23].

(3) The final and most important fact is that injection of antiplasmodium sera can provoke attenuation or even true cure [7, 8, 12]. Antibodies of maternal origin, moreover, have protective action in newborn babies [6]. These results alone suggested that the protective role of serum antibodies may be very important.

IV. Conclusion

Present-day conceptions with regard to antimalarial immunity may seem to consist entirely of contradictions. Instead of giving a solution, each new series of experiments seem, on the contrary, to raise additional questions. This is no doubt due to the complexity of the problem and to the multiple factors (humoral, cellular, nonspecific) which arise in immunity. Our experimental models, moreover, are still imperfect. Splenectomy, for example, which provokes strong immunosuppressive action, in fact acts at different levels of this immunity. It also causes blood decrease which in itself may encourage the installation or development of malaria. Nor do present-day serological methods enable us to titrate all antibodies directed against plasmodia. These parasites are in reality an antigenic mosaic and it is probable that all these antigens do not have the same 'vaccinating' power. This is suggested by certain of McGregor's works in whose opinion only antibodies aimed at thermolabile plasmodial antigens (La antigens) are possible protectors [18].

While awaiting the possibility of making specific titrations of these antibodies, numerous experimental situations remain to be explored. In this work we chose to observe the serology of animals in which splenectomy reduces the immunologic capacity. It would doubtless be particularly interesting to carry out the reverse experiment, that is, to observe variations in immunity in animals deprived of serum antibodies.

In short, all we can say at present is that if serum antibodies play a role in the immunology of malaria, it is certainly only partial, and it is difficult to prove its reality and appreciate its importance. Any conclusion drawn as to antimalarial immunity must, therefore, be extremely prudent. We can only accumulate the experimental results and record their sometimes conflicting evidence, but it is certainly still too soon to make a coherent synthesis of the data.

References

1 AMBROISE-THOMAS, P. et KIEN TRUONG, T.: Nouvelle technique de micro-prélèvements sanguins pour la réaction d'immuno-fluorescence indirecte. Bull. Ass. Dipl. Microbiol., Nancy *112:* 29–33 (1968).

2 AMBROISE-THOMAS, P.: Etude séro-immunologique de dix parasitoses par les techniques d'immuno-fluorescence; thèse Lyon (1969).

3 AMBROISE-THOMAS, P.: Le rôle de la rate dans l'équilibre hôte-parasite; thèse Lyon (1969).

4 AMBROISE-THOMAS, P.; KIEN TRUONG, T. et SALIOU, P.: Evolution des anticorps fluorescents au cours du paludisme expérimental des singes à *Plasmodium cynomolgi bastianellii.* Bull. Org. mond. Santé *44:* 719–728 (1971).

5 BROWN, K.N. and BROWN, I.N.: Immunity to malaria. Antigenic variations in chronic infections of *Plasmodium knowlesi.* Nature *208:* 1286–1288 (1965).

6 BRUCE-CHWATT, L.J.: Congenital transmission of immunity in malaria; in Immunity to protozoa, pp. 89–108 (Blackwell, Oxford 1963).

7 COHEN, S., MCGREGOR, I.A., and CARRINGTON, S.: Gamma-globulin and acquired immunity to human malaria. Nature *192:* 733–737 (1961).

8 COHEN, S. and MCGREGOR, I.A.: Gamma-globulins and acquired immunity to malaria; in Immunity to protozoa, pp. 123–159 (Blackwell, Oxford 1963).

9 COLLINS, W.E.; JEFFERY, G.M.; GUINN, E.G., and SKINNER, J.C.: Fluorescent antibody studies in human malaria. IV. Cross-reactions between human and simian malaria. Amer. J. trop. Med. Hyg. *15:* 11–15 (1966).

10 COLLINS, W.E.; SKINNER, J.C.; CONTACOS, P.G., and GUINN, E.G.: Fluorescent antibody studies in simian malaria. II. Development of antibodies to *Plasmodium cynomolgi.* Amer. J. trop. Med. Hyg. *16:* 267–272 (1967).

11 CONRAD, M.E. and DENNIS, L.H.: Splenic function in experimental malaria. Amer. J. trop. Med. Hyg. *17:* 170–172 (1968).

12 FABIANI, G. et FULCHIRON, G.: Demonstration *in vivo* de l'existence d'un pouvoir protecteur dans le sérum de rats guéris du paludisme expérimental. C.R. Soc. Biol. *147:* 99–103 (1953).

13 FABIANI, G.: Le rôle de la rate dans l'immunité anti-paludéenne. Bull. Soc. Path. exot. *59:* 605–647 (1966).

14 FABIANI, G.: Le rôle de la rate dans l'immunité anti-microbienne. Méd. Hyg. *26:* 185–186 (1968).

15 FABIANI, G.: Le paludisme et ses particularités immunologiques. Bull. Inst. Pasteur *67:* 5–29 (1969).

16 GARIN, J.P., AMBROISE-THOMAS, P., KIEN TRUONG, T. et SALIOU. P.: Evolution des anticorps fluorescents au cours du paludisme expérimental humain par malariathérapie à *Plasmodium vivax*. Bull. Org. mond. Santé *44:* 689–699 (1971).

17 GARNHAM, P.C.C.: An introduction to protozoal immunity; in Immunity to protozoa, pp. 3–21 (Blackwell, Oxford 1963).

18 MCGREGOR, I.A. and WILSON, R.J.M.: Gel-diffusion and immunity to malaria. J. Parasit. *56:* 66 (1970).

19 OMS: Immunologie du paludisme. Rapport technique No 396 (OMS, Genève 1968).

20 SCHINDLER, R.; SCHRÖDER, G. und STIEGER, R.: Untersuchungen über Immunität und serologische Reaktion bei Affen nach einer Infektion mit *Plasmodium cynomolgi bastianellii*. Z. tropenmed. Parasit. *21:* 239–245 (1970).

21 VERINE, H.; AMBROISE-THOMAS, P.; KIEN TRUONG, T. et MURAT, J.: La splénectomie chez *Macaca Irus*. Bull. Soc. Sci. vét., Lyon *72:* 177–183 (1970).

22 VOLLER, A. and ROSSAN, R.N.: Immunological studies with simian malaria. I. Antigenic variants of *Plasmodium cynomolgi bastianellii*. Trans. roy. Soc. trop. Med. Hyg. *63:* 45–56 (1969).

23 VOLLER, A.: The detection and measurement of malaria antibodies. Trans. roy. Soc. trop. Med. Hyg. *65:* 111–124 (1971).

Authors' addresses: PIERRE AMBROISE-THOMAS and Mrs. ANDRÉE GOULLIER, Laboratoire de Parasitologie et Pathologie Exotique, Faculté de Médecine de Grenoble, *F-38700 La Tronche;* THAI, KIEN-TRUONG, Laboratoire de Parasitologie, Faculté de Médecine de Lyon, *F-69000 Lyon;* HENRI VERINE, 6, rue du Parc, *F-69200 Vénissieux;* CHARLES DESCOURS, Centre hospitalier régional de Grenoble, *F-38700 La Tronche* (France)

Medical Primatology 1972. Proc. 3rd Conf. exp. Med. Surg. Primates, Lyon 1972, part III, pp. 22–30 (Karger, Basel 1972)

Isolation and Characterization of a New Herpesvirus from Owl Monkeys *(Aotus trivirgatus)*

A Preliminary Report[1]

H. H. Barahona, L. V. Meléndez, N. W. King, M. D. Daniel, C. E. O. Fraser and A. C. Preville

New England Regional Primate Research Center, Harvard Medical School, Southborough, Mass.

Introduction

Information on several owl monkey *(Aotus trivirgatus)* herpesvirus isolates has been presented in previous reports [1, 9–11]. Recently, one of these agents was more extensively studied and characterized [2]. The virus was designated as *Herpesvirus aotus* type 1. This paper presents preliminary information on a second herpesvirus from the owl monkey. The name *H. aotus* type 2 has been suggested for this new herpesvirus.

Materials and Methods

Standard procedures were followed for the physicochemical characterization of the agent (filtration, ether, heat, etc.). The nucleic acid type of the virus was determined by infecting cells treated with medium containing 40 μg/ml of 5-BUDR.

Primary and continuous cell cultures of owl monkey kidney (OMK) were used for these studies. The *in vitro* cell host range of the virus was investigated in the cell cultures listed under Results. Vero cells and squirrel monkey kidney cells were employed for plaque titrations. The plaque assay method and the overlay medium employed have been described elsewhere [3].

The electron microscopic observation of the virions was done in thin sections of infected cells doubly stained with uranyl acetate and lead citrate.

1 Supported by USPHS, NIH grant RR 00168-10.

Specific antisera against *H. aotus* type 2 was prepared in goats, and hyperimmune sera against other known herpesviruses were standard antisera prepared in our laboratory. The method of constant serum and varying viral dilutions was employed in these serological studies.

The acridine orange (AO) and the indirect fluorescent antibody staining have been described elsewhere [5, 14].

Results

Virus Isolation and Cultural Characteristics

The virus was obtained from the 11th transfer of an owl monkey kidney cell culture that was established 80 days prior to the isolation of the agent. When the cellular monolayer was fully grown, it developed focal areas of alteration which contained bizarre, refractile cells with long protrusions. These areas of cytopathic effect enlarged slowly to involve most of the monolayer in 15 days. Hematoxylin and eosin (HE) stained preparations of these cultures demonstrated the presence of typical Cowdry type A intranuclear inclusions (fig.1). Small polykaryocytes were also observed in these areas.

Table I. Comparative cell culture host range of *H. aotus* type 1 and *H. aotus* type 2

Cell cultures	Viruses	
	H. aotus type 1	*H. aotus* type 2
Owl monkey kidney	+	+
Owl monkey cornea	+	[1]
Cebus monkey kidney	±[2]	+
Squirrel monkey kidney[3]	–	+
Squirrel monkey kidney[4]	±	+
Vero[5]	±	+
Human cells	±	–
Rabbit kidney	–	+
Goat cells	–	+
Hamster heart	–	–

1 Not tested.
2 Grows poorly.
3 LLC-MK_4 line.
4 Primate Center line.
5 African green monkey kidney cell line.

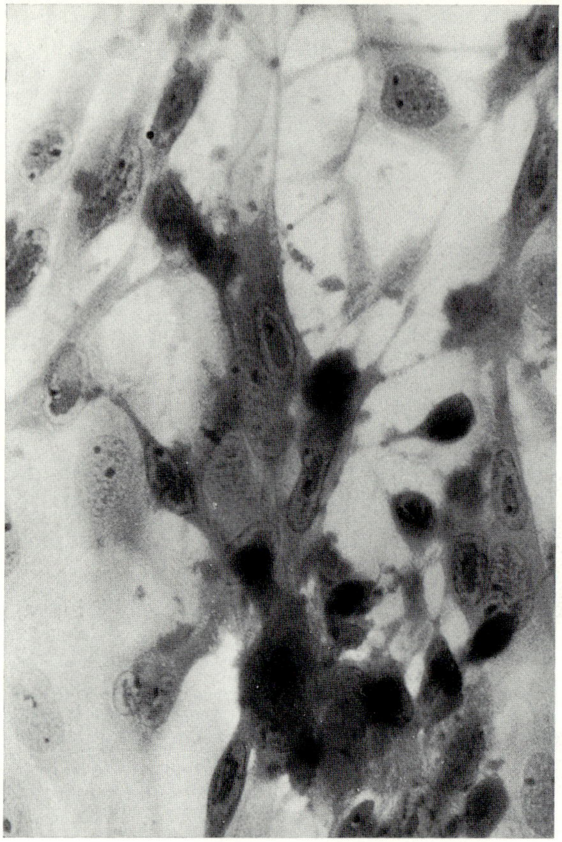

Fig. 1. Focal area of cell destruction showing characteristic type A intranuclear inclusions. OMK infected cells stained with HE. ×230.

As shown in table I, *H. aotus* type 2 has a relatively wide *in vitro* host range when compared with the cellular host range of *H. aotus* type 1. With the exception of whole human embryo cells, the virus grew well in all the cells of primate origin so far tested. It also grew well in rabbit kidney cells (RK) and goat cells (GC).

The virus was capable of forming plaques only in Vero cells. The plaques appeared on the 11th day as pinpoint sized foci and became clearly discernible on the 19th day and ranged in size from 0.5 to 1.0 mm [4].

The results of growth curve experiments done in OMK cells, indicated that *H. aotus* type 2 is readily released in infectious form from the cells.

Physical and Chemical Characteristics

The virus has been classified as a herpesvirus based on its physicochemical and electron microscopic characteristics (table II). The nucleic acid type of the virus was determined by indirect procedures to be deoxyribonucleic acid (DNA). Titration of the virus in cells pretreated with the thymidine analog 5-BUDR, showed a 2.0-log reduction in titer when compared with the titer obtained in untreated controls. Infected cultures stained with AO, revealed the presence of green DNA-type inclusion in the nuclei. The infectivity of the agent was shown to be destroyed by ether and heat. Filtration experiments indicated that the virions were larger than 100 nm and smaller than 220 nm. An average diameter of 156 nm for the mature enveloped virions was determined by electron microscopic observations.

Table II. Physicochemical and morphological characteristics of *H. aotus* type 2

Nucleic acid	DNA
Envelope	+
Ether sensitivity	+
Heat labile	+
Size of mature virions	148–160 nm
Size of naked capsids	105 ± 1 nm

In thin sections of infected cells, virus particles in various stages of development were observed in the nuclei, cytoplasm and extracellular spaces. Nonenveloped nuclear particles were commonly found in association with a moderately dense staining, granular inclusion (fig. 2). These nuclear particles were roughly hexagonal in profile, 105 ± 1 nm in diameter, consisted of 'empty' viral capsids and others with a dense core material. The core material was distributed in several distinct patterns within the capsid (fig. 2). In some it appeared as a single, centrally placed ovoid mass, in others it was in the form of an inner shell concentric with the capsid and in still others it occurred as small scattered clumps distributed radially subjacent to the capsid coat. Particles were found budding through the inner leaflet of the nuclear membrane. Enveloped capsids were found in the cisternae of the endoplasmic reticulum and in the extracellular space (fig. 3). These enveloped virions were 148–160 nm in diameter. The cytoplasm of some infected cells contained elongate crystalline structures which appeared in lamellar configuration (fig. 4). These structures were composed of a moderately dense staining matrial and were up to 5–6 μm in diameter.

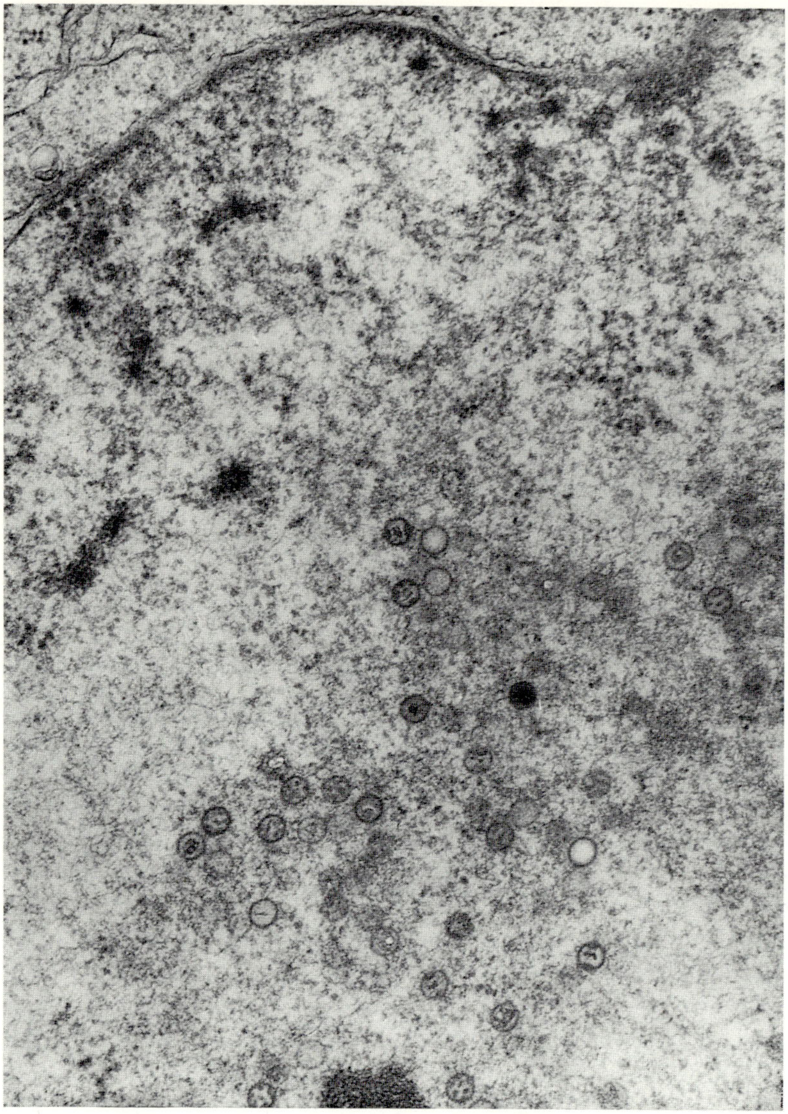

Fig. 2. Nucleus of an infected OMK cell showing an inclusion containing herpesvirus nucleocapsids in various stages of development. × 33,100.

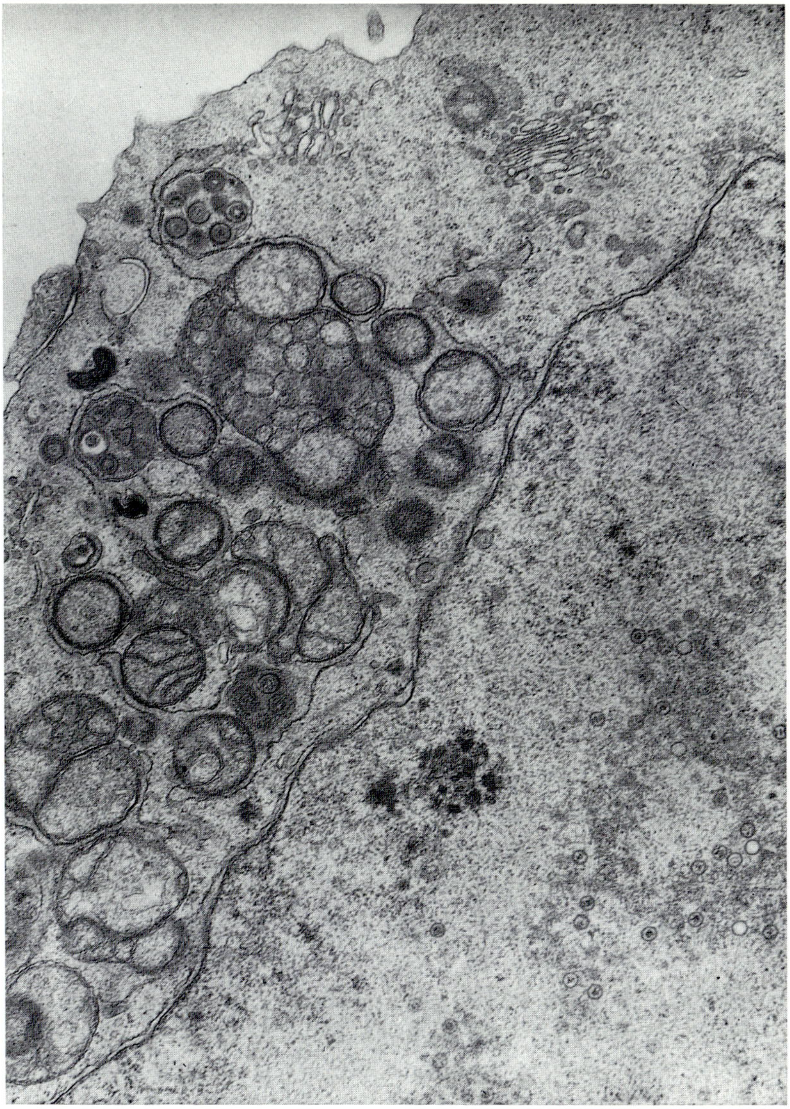

Fig. 3. Nonenveloped nuclear particles and enveloped cytoplasmic virions within dilated cisternae of the endoplasmic reticulum. × 17,600.

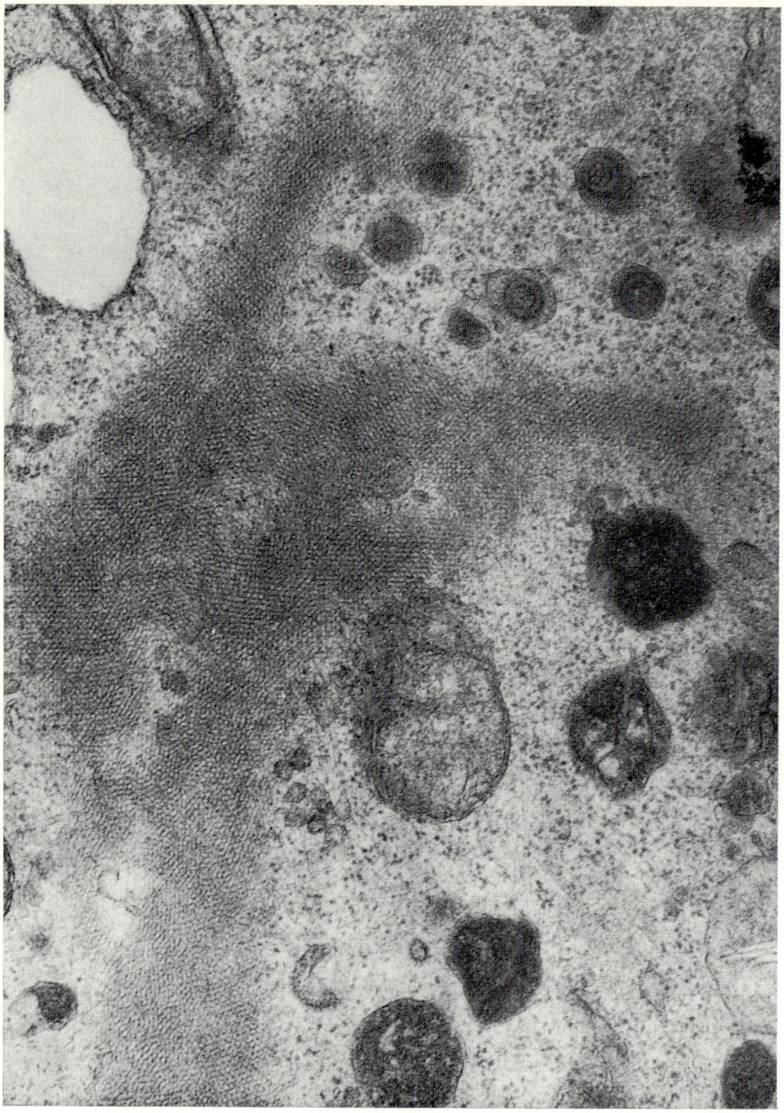

Fig. 4. Cytoplasmic elongate crystalline lamella and enveloped virions. × 33,100.

Serological Relationships with other Herpesviruses

The infectivity of *H. aotus* type 2 was not neutralized by specific antisera against *H. simplex, H. tamarinus, H. simiae, H. saimiri, H. aotus* type 1, owl monkey kidney isolate 372-70 and infectious bovine rhinotracheitis. *H. aotus* type 2 antisera prepared in goats failed to neutralize these viruses. No cross-reaction was found by indirect immunofluorescent test between *H. aotus* type 2 and *H. saimiri, H. ateles, H. tamarinus* and *H. simplex* type 1.

Discussion

The biological, physicochemical and morphological features of the agent described in this report are consistent with those of the herpesvirus group. It is a DNA virus, ether and heat sensitive, and the mature extracellular virus particles average 156 nm in diameter. In HE stained infected cells typical type A intranuclear inclusions are observed. Serological studies indicate that the virus is unrelated antigenically to a number of herpesviruses. Among these viruses are included several new herpesviruses from New World monkeys that have been recently described [6–8, 12, 13]. However, it was particularly important to establish a clear differentiation between *H. aotus* type 1 [2] and *H. aotus* type 2. Both viruses were isolated from the cultured cells of apparently normal owl monkeys, but differ in several of their characteristics.

H. aotus type 1, so far has been capable of growing only in cells of primate origin. *H. aotus* type 2 grows well in cells of primate origin as well as in RK and GC cultures (table I). *H. aotus* type 2 forms plaques in Vero cells whereas *H. aotus* type 1 does not [2, 4].

In electron microscopic preparations elongated lamellar crystalline structures have been observed in the cytoplasm of OMK cells infected with *H. aotus* type 2. No such structures have been found in the same type of cells infected with *H. aotus* type 1.

These differences plus the finding that these two viruses are unrelated antigenically would indicate that *H. aotus* type 2 is a new herpesvirus.

Acknowledgements

We greatly appreciate the technical assistance of DEBORAH FELMLEE and D. JACKMAN. We are also indebted to Mrs. MARJORIE VALLEE for typing this paper.

References

1 BARAHONA, H.H.; DANIEL, M.D.; MELÉNDEZ, L.V.; KING, N.W.; FRASER, C.E.O., GARCIA, F.G.: Herpesviruses from the owl monkey *(Aotus trivirgatus)*. Symp. Viruses South American Monkeys, Mexico City 1971. J.nat.Cancer Inst. *49:* 219–224 (1972).

2 DANIEL, M.D.; MELÉNDEZ, L.V.; KING, N.W.; FRASER, C.E.O.; BARAHONA, H.H.; HUNT, R.D., and GARCIA, F.G.: *Herpesvirus aotus:* A latent herpesvirus from owl monkeys *(Aotus trivirgatus)*. Isolation and characterization. Proc.Soc.exp.Biol.Med. *138:* 835–845 (1971).

3 DANIEL, M.D.; RABIN, H.; BARAHONA, H.H., and MELÉNDEZ, L.V.: *Herpesvirus saimiri.* III. Studies on plaque formation under multiagar overlay, starch and methylcellulose in various primate cell cultures. Proc.Soc.exp.Biol.Med. *136:* 1192–1196 (1971).

4 DANIEL, M.D.; MELÉNDEZ, L.V., and BARAHONA, H.H.: Plaque characterization of viruses from South American non-human primates. Symp. Viruses South American Monkeys, Mexico City 1971. J.nat.Cancer Inst. *49:* 239–249 (1972).

5 FRASER, C.E.O.; MELÉNDEZ, L.V.; BARAHONA, H.H., and DANIEL, M.D.: The effect of Poly I:C on fluorescent and neutralizing antibodies to *Herpesvirus saimiri* in goats. Int.J.Cancer *7:* 397–402 (1971).

6 HOLMES, A.W.; CALDWELL, R.G.; DEDMON, R.E., and DEINHARDT, F.: Isolation and characterization of a new herpesvirus. J.Immunol. *92:* 602–610 (1964).

7 HULL, R.N.: The simian viruses; in Virology monographs, vol. 2, pp. 1–66 (Springer, New York 1968).

8 MELÉNDEZ, L.V.; DANIEL, M.D.; HUNT, R.D., and GARCIA, F.G.: An apparently new herpesvirus from primary kidney cultures of the squirrel monkey *(Saimiri sciureus)*. Lab.Anim.Care *18:* 374–381 (1968).

9 MELÉNDEZ, L.V.; HUNT, R.D.; DANIEL, M.D., and TRUM, B.F.: New World monkeys, herpesviruses and cancer; in BALNER and BEVERIDGE Infections and immunosuppression in sub-human primates, pp. 111–117 (Munksgaard, Copenhagen 1970).

10 MELÉNDEZ, L.V. and DANIEL, MD..: Herpesviruses from South American monkeys; in GOLDSMITH and MOOR-JANKOWSKI Medical primatology 1970, pp. 686–693 (Karger, Basel 1971).

11 MELÉNDEZ, L.V.; DANIEL, M.D.; BARAHONA, H.H.; FRASER, C.E.O.; HUNT, R.D., and GARCIA, F.G.: New herpesviruses from South American monkeys. Preliminary report. Lab.Anim.Sci. *21:* 1050–1054 (1971).

12 MELÉNDEZ, L.V.; CASTELLANOS, H.; BARAHONA, H.H.; DANIEL, M.D.; HUNT, R.D.; FRASER, C.E.O.; GARCIA, F.G., and KING, N.W.: Two new herpesviruses from spider monkeys *(Ateles geofroyii)*. Symp. Viruses South American Monkeys, Mexico City 1971. J.nat.Cancer Inst. *49:* 233–238 (1972).

13 MELNICK, J.L.; MIDULLA, M.; WIMBERLY, Il.; BARRERA-ORO, J.G., and LEVY, B.M.: A new member of the herpesvirus group isolated from South American marmosets. J.Immunol. *92:* 595–601 (1964).

14 POLLARD, M. and STARR, T.J.: Study of intracellular virus with acridine orange fluorochrome; in Progr.med.Virol., vol. 4, pp. 54–67 (Karger, Basel 1962).

Authors' address: Dr. H.H. BARAHONA, Dr. L.V. MELÉNDEZ, Dr. N.W. KING, Dr. M.D. DANIEL, Dr. C.E.O. FRASER and Dr. A.C. PREVILLE, New England Regional Primate Research Center, Harvard Medical School, 1 Pine Hill Drive, *Southborough, MA 01772* (USA)

Medical Primatology 1972. Proc. 3rd Conf. exp. Med. Surg. Primates, Lyon 1972, part III, pp. 31–34 (Karger, Basel 1972)

Nonhuman Primates and Treponematoses

C. Bouloux and P. Cirera

In 1928, Schobl [cited by Hackett, 1963] reported his results on yaws experimentally induced in Philippine monkeys, showing that *T. pertenue* caused the disease. Additional studies were summarized by Hasselman [cited by Hackett, 1963] and Schobl and Hasselman [cited by Hackett, 1963]. In 1963, Fribourg-Blanc *et al.* successfully showed the presence of fluorescent antitreponemic antibodies in sera of baboons. Fribourg-Blanc and Mollaret [1968] isolated and identified *T. pertenue* from certain monkeys indigenous to Africa. In 1968, Thivolet *et al.* noted the existence of antitreponemic antibodies in sera from monkeys of various origins. Sepetjian *et al.* [1969] assigned to the treponema isolated by Fribourg-Blanc *et al.* [1963] the provisional name of Treponema F. B. In the United States Kuhn and coworkers [1968] called attention to the existence, in nonhuman primates, of antibodies which react positively to the treponemic and lipidic antigens of syphilis. Brown *et al.* [1970] and Kuhn *et al.* [1968] have made a special study of experimental treponematosis in the chimpanzee – notably syphilis and pinta. This report is concerned with a survey for treponematoses in baboon sera.

Material and Methods

437 baboons sera were obtained from the following sources:

(1) 130 sera received from Marseilles, of which 122 *Papio papio* were captured in Senegal (Casamance) and eight *Papio hamadryas* came from Ethiopia. These animals had been in captivity for a short period before being sampled.

(2) Sixty sera from *Papio cynocephalus* and *Papio anubis* kept in captivity in Paris with some F_1 and F_2 generations.

(3) 247 sera from two *Papio papio* groups from Senegal captured and sampled during a field expedition in Niokholo Koba National Park.

Each serum sample was submitted to the following three reactions:

(1) Kline reaction (MFT) with cardiolipidic antigen from the Pasteur Institute, Paris.

(2) Complement fixation test with Reiter proteinic antigen from the Pasteur Inst., Paris.

(3) Complement fixation test with Kolmer cardiolipidic antigen from the Pasteur Institute, Paris.

Hemolysin reactions were carried out by the Kolmer method in accordance with the procedure followed at the Pasteur Institute, Paris.

Results on these sera as examined by all three procedures are shown in table I.

Table I. Codification of results for the interpretation of serological reactions for treponematoses

Code	Type of reaction	Results					
		Marseille		Senegal		Paris	
		number 130	%	number 247	%	number 60	%
R	reactive	6	4.6	9	3.5	0	0
PR	probably reactive	14	10.7	29	11.7	2	3.3
B	borderline	1	0.7	1	0.4	0	0
NS	nonspecific	29	22.3	48	19.4	7	11.6
Ac	anticomplementary	3	2.1	46	18.7	1	1.6
Ne	negative	84	59.6	114	46.3	50	83.5

R = 3 reactions $\geq +$.
PR = 2 reactions $\geq +$ and 1 reaction $\leq \pm$.
B = 1 reaction $= +$ and 1 reaction $\leq \pm$.
NS = 2 reactions $\leq +$ and 1 reaction $\geq +$.

Results

The baboons of the Marseilles and Senegal groups were most affected by treponematosis if the reactive and probably reactive results are grouped (15.3% for each group).

On the other hand, the baboons of the Paris group seem to be the least affected with only 3.3% showing any reactivity. As indicated above, the baboons from Senegal were captured in the wild and sampled immediately afterwards, and the Marseilles group were sampled soon after their arrival at the laboratory. Most of the monkeys of the Paris group, if not all, have, on the contrary, lived in captivity from birth.

Discussion

Interpretation of the seroreactive sera does not raise any special problem. They probably result from infection with pathogenic treponemas. The other reactions are more difficult to interpret and are presented merely as indicative of the results obtained. We have chosen to group the 'probably reactive' group as positive and the 'borderline' as nonspecific. We have also presented them separately in the table as this allows for a more descriptive picture of the results.

The nonspecific results may be due to nonpathogenic treponemas possessing group antigens capable of provoking the appearance of cross-reacting antibodies with antigens used in treponemic serology. Indeed, the work of VELDKAMP [cited by HACKETT, 1963] and of DEBRUIJN [1963] has shown that *T. zuelzerae,* isolated and identified by VELDKAMP and studied by DEBRUIJN possesses a proteinic antigen specific for the *T. reiteri* group which is closely related to *T. pallidum.* These authors have also studied, from the epidemiological viewpoint, the serological response of a number of monkeys captured either in a zone in which yaws is endemic or in a zone in which syphilis is endemic. Of 20 samples of sera coming from the yaws endemic zone, 17 (85%) showed positive immunofluorescent reactions. The 91 sera from the syphilis endemic zone, on the other hand, did not react. This would confirm the suggestion of KUHN [1971] which indicated that *T. pertenue* (yaws) is responsible for natural treponematosis in monkeys and is in agreement with the data reported here. It still remains to find out if the treponematosis of the monkey caused by *T. pertenue* can be transmitted to man. To our knowledge this problem has yet to be solved. We have had the opportunity to carry out population studies in Senegal in two human groups living in the same region as the baboons reported here. We found approximately 30% of these individuals to be reactive. It is not our purpose to propose a common link between the two – it remains to be seen whether the same treponema is responsible.

References

BROWN, W.J.; KUHN, U.S.G.; TOLLIVER, E.A., and NORINS, L.C.: Experimental syphilis in the chimpanzee. Immunoglobin class of early antibodies reactive with *Treponema pallidum.* Brit. J. vener. Dis. *46:* 198 (1970).

FRIBOURG-BLANC, A.; NIEL, G. et MOLLARET, H.H.: Sur quelques aspects immunologiques du cynocéphale africain. Bull. Soc. Path. exot. *56:* 474 (1963).

FRIBOURG-BLANC, A. et MOLLARET, H.H.: La tréponématose naturelle du singe africain. Not publ. WHO/VDT/RES/68.135 (1968).

HACKETT, C.S.: On the origin of the human treponematoses (Pinta, Yaws, endemic syphilis and venereal syphilis). Bull. Wld Hlth Org. *29:* 7–41 (1963).

KUHN, U.S.G.: Humoral aspects of treponematoses of chimpanzees; in GOLDSMITH and MOOR-JANKOWSKI Medical primatology 1970, pp. 761–765 (Karger, Basel 1971).

KUHN, U.S.G.; BROWN, W., and FALCONE, V.H.: Seroreactivity of nonhuman primates in treponemal and nontreponemal antigentests for syphilis. Not publ. WHO/VDT/RES/68.137 (1968).

KUHN, U.S.G.; VARELA, G.; CHANDLER, F.W., jr., and OSUNA, G.G.: Experimental pinta in the chimpanzee. J. amer. med. Ass. *206* (1968).

SEPETJIAN, M.; TISSOT GUERRAZ. F.; SALUSSOLA, D.; THIVOLET, J. et MONIER, J.G.: Contribution à l'étude du tréponème isolé du singe par Fribourg-Blanc. Bull. Org. mond. Santé *40:* 141 (1969).

THIVOLET, J.; SEPETJIAN, M. et TISSOT GUERRAZ, F.: Recherche d'anticorps tréponémiques dans 667 sérums de singes d'origines diverses. Not publ. WHO/VDT/RES/68.136 (1968).

Authors' address: C. BOULOUX and P. CIRERA, Centre de Transfusion sanguine, d'Hématologie et de Génétique humaine Charles-Lefebvre, Service de sérologie, Centre d'Hémotypologie du CNRS, CHU Purpan, Avenue de Grande-Bretagne, *F-31000 Toulouse* (France)

Medical Primatology 1972. Proc. 3rd Conf. exp. Med. Surg. Primates, Lyon 1972, part III, pp. 35–38 (Karger, Basel 1972)

Pathogenic Enterobacteriaceae of Free-Living Baboons *(Papio ursinus)*

H. D. Brede

Department of Medical Microbiology, University of Stellenbosch and Tygerberg Hospital, Tiervlei, C.P.

Routine examination of the intestinal flora of 851 baboons by taking rectal swabs soon after capture proved a high incidence of pathogenic organisms. The carrier rate of Salmonellae, Shigellae and enteropathogenic *E. coli* is shown in tables I–III. It is striking that a limited number of Salmonellae and Shigellae predominates.

Table I. Salmonellae isolated from 851 free-living baboons

Salmonellae	Carrier, %	Number of baboons
S. typhimurium	1.41	12
S. isangi	0.12	1
S. grabouw	0.12	1
S. sundsvall	10.93	93
S. cerro	0.12	1
Undefined rough and untypable	1.05	9
Total	13.75	117

Contrary to the spectrum of Salmonellae occurring in human beings in the South Western Cape which consists of over 100 different types [1], baboons show a high prevalence of only a few types which have not been of importance to humans. This accentuates again the group specific bacterial flora of primates. Of 851 free-living baboons the total *Salmonella* carrier rate after capture was 13,75%. Not one of the animals appeared ill. We conclude that the 1.4-percent carrier rate for *S. typhimurium* can be accepted as a real carrier rate, but that the high incidence of *Salmonella sundsvall* (Kauffmann-White scheme group H, formula: 1, 6, 14, 25:z:e, n, x) indicates endosymbio-

Table II. Shigellae isolated from the same 851 free-living baboons

Shigellae	Carrier, %	Number of baboons
S. flexneri II	5.99	51
S. flexneri III	0.12	1
S. flexneri IV	5.17	44
S. flexneri V	5.28	45
S. schmitzi	2.0	17
S. sonnei	0.82	7
Total	19.38	165

Table III. Enteropathogenic *E. coli* isolated from 851 free-living baboons

Type of enteropathogenic *E. coli*	Carrier, %	Number of baboons
026	4.44	37
028	0.12	1
055	8.28	69
086	1.56	13
0111	0.72	6
0119	6.12	51
0125	2.64	22
0126	2.00	17
0127	0.72	6
0128	2.64	22
026+0125	0.24	2
026+0126	0.24	2
055+0119	0.12	1
0111+0126	0.12	1
0111+0119	0.12	1
0119+0125	0.12	1
0125+0126	0.12	1
Total	30.32	253

sis of this type in the South African baboon. *S. sundsvall* was first described and detected by OLIN and ALIN [3] in Sweden from a human patient suffering from gastroenteritis. KELTERBORN [4] mentions further isolations from humans in the USA, Mexico, Israel and Germany, from animals and foodstuffs in Morocco and the Netherlands. In 12 years we isolated *S. sundsvall* only from three human beings suffering from gastroenteritis without known contact to baboons. Under stress in captivity, *S. sundsvall* triggers gastroenteritis and bacteraemia in baboons undergoing immunosuppressive therapy.

S.grabouw is the only type belonging to the *Salmonella* subgenus II in our material. This type was detected in South Africa and first isolated from a human with gastroenteritis [2]. The nonhuman primate is as susceptible to *Salmonella* subgenus II infections as human beings, especially under stress and immunosuppressive therapy.

The incidence of Shigellae in the same 851 baboons (table II) was 19.38 %. The types detected correspond well with findings of other authors. *Shigella flexneri* infections especially types II, IV and V dominated in our material as well as in Sukhumi, and at the Nuffield Institute of Comparative Medicine [5]. Almost all primates, especially the gibbons and the Cercopithecoidea, can be carriers of shigellae, usually of the Flexner group, sometimes also of the Schmitz and Sonne group (table II). *Shigella* can cause overt disease at any time, under adverse conditions. Shigellae can be carried for life and are difficult to eliminate.

Approximately 30.0 % of our baboons carried enteropathogenic *E.coli* types at arrival in our colony. The most prominent types were 055, 0119, 026 (table III). All these baboons appeared healthy. Enteropathogenic *E.coli* created problems under immunosuppressive therapy in gaining pathogenicity even in adult baboons. Even more disturbing are the chances of unwanted immune reactions due to heterogenetic antigens shared by *E.coli* and by the cell membranes of different animal species, thus endowing the passive carriers with new serological specificities [6].

Acknowledgement

This investigation was partly supported by a grant for current expenses from the Medical Research Council of the Republic of South Africa.

References

1 Brede, H.D.: Les salmonelloses au sud de l'Afrique; dans Van Oye The world problem of salmonellosis, pp.379–393 (Junk, Den Haag 1964).
2 Brede, H.D.: Salmonella grabouw = 11:g, m, s, t:z 39, a new species. J.Bact. *87:* 479–480 (1964).
3 Olin, G. und Alin, K.: Ein neuer Salmonellatyp *(S.sundsvall)* in Schweden nachgewiesen. Acta path.microbiol.scand. *20:* 607–614 (1943).
4 Kelterborn, E.: Salmonella species, p.359 (Junk, Den Haag 1967).
5 Fiennes, R.N.T-W-: Stress and the latent pathogen; in Balner and Beveridge In-

fections and immunosuppression in subhuman primates, pp. 149–154 (Munksgaard, Copenhagen 1970).

6 WHANG, H. Y. and NETER, E.: Immunological studies of a heterogenetic enterobacterial antigen (Kunin). J. Bact. *84:* 1245–1250 (1962).

Author's address: Prof. Dr. med. H. D. BREDE, Department of Medical Microbiology, University of Stellenbosch and Tygerberg Hospital, *Tiervlei, C.P.* (South Africa)

Medical Primatology 1972. Proc. 3rd Conf. exp. Med. Surg. Primates, Lyon 1972, part III, pp. 39–44 (Karger, Basel 1972)

Infectious Agents and the Management of Simians in a Medical Research Institute

C. R. Coid

Clinical Research Centre, Harrow, Middlesex

In many institutes the accommodation provided for laboratory primates is self-contained with all facilities necessary for the proper management of the animals. However, there are a number of institutes where, for reasons of economy, the supporting services have had to be centralised and this communication describes the procedures for managing simians in an animal facility which also contains many other different species of experimental animals and communal ancilliary services.

The basic principles of animal management applicable to the common species of laboratory animals for medical research also apply to the management of simians. There are, however, additional factors which must be considered and the most important is that many simians used in laboratories today may carry and transmit infectious agents, not only to their own kind, but also to man and other species. It is apparent, therefore, that systems of management employed must take into consideration the nature and pathogenesis of the micro-organisms likely to be involved, and their modes of transmission.

Principal Pathogenic Micro-Organisms of Simians

The principal bacterial infections of nonhuman primates which present a hazard to man are those caused by *Mycobacterium tuberculosis, Shigella* and *Salmonella.*

Tuberculosis is a relatively common disease in *Macaca mulatta.* A survey of the literature tabulated by Ruch [21] shows that the disease in monkeys is caused mainly by the bovine and human type of organisms, both of which cause infections in man. Pulmonary lesions in monkeys frequently cavitate and bacteria may be expelled by coughing. Such animals must, of course, be considered a serious hazard to personnel and other monkeys in contact.

The spread of *Shigella* infection to a human from simian species has been documented by CARPENTER and SANDIFORD [3]. The incident occurred when a child eating an ice cream was watching monkeys in a 'pets corner' of a large store. One of the animals put out its paw and touched the ice cream; the child licked it before the mother could throw it away. Two days later the child appeared off colour and after four days the faeces contained blood and mucus. *Sh. flexneri* 103Z was isolated from the child and also from the faeces on the floor of the monkey cage. Other cases of *Shigella* infections associated with monkeys have also been documented [7, 18, 21].

Many species of *Salmonella* have been isolated frequently from simians [20, 21] and transmission to handlers and to other species of animals must be considered a possibility. Recently it has been reported [23] that *Salmonella oranienburg,* isolated from a child was traced to a spider monkey in a local pet store managed by the child's mother.

Certain intestinal protozoa and nematodes may also be infectious to man and to other species of laboratory animals. Three organisms considered by NEAL [14] to be a handling hazard are *Entamoeba histolytica, Giardia intestinalis* and *Balantidium coli.*

Toxoplasmosis and mycotic infections occur not infrequently in simians [21] and the possibility that these infections may be transmitted to humans cannot be ignored.

The most serious microbial hazards to personnel are those created by the viruses. The principal agents known to cause disease are rabies [2, 19], *Herpesvirus simiae* [22] and the 'Marburg' agent of vervet monkeys [25].

Of 15 workers who died from *Herpesvirus simiae* infection, seven had been scratched or bitten by monkeys [15] and in the case of the 'Marburg' agent of vervet monkeys it seems possible that infection could have occurred through the unbroken skin [25]. It is also important to note that *Herpesvirus simiae,* which appears to be of low pathogenicity for monkeys, belongs to the same group as *Herpesvirus hominis* which, when latent, may be activated by various stimuli [1]. During experiments in which monkeys were given immunosuppressive treatment with antilymphocyte serum [26], these workers suggested that viral infections in the animals might have been due to *Herpesvirus simiae.* After injection of antileucocytic serum [COID and BURGOS, unpubl. obs.] a herpes-like vesicle on the lip of a treated animal of the species *Macaca fascicularis* was observed.

There are many other viral agents to be found in simians and a review of some outbreaks of viral diseases in nonhuman primates is given by ESPAÑA [9]. From the point of view of practical management it is probable that the precautionary measures adopted to reduce the risks from the micro-organisms previously mentioned should be adequate to control other organisms found in simians.

Management

From the information available about the various kinds of micro-organisms found in simians, it is apparent that an attempt must be made to reduce, and where possible, eliminate pathogens from animals which have been obtained recently from the wild state. This may be achieved by the administration of suitable antibiotics which reduce the pathogen burden and improve the conditions of the animals [4, 28]. It is also necessary that precautions are taken when handling simians or their tissues to prevent bites, abrasions and contamination of the skin or eyes with infected material.

Procedures for the care and management of simians during the quarantine period, aimed at improving the health, have been discussed at some length in recent years [12, 30], and in Britain official legislation has now been introduced making the quarantining of simians a statutory requirement.

Following acceptance by the British Parliament of the Report of the Committee of Inquiry on Rabies [17], 'The Rabies (Importation of Mammals) Order 1971' [16] was introduced and became operative on January 10, 1972. The importation of many species of animals is now strictly controlled so that the introduction of rabies into Britain may be prevented. Such animals are subject to six months quarantine but vampire bats must be quarantined for life.

The 'official' quarantine regulations imposed by the Ministry of Agriculture are applied for the control of rabies but undoubtedly these practices, required by law, also contribute towards the control of infectious agents in addition to rabies virus. However, it is also necessary to apply 'domestic' quarantine procedures to deal with the control of other infectious agents along the lines recommended in the Laboratory Animal Handbook 4 [12], and the World Health Organization Technical Report Series No. 470 [30].

The rooms for holding new arrivals in quarantine should be well separated from those housing conditioned healthy animals. Each room or suite of rooms for holding simians should preferably be self-contained with its own ancilliary accommodation [5]. However, satisfactory procedures can also be implemented provided there is storage space and changing area where outer protective clothing may be obtained before entering the quarantine. At the end of the quarantine period the rooms should be disinfected before removing equipment, such as cages for cleaning.

The permanent rooms used for holding simians should also have adjacent space provided for protective clothing and storage of equipment. After simians have completed their quarantine period and are in overt good health, careful handling procedures and safety precautions should still be followed [6]. The safety procedures, which are more elaborate than those usually adopted for normal and apparently healthy animals, are justified because of the possible recrudescence of latent infections, particularly under conditions of experimental stress [6, 11, 27].

Control of Infection by Breeding

Experience in many institutes throughout the world has shown that breeding simians in captivity under controlled conditions results in the production of good quality healthy animals free from the common pathogens. Recently it has also been reported that the incidence of herpesvirus infection is much reduced in captive-bred animals [8]. However, it is well to remember that herpesvirus and other virus infections [10, 13, 24] and toxoplasmosis [29] may be acquired *in utero,* and that laboratory breeding may not eliminate every kind of pathogen.

References

1 ANDREWES, C. and PEREIRA, H.G.: In Viruses of vertebrates, 2nd ed., p.284 (Bailliere, Tindall & Cassell, London 1967).

2 BOULGER, L.R.: Natural rabies in a laboratory monkey. Lancet *i:* 941 (1966).

3 CARPENTER, K.P. and SANDIFORD, B.R.: Epidemiology of a human case of bacillary dysentery due to infection by *Shigella Flexneri* 103Z. Brit. med. J. *i:* 142 (1952).

4 COID, C.R.: The effect of oral administration of therapeutic doses of chlortetracycline and oxytetracycline on the growth of rhesus monkeys. Vet. Rec. *70:* 726 (1958).

5 COID, C.R.: Building design in relation to function of a laboratory primate unit. Lab. Anim. Symp. *1:* 113 (1968).

6 COID, C.R.: Management in relation to safety in a laboratory primate unit; in PERKINS

and O'DONOGHUE Laboratory animal handbooks, vol. 4, p. 213 (Laboratory Animals Ltd., London 1969).
7 COOK, R.: Simian Shigellosis; in PERKINS and O'DONOGHUE Laboratory animal handbooks, vol. 4, p. 83 (Laboratory Animals Ltd., London 1969).
8 DI GIACOMO, R.F. and SHAH, K.V.: Virtual absence of infection with *herpesvirus simiae* in colony-reared rhesus monkeys *(Macaca mulatta)*, with a literature review on antibody prevalence in natural and laboratory rhesus populations. Lab. anim. Sci. *22:* 61 (1972).
9 ESPAÑA, C.: Review of some outbreaks of viral disease in captive nonhuman primates. Lab. anim. Sci. *21:* 1023 (1971).
10 FENNER, F.: In The biology of animal viruses, vol. 2, p. 525 (Academic Press, New York 1968).
11 FIENNES, R.N. T-W: Stress and the latent pathogen; in BALNER and BEVERIDGE Infections and immunosuppression in subhuman primates, p. 149 (Munksgaard, Copenhagen and Williams & Wilkins, Baltimore 1970).
12 Proposed procedure for the housing and handling of simians to decrease the transmission of disease to man: in PERKINS and O'DONOGHUE Laboratory Animal Handbooks, vol. 4, p. 255 (Laboratory Animals Ltd., London 1969).
13 MONIF, G.R.G.: Viral infections of the human fetus (Collier-Macmillan, London 1969).
14 NEAL, R.A.: Intestinal protozoa of simians as a handling hazard; in PERKINS and O'DONOGHUE Laboratory animal handbooks, vol. 4, p. 77 (Laboratory Animals Ltd., London 1969).
15 PERKINS, F.T. and HARTLEY, E.G.: Precautions against B virus infection. Brit. med. J. *i:* 899 (1966).
16 Rabies (Importation of Mammals) Order 1971. S.I. No. 2045 (Her Majesty's Stationery Office, London 1971).
17 Report of the Committee of Inquiry on Rabies: Cmnd. 4696 (Her Majesty's Stationery Office, London 1971).
18 REWELL, R.E.: Outbreak of *Shigella schmitzii* infection in men and apes. Lancet *i:* 220 (1949).
19 RICHARDSON, J.H. and HUMPHREY, G.L.: Rabies in imported nonhuman primates. Lab. anim. Sci. *21:* 1083 (1971).
20 ROWE, B.: Salmonellosis in simians and other non-human primates; in PERKINS and O'DONOGHUE Laboratory animal handbooks, vol. 4, p. 63 (Laboratory Animals Ltd., London 1969).
21 RUCH, T.C.: Diseases of laboratory primates (Saunders, Philadelphia/London 1959).
22 SABIN, A.B. and WRIGHT, A.M.: Acute ascending myelitis following a monkey bite, with the isolation of a virus capable of reproducing the disease. J. exp. Med. *59:* 115 (1934).
23 SCHRIER, A.M.: Pet spider monkey transmits Shigellosis and Salmonellosis to humans; in Laboratory primate newsletter, vol. 10, p. 12 (Brown University, Providence, R. 1. at 1971).
24 SEVER, J.L.: Virus infections and malformations. Fed. Proc. *30:* 114 (1971).
25 SMITH, C.E.G.; SIMPSON, D.I.H.; BOWEN, E.T.W., and ZLOTNIK, I.: Fatal human disease from vervet monkeys. Lancet *ii:* 1119 (1967).

26 Bekkum, D.W. van; Ledney, G.D.; Balner, H.; Putten, L.M. van, and Vries, M.J. de: In Wolstenholme and O'Connor Antilymphocytic Serum. CIBA Study Group, No.29, p.110 (1967).

27 Bekkum, D.W. Van: Immunosuppressive regimens. Hazards to experimental animals and personnel. An introduction; in Balner and Beveridge Infections and immunosuppression in subhuman primates, p.195 (Munksgaard, Copenhagen and Williams & Wilkins, Baltimore 1970).

28 Waaij, D. van der; Vries, J.M. de, and Lekkerkerk, J.E.C.: Eliminating bacteria from monkeys with antibiotics; in Balner and Beveridge Infections and immunosuppression in subhuman primates, p.21 (Munksgaard, Copenhagen and Williams & Wilkins, Baltimore 1970).

29 White, L.T. and Sever, J.L.: Etiologic agents; in Rubin Handbook of congenital malformations, p.353 (Saunders, Philadelphia/London 1967).

30 World Health Organization Technical Report Series No.470: Health aspects of the supply and use of non-human primates for biomedical purposes (World Health Organization, Geneva 1970).

Author's address: Dr. C.R. Coid, Clinical Research Centre, Watford Road, Harrow, *Middlesex HA1 3UJ* (England)

Medical Primatology 1972. Proc. 3rd Conf. exp. Med. Surg. Primates, Lyon 1972, part III, pp. 45–53 (Karger, Basel 1972)

Transmission of Human Hepatitis B Virus Infection to the Chimpanzee

J. Desmyter, W. T. Liu, P. de Somer and J. Mortelmans

Rega Institute for Medical Research, University of Leuven, Leuven and Institute of Tropical Medicine, Antwerp

Introduction

Australia antigen (SH antigen, HAA, hepatitis B antigen) is specifically associated with human viral hepatitis type B [4, 15]. The antigen and the virus-like characteristic particles which carry it [6, 8] have been found in non-human primates in addition to man, but not in other animals. With immuno-diffusion and complement fixation, Australia antigen was found in approximately 3 % of anthropoid apes, antibodies in about the same percentage, and lower primates were negative [5, 8, 11–13, 15–18). However, Blumberg's group [2–4] mentioned the finding of Australia antigen in spider monkeys, vervets and marmosets in addition to apes. The spontaneous occurrence of Australia antigen or antibody in a nonhuman primate species evidently points towards the possibility that this species is susceptible to the virus of human viral hepatitis type B.

In the present study, we report on the administration of Australia antigen-positive human serum to five chimpanzees. The results indicate that active infection with human hepatitis B virus, and not merely immunization against Australia antigen [11], does occur in this species. Evidence is also given that the natural distribution of Australia antigen and antibodies in chimpanzees follows an infectious pattern. Additional reasons are given why Australia antigen in chimpanzees and in man, and the viral agent to which they relate, are probably identical. The studies indicate that, until more becomes known about the lower monkey species, the chimpanzee is the animal of choice for experimental studies on human hepatitis B virus which cannot be carried out in man.

Materials and Methods

Chimpanzees were housed in two colonies. All animals had been in captivity for at least one year, and were at least two years of age. Studies pertaining to the natural distribution of Australia antigen and antibodies were performed prior to the experimental introduction of human hepatitis B virus in one colony (colony A).

The Ouchterlony test (double immunodiffusion), counterelectrophoresis (immune precipitation electrophoresis), complement fixation, and (immune) electron microscopy were performed, with minor adaptations, as described by BLUMBERG, PESENDORFER, TAYLOR, ZUCKERMAN *et al.* in a WHO memorandum [1]. Serum transaminase (SGPT) levels were determined according to the Rietmann-Frankel method. Blood and biopsies were taken from chimpanzees under phencyclidine hydrochloride (Sernylan®) anesthesia.

Results

The serum of a hemophiliac who became a chronic carrier of Australia antigen following acute hepatitis was used as a source of virus. Contagiousness of this material was suggested by the fact that his wife developed antigen-positive hepatitis three months after he provided blood for the experiment. The serum was pelleted at 100,000 *g* for 2 h, washed with phosphate-buffered saline, pelleted and washed again, and injected into five chimpanzees of colony A. Each animal received the equivalent of 20 ml of serum containing Australia antigen at a titer of 1,024 by complement fixation. Equal amounts of the inoculum were injected simultaneously in the liver and i.v.

The results (table I) show that four different reaction patterns were observed in the five chimpanzees. Animal A had no antigen or antibody before exposure, and reacted with antibody after eight weeks. This could be due to infection, or to primary or secondary immunization without infection. The late appearance of antibody suggests, but does not prove, that infection occurred.

Chimpanzee B had antibody as detected by counterelectrophoresis, complement fixation and immune electron microscopy ten weeks before exposure, but not at the time of exposure. Antibody was first detected 13 weeks after exposure. Antigen appeared after 19 weeks. By week 15, antibody ceased to be detectable by complement fixation. It was replaced by a slight anticomplementary effect, suggesting the presence of antigen-antibody complexes. When this effect was present, antibody could usually be detected by counterelectrophoresis. By week 23, a high antigen titer was present, and counterelectrophoresis revealed specific precipitation lines both for antigen and antibody. With electron microscopy, spontaneous aggregates essentially consist-

Table I. Australia antigen and antibody response in chimpanzees following injection of antigen-positive human serum

Weeks before/after exposure	Chimpanzees							
	A		B		C		D+E	
	Ag	Ab	Ag	Ab	Ag	Ab	Ag	Ab
–30	–	–			–	8	–	–
–26	–	–			–	8		
–10	–	–	–	2	–	8	–	–
– 2					–	2		
– 0	–	–	–	–	–	2	–	–
1	–	–	–	–			–	–
2	–	–	–	–	–	128	–	–
3			–	–			–	–
4	–	–	–	–	–	64	–	–
5	–	–	–	–	–	64		
6	–	–	–	–	–	32	–	–
7	–	–						
8	8	4	–	–			–	–
9							–	–
10							–	–
12	–	4	–	–	–	16	–	–
13	–	4	–	8				
14	–	8	–	8				
15	–	2	–	AC4; CE–			–	–
16	–	2	–	AC4; CE+	–	8		
17	–	2	–	–			–	–
19	–	2	4	–			–	–
21	–	–					–	–
22	–	–						
23		2	128; CE+	AC4; CE+			–	–
25	–	–	512; CE+	AC4; CE+			–	–
				EM: aggregates				
27	–	–						

Ag = Australia antigen; Ab = Australia antibody; AC = anticomplementary; CE = counterelectrophoresis; EM = electron microscopy; – = no antigen or antibody. All sera tested with complement fixation (CF) and CE. The CF titer is given.

ing of the small particle of Australia antigen were demonstrated easily. The simultaneous presence of antigen and antibody, extending over a period of at least ten weeks, was established by four criteria: alternation of antigen and antibody, the anticomplementary effect [18], presence of antigen and antibody in single serum samples, and the presence of aggregates. Evidence of liver damage was obtained after week 16. There was some infiltration of the portal fields with mononuclear and polynuclear leukocytes after, but not before this date. Transaminase (SGPT) levels raised to 90 units, while early sera of this animal and all other sera of the other four chimpanzees remained within normal levels (35 units or less).

Chimpanzee C had antibody at the time of exposure, and reacted with an immediate booster response resulting in higher titers of antibody than observed in spontaneously positive chimpanzees (128 vs. 2–32 in other studies). No antigen was detected, including by electron microscopy.

Chimpanzees D and E were free of antigen and antibody before exposure, and remained so for the course of the study.

Presence of Australia Antigen in Untreated Chimpanzees

Sera were obtained from 48 nonanthropoid primates (13 *C. aethiops,* 14 *M. mulatta,* and 12 other species) [7]. Two orangutans, two gorillas, three dwarf chimpanzees, and 50 chimpanzees were also examined. No antigen was detected except in one chimpanzee, and no antibody was detected except in six chimpanzees. With double immunodiffusion, counterelectrophoresis, and complement fixation, the same cases of circulating antigen and antibody were detected. No additional positives were found when chimpanzee Australia antigen was used to detect antibodies in the 105 animals using complement fixation and counterelectrophoresis. No additional positives were found when chimpanzee Australia antiserum was used to detect Australia antigen. Chimpanzees positive for Australia antigen and antibodies had not been treated to our knowledge with human or animal blood or tissue transplants. Serum transaminase levels were within the normal range.

As reported elsewhere, Australia antigen and antibodies in the chimpanzee and in man could not be distinguished from each other [6]. In double immunodiffusion, chimpanzee antigen and antiserum gave reactions of identity with their human counterparts. Australia antigen and antibodies from human or chimpanzee origin could be used indifferently to titrate human and chimpanzee antibodies and antigen. A similar result has been reported by Maynard *et al.* [12]. Chimpanzee antigen contained large and tubular particles similar to those of man [6], in addition to the small particle which has been described previously [8]. All three particle types of the chimpanzee and those of man shared at least one common antigen, as shown by immune electron microscopy [6].

Infectious Patterns of Australia Antigenemia and Antibodies in Untreated Chimpanzees

Although spontaneous Australia antigen and antibodies have been described in chimpanzees, their association with infection and liver pathology have remained far from clear. The following results indicate an infectious pattern in the occurrence of antigen and antibodies in the chimpanzee. They were obtained prior to our administration of Australia antigen-positive serum in a number of chimpanzees, as mentioned above.

Our 50 chimpanzees were housed in two colonies, entirely separate from each other and staffed with different personnel. All six antibody-positive animals were part of small colony A, which consisted of 15 animals (table II). This clustering of antibody-positive animals was not due to chance, as shown by statistical analysis. In addition, the only antigen-positive animal also belonged to colony A. Among six persons who were in charge of the immediate care of animals in colony A, one was a symptom-free carrier of Australia antigen, which may have resulted from acute hepatitis three years before the initiation of the study.

Table II. Antibodies to Australia antigen in two colonies of chimpanzees

Antibodies	Positive	Negative	Total chimpanzees
Colony A	6	9	15
Colony B	0	35	35
Total chimpanzees	6	44	50

$p < 0.01$ (Fisher's test).

Positive titers of antibody in colony A varied between 1:2 and 1:8 by complement fixation during an observation period of ten months. Titers by counterelectrophoresis were generally twice as low. Evidence of antibody was lost in two chimpanzees after a period of two to six months, using the same methods. In two others, titers decreased two- or fourfold. In another animal, the decrease of antibody was equivocal. The sixth chimpanzee died in the course of the study. The specificity of the decrease of antibody titers was ascertained by simultaneous testing of serum samples and by the parallel results which were obtained using two different assay methods [7].

The limitation of Australia antigen and antibody to one colony, and the simultaneous drop of antibody titers suggested that we were dealing with a single antigenic stimulation, which may have intervened in colony A shortly before the beginning of our study. In other words, we were probably dealing with a single outbreak of infection by the virus associated with Australia antigen. How it was introduced or spread is not known. Fecal contact could encompass all cases, although other modes of transmission are also possible.

Discussion

The reaction patterns found after challenge of chimpanzees with human Australia antigen-positive serum were extremely varied. Each, however, is compatible with the course of reinfection with hepatitis B virus as observed in man. We, therefore, suggest that most or all chimpanzees used by us had some degree of acquired immunity at the time of attempted transmission. This immunity did not prevent infection, however.

Chimpanzee A (table I), with antibody appearing after more than four weeks, could be classified according to PRINCE *et al.* [14] as a primary responder, implying no previous contact with the virus. However, this slow reaction pattern is also in agreement with the slow appearance of Australia antibodies in children challenged with live hepatitis virus, after immunization with heated antigen-positive serum [10]. Immunization in chimpanzee A thus could be secondary as well as primary. Whether this reaction pattern is accompanied by viral replication is not clear, but the late appearance of antibodies suggests active infection.

In chimpanzee B, which had antibody weeks before but not at exposure, alternation of antigen and antibodies is quite similar to human reinfection by MS-2 virus observed by KRUGMAN and GILES [9]. Histological and transaminase changes were slight, but distinct. They were perhaps related to the presence of antigen-antibody complexes, which were abundant in the late sera from this animal and practically absent in the spontaneous chimpanzee carrier of Australia antigen [6]. None of the 45 untreated chimpanzees of our study acquired antigen or antibodies during an observation period of more than one year. The acquisition of active antigenemia and liver damage by chimpanzee B were, therefore, due to experimental (re)infection, and not to intercurrent spontaneous reinfection or to reactivation of its original infection.

Chimpanzee C, with antibody at the time of challenge, reacted with high-titered antibody within two weeks, indicating an anamnestic response. This early type of response typically occurs in immune individuals [14].

Chimpanzees C and D apparently did not become infected or immunized. A definitive judgment on this absence of reaction needs to be postponed until the sera have been examined with more sensitive methods for antigen and antibody detection. PURCELL [personnel commun.] reported antibodies detected by radioimmunoprecipitation in a majority of two-year-old chimpanzees. Studies with a radioimmunoassay for antigen detection (Abbott Laboratories) and passive hemagglutination for antibodies [19] are currently in progress.

It appears from these results that chimpanzees are susceptible to infection by human hepatitis B virus, that liver damage upon experimental infection is probably less pronounced than in man, and that infection is modified but not entirely suppressed by previous spontaneous experience of the chimpanzee with Australia antigen.

The association of spontaneously-acquired Australia antigen and antibodies with infection and liver disease in the chimpanzee has remained elusive. Applying identical methods in two different colonies of chimpanzees, we have shown that chimpanzees which were positive for antibody or antigen all clustered in one colony, and that antibody titers decreased progressively over a period of several months during which no animal acquired antigen or antibodies. This is strong evidence of an infectious epidemiological pattern similar to that of man. Liver damage was not observed in these chimpanzees.

The similarity of Australia antigen and antibodies in chimpanzees and in man was further stressed by an examination of their morphological and antigenic properties, as reported more extensively elsewhere [6].

In conclusion, Australia antigenemia and antibodies in the chimpanzee follow an infectious epidemiological pattern. The antigen is morphologically and antigenically similar, and probably identical with that of man. We have successfully attempted to transmit human hepatitis B virus infection to the chimpanzee. The usefulness of this animal as a model will be limited by its scarcity, and complicated by various degrees of naturally-acquired immunity, and low degree of liver pathology. Until another animal is found which can be reproducibly infected, the chimpanzee will prove an irreplaceable model for the study of various aspects of viral hepatitis type B.

Acknowledgements

We thank Dr. H. BALNER, TNO, Rijswijk, Netherlands, for providing us with chimpanzee sera.

References

1 ANON.: Viral hepatitis and test for the Australia (hepatitis-associated) antigen and antibody. Bull. Wld Hlth Org. *42:* 957 (1970).

2 BLUMBERG, B.S.: Australia antigen and leukemia. Comparative studies; in Proc. 6th Int. Symp. Comp. Leuk. Res. (1969).

3 BLUMBERG, B.S.; SUTNICK, A.I., and LONDON, W.T.: Hepatitis and leukemia. Their relation to Australia antigen. Bull. N.Y. Acad. Sci. *44:* 1566 (1968).

4 BLUMBERG, B.S.; SUTNICK, A.I.; LONDON, W.T., and MILLMAN, I.: The discovery of Australia antigen and its relation to viral hepatitis. Perspect. Virol. *7:* 223 (1971).

5 DEINHARDT, F.: Hepatitis in subhuman primates, and the hazards to man; in Infections and immunosuppression in subhuman primates, pp. 55–63 (Munksgaard, Copenhagen 1970).

6 DESMYTER, J.; LIU, W.T., and CREEMERS, J.: The large particle of Australia antigen. Amer. J. Dis. Child. *123:* 315 (1972).

7 DESMYTER, J.; LIU, W.T.; SOMER, P. DE, and MORTELMANS, J.: Primates as a model for human viral hepatitis. Transmission of infection by human hepatitis B virus. Vox Sang. (in press).

8 HIRSCHMAN, R.J.; SHULMAN, R.N.; BARKER, L.F., and SMITH, K.O.: Virus-like particles in sera of patients with infectious and serum hepatitis. J. amer. med. Ass. *208:* 1667 (1969).

9 KRUGMAN, S. and GILES, J.P.: Viral hepatitis. New light on an old disease. J. amer. med. Ass. *212:* 1019 (1970).

10 KRUGMAN, S.; GILES, J.P., and HAMMOND, J.: Viral hepatitis type B (MS-2 strain). Studies on active immunization. J. amer. med. Ass. *217:* 41 (1971).

11 LICHTER, E.A.: Chimpanzee antibodies to Australia antigen. Nature, Lond. *224:* 810 (1969).

12 MAYNARD, J.E.; BERQUIST, K.R.; HARTWELL, W.V., and KRUSHAK, D.H.: Viral hepatitis and studies of hepatitis associated antigen in chimpanzees. Canad. med. Ass. J. *106:* 473 (1972).

13 PRINCE, A.M.: Hepatitis associated antigen. Long-term persistence in chimpanzees; in GOLDSMITH and MOOR-JANKOWSKI Medical primatology 1970, p. 731 (Karger, Basel 1971).

14 PRINCE, A.M.; BROTMAN, B., and CHERUBIN, C.E.: Immune response in patients who received blood containing SH antigen. Amer. J. Dis. Child. *123:* 415 (1972).

15 PRINCE, A.M.; SZMUNESS, W.; HARGROVE, R.L.; JEFFRIES, G.H.; CHERUBIN, C.E., and KELLNER, A.: The serum hepatitis virus specific antigen. A status report. Perspect. Virol. *7:* 241 (1971).

16 RIVERS, S.L. and KEELING, M.: A study of the incidence of Australia antigen and antibody in nonhuman primates. Vox Sang. *19:* 270 (1970).

17 SHULMAN, N.R.: Hepatitis-associated antigen. Amer. J. Med. *49:* 669 (1970).
18 SHULMAN, N.R. and BARKER, L.F.: Virus-like antigen, antibody, and antigen-antibody complexes in hepatitis measured by complement fixation. Science *165:* 304 (1969).
19 VYAS, G.N. and SHULMAN, N.R.: Hemagglutination assay for antigen and antibody associated with viral hepatitis. Science *170:* 332 (1970).

Authors' addresses: Dr. JAN DESMYTER, Dr. WU TSE LIU and Dr. PIERRE DE SOMER, Rega Institute for Medical Research, University of Leuven, *Leuven,* Dr. JOSEPH MORTELMANS, Institute of Tropical Medicine, *Antwerp* (Belgium). Reprint requests to Dr. DESMYTER

Medical Primatology 1972. Proc. 3rd Conf. exp. Med. Surg. Primates, Lyon 1972, part III, pp. 54–57 (Karger, Basel 1972)

Nonhuman Primates in Cholera Experiments[1]

O. FELSENFELD and R. H. WOLF

Tulane University Delta Primate Research Center, Covington, La.

Several decades ago SANARELLI and his group [quoted from POLLITZER, 1959] introduced the use of nonhuman primates in the study of cholera. Unfortunately, at that time such animals were not readily available. Therefore, experimentation on monkeys and apes under controlled conditions had to be postponed until more animals kept in properly-equipped colonies became accessible. This opportunity arose during the extensive work on poliomyelitis in the 1950's. The recent increase of primate centers further enhanced the possibility of utilizing the nonhuman primate as a cholera model. With the support of the World Health Organization, a cholera study section was established at this Primate Center.

The selection of the proper primate species was difficult because, although nonhuman primates are apparently not infected with cholera in nature, large numbers of animals of many species had antitoxic and/or vibriocidal antibodies in their circulation. After extensive screening, macaques and most South American monkeys were found not useable for cholera experimentation while individual *Erythrocebus patas* and *Cercopithecus aethiops* were susceptible to orally-administered cholera vibrios. However, the supply of vervet monkeys became temporarily limited after the Marburg outbreak in 1967, and *Papio* and *Cercocebus* were not available in sufficient numbers or at acceptable cost. Prosimii were not tested. The susceptibility to cholera decreased with age; therefore, the number of chimpanzees available was

1 These experiments were supported by grant AI 07632 of the National Institutes of Health in Bethesda, Md.; by the World Health Organization; and by the Swiss Serum and Vaccine Institute in Bern.

Table I. 'Natural' cholera antitoxin and vibriocidal levels in the sera of some primates

Species	Number examined	Antitoxin levels[1]			Vibriocidal titers[2]		
		< 30	30	% positive	< 100	100	% positive
Pan troglodytes	50	38	12	24	43	7	14
Theropithecus gelada	20	17	2	10	18	2	10
Macaca speciosa	20	15	5	25	16	4	20
Macaca mulatta	60	23	37	61.7	29	31	51.7
Cercopithecus aethiops	50	39	11	22	38	12	24
Erythrocebus patas	100	82	18	18	85	15	15

1 Determined by ligated gut neutralization test.
2 Determined by the tube method.

always limited. Table I shows the result of the examination of 300 nonhuman primates for circulating cholera antitoxin and vibriocidal antibodies. These primates came from areas not invaded by cholera before their capture. Animals with > 30 rabbit ligated loop antitoxin units and/or > 100 vibriocidal antibody titers per milliliter serum were not used in cholera experiments.

In the course of the experiments six cholera strains were used, among them the Inaba 569 B strain of Dutta which is widely employed in cholera studies.

The infective dose was 10 ± 1 MID. It varied between approximately 10^6 and 10^9 vibrios, according to the strain, and was given after a 24-hour starvation by duodenal gavage. Only a limited (5–10) percent of the infected animals developed frank cholera symptoms. The others developed only mild diarrhea. This resembled closely observations in man. The principal goal of the studies was to evaluate local and generalized immunologic phenomena, particularly the enumeration of immunologically competent cells and the determination of immunoglobulin, antitoxin, vibriocidal and precipitating antibody levels, as well as testing new immunizing agents and their influence on the immunologic system. It was shown that patas and vervet monkeys, as well as chimpanzees, possess a semiautonomous gastrointestinal local defense mechanism that was strongly influenced by a 'center' in the cecum. The principal role of IgA was found to be antitoxic, whereas vibriocidal activity was mostly a function of IgG. IgM appeared to be active particularly during the early days after infection. The role of IgE class antibodies is under investigation. The defense afforded by circulating antibodies was of secondary nature. The results have been published in several communications [FELSEN-

FELD and GREER, 1968; FELSENFELD *et al.,* 1966a and b, 1967, 1968a and b, 1969].

The formation of local antibodies in the gastrointestinal tract, its plasma cell system and of the biliary system was studied by periodic collection of biopsy specimens. It was demonstrated that, if such surgery is properly performed, the organisms do not enter the tissues. Lymph nodes and lymphoid-plasma cell accumulations could be collected at about ten-day intervals without interfering with the response to cholera vibrios and their toxins. Implantation of segments of the jejunum with intact blood, nerve and lymph supply under the skin allowed the introduction of cholera vibrios and their derivatives into an isolated loop and permitted abbreviation of the effects on the animal *in toto* as well as locally. Studies of the biliary system with regards to antibody formation were also included [GREER *et al.,* 1968; KECLIK *et al.,* 1970]. Ligated intestinal loop experiments for testing fluid and electrolyte outflow were also possible but resulted in a higher mortality of the animals.

Nonhuman primates gave satisfactory results in the study of the fate of labeled antigens by the fluorescent antibody or the autoradiographic methods. Autoradiography also permitted the study of the formation and fate of secretory and excretory IgA in the intestines without sacrificing the animals [FELSENFELD and GREER, 1968; FELSENFELD *et al.,* 1967, 1968a and b].

The protective effect of immunizing agents was measured not only by the clinical picture and duration of vibrio excretion but also by determination of the enumerated immunologic phenomena. To date, heat treated and untreated routinely used cholera vaccines of various provenience and concentrations, the toxins and toxoids as prepared by Burrows, Ungar and others, vaccines with adjuvants, Watanabe's lipopolysaccharide, ribosomal vaccines and antigens prepared from attenuated organisms have been tested. Some of those that proved effective in monkeys and apes have been or are being already used in field trials in man [FELSENFELD *et al.,* 1968a, 1970].

While the routinely employed laboratory rodents are cheaper and easier to handle, nonhuman primates appear to afford a model that is phylogenetically much nearer to man. Their immunological response is more in accord with that of humans. Admittedly, nonhuman primates are more expensive, require more extensive care, and the collection of biopsy specimens can be performed only under aseptic conditions by an experienced surgeon. Animals without nonspecific or paraspecific antibody formation have to be selected with great care. Nevertheless the method deserves further exploitation, particularly in vaccine evaluations.

References

FELSENFELD, O. and GREER, W.E.: Vibriocidal activity, immune globulin producing cells, and immune globulin levels in *Theropithecus gelada* after administration of a *Vibrio cholerae* antigen. Immunology *14:* 319–324 (1968).

FELSENFELD, O.; FELSENFELD, A.D., and GREER, W.E.: Avidity of cholera antibody. Trans. roy. Soc. trop. Med. Hyg. *63:* 846–853 (1969).

FELSENFELD, O.; GREER, W.E., and FELSENFELD, A.D.: Cholera toxin neutralisation and some sites of immune globulin formation in *Cercopithecus aethiops*. Nature, Lond. *213:* 1249–1251 (1967).

FELSENFELD, O.; HILL, C.W., and GREER, W.E.: Response of *Cercopithecus aethiops* to cholera vibrio lipopolysaccharide and psychological stress. Trans. roy. Soc. trop. Med. Hyg. *60:* 514–518 (1966a).

FELSENFELD, O.; BURROWS, W., KASAI, G.J, and JIRICKA, Z.: Cellular immune response of nonhuman primates to crude type 2 cholera toxin. J. infect. Dis. *118:* 491–499 (1968a).

FELSENFELD, O.; FELSENFELD, A.D.; GREER, W.E., and HILL, C.W.: Relationship of some vibrio antibodies to serum immune globulins in man and in *Cercopithecus aethiops*. J. infect. Dis. *116:* 329–334 (1966b).

FELSENFELD, O.; GREER, W.E.; KIRTLEY, B., and JIRICKA, Z.: Cholera studies in nonhuman primates. Trans. roy. Soc. trop. Med. Hyg. *62:* 378–284 (1968b).

FELSENFELD, O.; STEGHERR-BARRIOS, A.; ALDOVA, A.; HOLMES, J., and PARROTT, M.W.: *In vitro* and *in vivo* studies of streptomycin-dependent cholera vibrios. Appl. Microbiol. *19:* 463–469 (1970).

GREER, W.E.; JIRICKA, Z., and FELSENFELD, O.: Gallbladder damage and prolonged excretion of cholera vibrios in *Erythrocebus patas*. Proc. Soc. exp. Biol. Med. *127:* 551–555 (1968).

KECLIK, M.; WOLF, R.H.; FELSENFELD, O., and SMETANA, H.F.: Gallbladder, immunoglobulins and antibodies in bile. Amer. J. Gastroent. *54:* 19–29 (1970).

POLLITZER, R.: Cholera. Wld. Hlth. Org. Techn. Papers Ser. No. 43 (World Health Organization, Geneva 1959).

Author's address: Dr. O. FELSENFELD, Tulane University Delta Primate Research Center, *Covington, LA 70433* (USA)

Medical Primatology 1972. Proc. 3rd Conf. exp. Med. Surg. Primates, Lyon 1972, part III, pp. 58–67 (Karger, Basel 1972)

Nonhuman Primate Zoonoses Surveillance in the United States

A. F. Kaufmann

Epidemiology Program, Center for Disease Control, Health Services and Mental Health Administration, US Department of Health, Education and Welfare, Atlanta, Ga.

Introduction

Spontaneous disease in captive nonhuman primates is widely recognized as a serious problem. The financial loss caused by such disease on a world-wide basis, while unknown, must be extraordinary based on the cost of the animals themselves, interruption in scientific investigations and invalidation of laboratory results. The public health impact and the drain on the dwindling supply of free-living animals are also important but poorly defined factors.

Despite the cost of disease in these animals, surprisingly little progress has been made in understanding the epidemiology of their diseases and developing rational disease control programs. In the United States, preventive medicine programs for nonhuman primates are limited for the most part to initial quarantine, tuberculosis screening and the questionable practice of antibiotic prophylaxis. Even this limited program is not uniformly followed. The length of the usual quarantine period in various laboratories ranges from essentially none to 90 days. The methods, efficacy and extent of tuberculosis screening also vary greatly among laboratories. The approximately 50,000 monkeys imported into the United States each year for sale as pets are neither routinely quarantined nor screened for potential human pathogens.

Surveillance is a basic requirement of any disease control program. Surveillance is essential to quantify the relative importance of any given disease as a cause of nonhuman primate morbidity and mortality. It provides information on age, sex and species specific attack rates, and whether the incidence of disease in a particular group of animals is unusual and may represent a specific colony management problem. Through determination of attack rates by time in colony, surveillance can indicate the quarantine period length necessary to exclude certain diseases from a colony. However, surveillance without communication is a limited tool. Effective rapid communication for the exchange of data on morbidity and mortality and other information on nonhuman primates is currently lacking. Material in scientific journals is often a year or more out-of-date because of the time involved in producing such publications. Also, personal communication between individual colonies is erratic. This has often resulted in duplication of effort by several investigators studying similar and concurrent disease outbreaks.

In 1970, the Center for Disease Control initiated the Primate Zoonoses Surveillance Program to obtain data on spontaneous disease incidence in captive nonhuman primates and the real risk to human health associated with handling these animals. The program is based on monthly reports submitted by selected centers in the United States that utilize large numbers of nonhuman primates. Analyses of the data are published in the quarterly CDC Primate Zoonoses Surveillance Report. In addition, the report includes informal notes on interesting current outbreaks, serologic surveys and other information derived from a variety of sources.

Surveillance of Disease in Nonhuman Primates

The participating centers submitted data on disease in 2,027 animals (2,379 diagnoses) in 1970 and 2,091 animals (2,478 diagnoses) in 1971. The average monthly population at risk was 7,069 animals in 1970 and 9,328 in 1971. The overall reported case-fatality ratio was 41.9% (850:2,027) in 1970 and 35.7% (747:2,091) in 1971.

The three leading causes of morbidity and mortality in both 1970 and 1971 were digestive, respiratory and traumatic diseases, in that order. The three leading causes of mortality were digestive, respiratory and generalized diseases. The relative frequency of organ system involvement by quarter was relatively constant in 1970 and 1971 (tables I and II). The observed variations were often the result of single outbreaks. For example, reported disease of the nervous system was relatively infrequent except in the fourth quarter of 1970, when it was the fourth leading cause of morbidity and mortality and the second leading cause of mortality. This variation was the result of an outbreak of an obscure neurologic disease associated with a picornavirus at one colony.

Table I. Organ system rank by frequency of involvement as a cause of reported non-human primate morbidity and mortality, 1970–1971

Organ system	1970				1971			
	Jan.-March	Apr.-June	July-Sept.	Oct.-Dec.	Jan.-March	Apr.-June	July-Sept.	Oct.-Dec.
Digestive	1[1]	1	1	1	1	1	1	1
Respiratory	2	4	3	3	3	2	3	4
Trauma[2]	3	2	2	2	2	3	2	2
Generalized	4	3	4	5	4	4	4	3
Urogenital	5	5	6	6	5	5	5	6
Integumentary	6	5	5	7	6	8	6	8
Musculoskeletal	7	8	9	9	7	8	8	8
Cardiovascular	8	6	7	8	8	6	7	5
Unspecified	9	7	10	10	9	9	10	8
Nervous	10	7	8	4	10	7	7	7
Neoplasia[2]	–[3]	9	11	11	11	9	9	9

1 Rank in this quarter.
2 All organ systems.
3 No cases reported in this quarter.

Table II. Organ system rank by frequency of involvement as a cause of reported non-human primate mortality, 1970–1971

Organ system	1970				1971			
	Jan.-March	Apr.-June	July-Sept.	Oct.-Dec.	Jan.-March	Apr.-June	July-Sept.	Oct.-Dec.
Digestive	1[1]	2	1	1	1	1	1	1
Respiratory	2	1	2	3	3	2	2	2
Generalized	3	3	3	4	2	3	3	3
Trauma[2]	4	4	4	5	4	5	5	4
Unspecified	5	6	7	7	5	8	8	8
Cardiovascular	6	5	5	6	6	4	7	6
Urogenital	7	7	6	6	5	6	4	5
Nervous	8	8	6	2	8	7	6	7
Integumentary	9	8	8	8	8	–[3]	9	10
Musculoskeletal	10	9	8	7	7	9	–[3]	9
Neoplasia[2]	–[3]	10	8	9	9	9	8	10

1 Rank in this quarter.
2 All organ systems.
3 No cases reported in this quarter.

The incidence of disease per 100 monkey months' residence in colony was 2.4 in 1970 and 1.9 in 1971. The decreased incidence in 1971 may be related to a general decrease in procurement of simians by the participating centers. Certain species, such as *Lagothrix* spp., *Aotus trivirgatus* and *Erythrocebus patas,* had a consistently higher disease incidence than other species (table III). The case-fatality ratio for all diseases was significantly higher in prosimians and New World monkeys than in Old World monkeys and great apes.

Infectious disease was a major problem in all the participating centers in 1970 and 1971. The pattern of occurrence of selected infectious disease entities

Table III. Relative incidence of disease and case-fatality ratios by animal species group, 1970–1971

Species group	Incidence[1]	Case-fatality ratio[2] and (%)	
I. Prosimians	0.6	32:39	(82.1)
II. All New World species	1.9	293:347	(84.4)
(1) lagothrix	8.2	3:6	(50.0)
(2) marmosets	4.8	48:52	(92.3)
(3) aotus	4.1	115:130	(88.5)
(4) other New World	2.6	22:27	(81.5)
(5) ateles	1.7	4:4	(100.0)
(6) saimiri	1.0	81:100	(81.0)
cebus	1.0	20:28	(71.4)
III. All Old World species	2.1	1,237:3,544	(34.9)
(1) *E. patas*	6.7	54:155	(34.8)
(2) *M. nemestrina*	2.8	205:497	(41.2)
(3) *M. mulatta*	2.2	726:2,161	(33.6)
(4) *M. fascicularis*	1.8	79:263	(30.0)
M. arctoides	1.8	37:124	(29.8)
(5) other Old World	1.5	43:96	(44.8)
(6) other macaque	1.1	68:156	(43.6)
(7) vervet	1.0	9:25	(36.0)
(8) baboons	0.9	16:47	(34.0)
IV. All great apes	3.7	31:179	(17.3)
(1) chimpanzees	4.0	26:146	(17.8)
(2) other great apes	2.9	5:33	(15.2)
V. All species[3]	2.1	1,597:4,118	(38.8)

1 Number of animals with reported disease/100 monkey months' residence in colony.
2 Number of fatal cases/total cases (%).
3 Includes three animals for which the species was not specified.

Table IV. Pattern of occurrence of selected infectious disease entities at the participating centers, 1970–1971

Sporadic cases	Endemic	Epizootic
(1) Systemic herpes virus infections	(1) Shigellosis[1]	(1) Varicella-like disease
(2) Varicella-like disease	(2) Salmonellosis[1]	(2) Measles (rubeola)
(3) Pneumococcal meningitis	(3) Enteropathogenic *E. coli* infections[1]	(3) Picornavirus-associated neurologic disease
(4) Pseudotuberculosis	(4) Parasitic enteritis	(4) Tuberculosis
(5) Tuberculosis		(5) 'Bloody nose syndrome'[2]
(6) *Mycobacterium avium/intracellulare* infections		(6) Lymphosarcoma (infectious?)
(7) Dermatophilosis		
(8) *Pneumocystis carinii* pneumonia		

1 Frequently present as severe outbreaks.
2 Etiology unknown but suspected to be viral.

is found in table IV. Diseases that caused major problems were shigellosis, measles, tuberculosis, varicella-like disease and picornavirus-associated neurologic disease.

Because of limitations of space, the present discussion of the surveillance data will be limited to brief comments on enteric and respiratory diseases.

Enteric Diseases

Diarrheal disease was the most commonly reported illness in both 1970 and 1971. The case-fatality ratio for diarrheal disease due to all causes was 39.7% (247:622) in 1970 and 35.0% (312:892) in 1971. The case-fatality ratio was high regardless of length of time in colony or age group (table V). Most cases were reported in adult animals (41.9%) and in animals in a colony 1–30 days (38.0%).

Shigellosis was the most frequently specified cause of diarrheal disease. Shigellosis appeared to be endemic in the participating centers; while it was frequently epizootic in animals during the first 90 days in colony, outbreaks were also common in long-term colonized animals as well. Outbreaks in nurseries for newborn animals were reported, reflecting the need for scrupulous hygiene in such areas. Most reported cases of shigellosis occurred in Old World monkeys. *Shigella flexneri* 4/4b was the most frequently specified

Table V. Case-fatality ratios for animals with diarrheal disease, 1970–1971

By time in colony				
1–30 days	31–90 days	91 days to 1 year	1 year +	Total[1]
244:576 (42.4)[2]	83:186 (44.6)	75:267 (28.1)	155:480 (32.3)	559:1,514 (36.9)
By age group				
Infant	Juvenile	Adult	Aged	Total[1]
62:215 (28.8)	253:633 (40.0)	226:634 (35.6)	12:18 (66.7)	559:1,514 (36.9)

1 Includes animals for which time in colony or age group were not specified.
2 Number of fatal cases/total cases (%).

infecting serotype (37.7%). The overall case-fatality ratio for reported shigellosis was 24.3% (92:379). The case-fatality ratio was highest for animals during the first 30 days in colony (28.7%) and for aged (83.3%) and mature (29.9%) animals.

Salmonella and enteropathogenic *Escherichia coli* infections were also noted to be endemic in many of the participating centers. Disease associated with these organisms was much less common than shigellosis, being reported only 20 and 25%, respectively, as frequently as shigellosis. The reported case-fatality ratio for *Salmonella* and enteropathogenic *E. coli* infections were 35.1% (27:77) and 26.3% (25:95), respectively. Infections occurred most frequently in animals in a colony more than one year and in mature animals. Group B *Salmonella* organisms were most frequently reported. Enteropathogenic *E. coli* infections were most frequent in the first 30 days of colonization and in mature animals. The most frequently reported infecting *E. coli* serotypes were 026, 055, and 0119.

Parasitic enteritis was reported in 97 animals in the two-year period. The case-fatality ratio was 21.6% (21:97). *Strongyloides* spp., *Entamoeba histolytica* and *Balantidium coli* were the most frequently reported etiologic agents. These infections were most common in mature animals maintained in a colony for more than one year.

One problem area in enteric disease of nonhuman primates is the frequent occurrence of multiple-drug resistant enterobacteria. This multiple resistance is due in part to indiscriminate use of antimicrobial agents for prophylactic and therapeutic treatment of the animals following importation. However, the finding of such resistances in newly arrived animals which reputedly had not received prior antimicrobial therapy suggests that other factors may be playing a role. One possible explanation is that the resistances may result from exposure to R-factors of human origin in the exporting country. There is some suggestive evidence that such a mechanism may be occurring in New World monkeys.

Respiratory Disease

Pneumonia was the second leading cause of morbidity and mortality at the participating centers in 1970–1971. A total of 411 cases, exclusive of pneumonia associated with systemic disease due to measles and herpesvirus infections, were reported. The reported case-fatality ratio was 83.9% (345:411) (table VI). Most cases (65.2%) occurred during the first 90 days in colony. There was no apparent seasonal periodicity to the occurrence of the reported cases. An etiology was specified for only 30% of the 411 cases. Over 25 different agents were specified, including *Streptococcus pneumoniae, Bordetella bronchiseptica, Klebsiella* spp., β-hemolytic streptococci, *Staphylococcus aureus* and *Pneumocystis carinii.* Any given agent was associated with only a small number of cases. In addition to these cases, pneumonia was observed in 102 of 127 (80.3%) animals infected with measles and in two of the 49 (4.1%) with herpesvirus infections.

Pneumonia of nonhuman primates is poorly understood. The high case-fatality ratio suggests that either therapy is relatively ineffective or that a large number of clinical cases go undetected. Many cases may be secondary to other disease processes. For example, 106 of the 411 cases were associated with severe diarrheal disease. The role of viral infections is poorly understood. Measles infections frequently cause a pneumonia, and undoubtedly other

Table VI. Case-fatality ratios for animals with pneumonia, 1970–1971[1]

By time in colony				
1–30 days	31–90 days	91 days to 1 year	1 year +	Total
172:190 (90.5)[2]	65:78 (83.3)	55:71 (77.5)	53:72 (73.6)	345:411 (83.9)
By age group				
Infant	Juvenile	Adult	Aged	Total
62:82 (75.6)	138:154 (89.6)	138:168 (82.1)	6:6 (100.0)	345:411 (83.9)

1 Excludes animals having pneumonia as a component of systemic infections due to measles or herpesviruses.
2 Number of fatal cases/total cases (%).

common viral diseases of nonhuman primates cause primary pneumonia; which ones we do not know.

Tuberculosis was a major problem in 1970–1971. Thirty-two cases of tuberculosis that resulted in death or necessitated sacrifice of the affected animals were reported. An additional 20 animals converted to tuberculin positive during an epizootic and were placed on antituberculosis therapy. The number of cases by species were: *Erythrocebus patas:* 1; *Gorilla gorilla:* 4; *Macaca fascicularis:* 1; *M. mulatta:* 23; *M. nemestrina;* 1; *Pan troglodytes:* 12; and *Pongo pygmaeus:* 10.

Available data indicate a great need for improved diagnostic procedures. Many of the reported cases were not detected during the quarantine period even though methods equivalent to or better than currently recommended procedures were used by the reporting centers. Fourteen of the 32 animals that died had been in a colony one to 30 days, three for 31–90 days, seven for 91 days to one year, and eight for more than one year prior to diagnosis. Eleven of the 32 fatal cases had originated in another primate colony; the rest were imported. An epizootic of tuberculosis in one colony apparently resulted from introduction of a tuberculous chimpanzee. This animal was not detected by routine tuberculin screening during the quarantine period, and its disease was recognized only at necropsy seven months after purchase.

Surveillance of Human Disease Associated with Nonhuman Primate Contact

Illness and injuries in persons having direct contact with nonhuman primates at the participating centers are summarized in table VII. In 1970–1971, 22 tuberculin conversions, 86 cases of gastroenteritis and five monkey bites were reported. The true occurrence of such disease at the participating

Table VII. Reported illness and injuries in humans having close contact with nonhuman primates in the participating centers, 1970–1971

Year	Number with direct contact	Tuberculin convertors	Gastro-enteritis	Monkey bites
1970	350[1]	6	61	2
1971	500	16	25	3

1 Estimated number of individuals included on one or more monthly reports during the year.

centers is known to be greater because all centers do not actively report human disease.

The frequency of tuberculin conversion is much higher than would be caused by chance alone in the small study population. In the United States, the estimated annual rate for new human tuberculosis infections as measured by tuberculin conversions and the detection of active cases in 3 per 10,000. The infection rate in the human population under surveillance at the participating centers was 171 per 10,000 in 1970 and 320 per 10,000 in 1971. These rates indicate a need for intensified tuberculosis control programs for all persons handling nonhuman primates.

In addition to cases reported by the participating centers, numerous other instances of nonhuman primate-associated disease were noted by state and local health departments in the United States in 1970–1971. One case of active tuberculosis [4] and four tuberculin conversions associated with exposure to tuberculous nonhuman primates were reported. Five outbreaks of chimpanzee-associated hepatitis that resulted in 38 cases of human disease were reported by three states [2, 4]. A fatal case of human shigellosis due to *S.flexneri* 2a acquired from a pet spider monkey occurred in 1970 [5]. A related spider monkey associated outbreak in another state occurred in the same year [1]. The latter outbreak resulted in five cases of diarrheal illness in a single family, three *S.flexneri* 2a infections, one *Salmonella oranienburg* infection, and one infection which was not cultured.

Nonhuman primate bites often result in serious complications because of their septic nature. In addition to the associated pain and possible disfiguration, transmission of serious viral diseases, such as herpesvirus infections and rabies, may result. The incidence of such bites in the relatively small population directly exposed to nonhuman primates is unknown but must be high. In the period 1967–1971, 542 cases of humans bitten by nonhuman primates were reported to the New York City Health Department [3]. Most of the reported bites were inflicted by pet (68.1%) and stray (14.9%) monkeys. The incidence of such bites in New York City alone indicates that at least several thousand cases must occur annually in the United States.

The data reported to the Center for Disease Control indicates that human disease resulting from nonhuman primate contact is a real problem in the small population at risk. Better data is needed to adequately quantify its magnitude, particularly for persons exposed to pet monkeys. However, available evidence clearly demonstrates the need for intensified hepatitis and tuberculosis control programs, as well as a continuing education program on the associated health risks for persons exposed to these animals.

Acknowledgements

The success of any surveillance program depends on the collaboration of the individual participants. Nine centers participated in the Primate Zoonoses Surveillance Program in 1970–1971: Delta Regional Primate Center, Tulane University, Covington, La.; National Center for Primate Biology, University of California, Davis, Calif.; New England Regional Primate Research Center, Harvard University, Southborough, Mass.; Oregon Regional Primate Research Center, University of Oregon, Beaverton, Oreg.; Washington Regional Primate Research Center, University of Washington, Seattle, Wash.; Wisconsin Regional Primate Center, University of Wisconsin, Madison, Wisc.; Yerkes Regional Primate Research Center, Emory University, Atlanta, Ga.; Laboratory Division, Center for Disease Control, Atlanta, Ga.; and Research Animal Branch, USAF School of Aerospace Medicine, Brooks Air Force Base, Tex.

References

1 Anderson, H.W.; Peterson, D.R., and Watkins, R.B.: Human shigellosis and salmonellosis acquired from a spider monkey. Primate Zoonoses Surveillance Report No. 6. Center for Disease Control, Health Services and Mental Health Administration, Atlanta, Ga. (1971).

2 Anon.: Review of nonhuman primate-associated hepatitis. Primate Zoonoses Surveillance Report No. 6, Center for Disease Control, Health Services and Mental Health Administration, Atlanta, Ga. (1971).

3 Bernstein, G.: Vector Control Consultant, City of New York Department of Health, New York (personal commun., 1972).

4 Capucci, D.: Public Health Veterinarian, California State Department of Public Health, Berkeley, Calif. (personal commun., 1972).

5 Lamm, S.H.; Nadel, M.; Jakowski. R.M., and Hart, J.C.: A fatal case of human shigellosis associated with a pet spider monkey. Primate Zoonoses Surveillance Report No. 4, Center for Disease Control, Health Services and Mental Health Administration, Atlanta, Ga. (1971).

Author's address: Arnold F. Kaufmann, Epidemiology Program, Center for Disease Control, Health Services and Mental Health Administration, US Department of Health, Education and Welfare, *Atlanta, GA 30333* (USA)

Medical Primatology 1972. Proc. 3rd Conf. exp. Med. Surg. Primates, Lyon 1972, part III, pp. 68–72 (Karger, Basel 1972)

Diseases of Marmosets

W. R. Kingston

Fisons Ltd., Pharmaceutical Division, Hillcrest Research Station, Belton, Loughborough, Leicestershire

We have maintained a breeding colony of marmosets and tamarins, mainly *Callithrix jacchus* together with small numbers of other species since 1965. Over the same period we have imported some 800 animals for experimental purposes. I give below an account of the disease problems encountered in both the stabilised breeding colony and the imported stock, but must point out that the major cause of losses in both groups although both presenting typical symptoms have not been identified. We do not have facilities for virus identification so our investigations have been more or less confined to bacteria and limited biochemistry and haematology.

Imported Stock

The picture here, apart from the obvious dehydration and malnutrition problems common to all newly-imported primates, is one of extreme variation between batches although they have all come from the same supplier and importer and at all times of the year. The vast majority of the shipments have arrived in reasonably good condition. At the end of our internal eight-week quarantine and conditioning period the survival rate was in excess of 90%. Subsequently the animals remained free of disease and in good general health until sacrifice, i.e. in some cases as long as two years. Occasional batches, however, although looking and behaving quite normally in other respects, have shown a considerable darkening in colour of the bare facial skin in many of the animals. Within a few days these have begun to die and as many as eighty of a batch of one hundred have died within four or five weeks. No significant bacteria have been found in cultures of faeces, urine and blood and *post mortem* examination and limited histology have not revealed anything of apparent significance. Oral and systemic antibiotic therapy using a wide range of products have failed to prevent these deaths except that chloramphenicol (Intramycetin, Parke Davies) may have saved a few of the animals we expected to die. Survivors have subsequently remained in good health but due to relatively large numbers of animals housed in gang cages it is impossible to say with certainty if any of these had shown the darkened skin and lost it on recovery, but that phenomenon was certainly present in all the animals that died.

Apart from this one syndrome imported *C. jacchus* have not presented a serious disease problem and were relatively free of the acanthocephalid worm *Prosthenorchis elegans.* Unidentified microfilaria are frequently found in the blood of these animals but do not appear to present a health problem.

With regard to the other species, we have not seen the darkened skin syndrome in any of these, but the principal problem was due to the abovementioned acanthocephalid which has been the apparent cause of death of a number of animals, particularly in *Saguinus nigricollis,* an otherwise very robust species. The ICI product, 'Promintic', administered i.p., will eliminate this worm but causes considerable trauma to the host.

Breeding Colony

Established breeding pairs, some of which have been breeding steadily for almost seven years, remain remarkably free from illness of any kind and this is equally true of young animals up to the time of weaning which we now do just prior to the birth of the next litter at 20 weeks of age. (Our *jacchus* pairs are now regularly producing twins at an average interval of 22–23 weeks following a *post partum* oestrus which must occur within 14 days of parturition, allowing for a gestation of 20 weeks). The disease vulnerable group are the post-weaned young up to the age of 12 months, in which group we have had considerable losses.

In 1967 we foolishly introduced some newly-imported animals into the breeding colony. Within a fortnight we had lost 16 young with an uncontrollable enteritis. Stool cultures revealed a very high count of a *Shigella* which failed in most cases to respond to antibiotic therapy. None of the adults were involved and we have not seen anything approaching it since; in fact the incidence of enteric disease appears to be remarkably low in *Callithricidae* as compared with other primates.

The other problem, the aetiology of which is still unknown to us, has occurred from time to time over the past five years and has caused the death of large numbers of young animals. The first visible symptom is a considerable oedematous swelling in the gular region which, although varying from day to day, is persistent and occasionally spreads to the abdominal area. For some days or weeks this appears to give only mechanical problems to the animals which retain normal appetite and activity. In some cases it disappears uneventfully, but in the majority it is followed by a gradual deterioration of the general condition of the animal, progressive weight loss and eventual death in anything from four to 20 weeks. Bacterial cultures show nothing significant, and fluid drawn from the swelling sac is colourless, cell free and apparently bacteriologically sterile. There are no macroscopic lesions on *post mortem* and histology, although very limited, gave negative results.

It was thought that toxoplasmosis might be the cause, and this was investigated on our behalf by Prof. J. K. A. BEVEREY of the University of Sheffield, but gave negative results. A suggested course of treatment of oral sulphadimidine, i. m. chloramphenicol and vitamin B_{12} appears to have cured some of the animals but whether any one of these was effective or there was a synergistic effect is not known. It is difficult to say whether the condition is infectious because although we have had an incidence as high as three or four in a cage of five, we have also had only one animal ill in a group and one of a set of twins. Apart from these two ailments we have had no other disease problems of any significance at all.

Zoonoses

A fairly comprehensive and sustained review of the literature very much helped by the excellent primate reference service of the University of Washington [TERRY, 1973], has so far not indicated any known transfer of disease from *Callithricidae* to man. The isolation of a new herpesvirus from marmosets [HOLMES, 1963; MELNICK *et al.*, 1964] and an inclusion body hepatitis [SAUER and BISHOP, 1963] certainly suggests caution. In view of the fact that the animals share the same habitat as the vampire bats, the possibility of rabies must be considered. Filaria are commonly found in these animals as are trypanosomes and yellow fever virus. The susceptibility to experimental infection with viral hepatitis [DEINHARDT *et al.*, 1967] suggests another possible hazard. All that can safely be said on the risks of these animals to man is that they have not so far been implicated. Although their small size makes them less of a physical danger than the larger monkeys, wild caught specimens should still be considered a potentially dangerous animal and the usual safety precautions strictly followed.

Anthroponoses

Apart from the viral hepatitis mentioned above, the heavy mortality induced by measles in the colony maintained by the University of Texas Dental Science Institute [Levy and Mirkovic, 1971] is one proved human disease to which marmosets are vulnerable. Investigations by Dr. F. T. Perkins on the feasibility of innoculation against this disease suggest that it may well be possible and worthwhile, but the tests were limited by the small number of available animals and should be extended before being used on a large scale. These animals are known to be very resistant to infection with tuberculosis of human, bovine or avian strains, although tuberculosis has been reported from zoological gardens. We have a subjective opinion that we lost a few animals with respiratory disease immediately following an 'influenza cold' in one of the staff but lack proof of this. From the above evidence alone, however, we insist on face masks being worn by all personnel entering the marmoset room. The work of Deinhardt [1966] in induction of neoplasms in neonatal tamarins with Rous sarcoma virus; the induction of lymphomas and lymphocytic leukaemias in young and adult marmosets with *Herpesvirus saimiri* [Wolfe, 1971] suggests that these animals are very suitable for investigation into suspected human viral oncogens, particularly since neonatal animals can quite easily and regularly be provided at relatively low cost.

Finally, the unique embryology and concomitant partial immunological tolerance of the normal dizygotic twins, plus the known possession of human type reaginic antibodies must surely make these animals of outstanding interest for a wide range of investigations in immunology including graft and transplant rejection and allergic diseases. The ease and predictability with which they can be bred are of potential value in teratology.

References

Deinhardt, F.: Neoplasms induced by Rous sarcoma virus in New World monkeys. Nature *210:* 443 (1966).

Deinhardt, F., Holmes, A. W.; Capps, R. B., and Popper, H.: Studies on the transmission of human viral hepatitis to marmoset monkeys. J.exp. Med. *125:* 673–688 (1967).

HOLMES, A.W.; DEDMON, R.E., and DEINHARDT, F.: Isolation of a new herpes-like virus from South American marmosets. Fed. Proc. *22:* 334 (1963).

LEVY, B.M. and MIRKOVIC, R.R.: An epizootic of measles in a marmoset colony. Lab. anim. Sci. *21:* 33–39 (1971).

MELNICK, J.L.; MIDULLA, M.; WIMBERLEY, I.; BARNERA-ORO, J.G., and LEVY, B.M.: A new member of the herpes virus group isolated from South American marmosets. J. Immunol. *92:* 596–601 (1964).

SAUER, R.M. and BISHOP, R.W.: Inclusion body hepatitis in marmosets. Lab. anim. Care *13:* 790–792 (1963).

TERRY, M.: Primate Information Center as a Tertiary Communication Service; in GOLDSMITH and MOOR-JANKOWSKI Medical Primatology 1972, part I, pp. 198–200 (Karger, Basel 1972).

WOLFE, L.G.; FALK, L.A., and DEINHARDT, F.: Oncogenicity of *Herpesvirus saimiri* in marmoset monkeys. J. Nat. Cancer Inst. *47:* 1145–1162 (1971).

Author's address: Mr. W.R. KINGSTON, Fisons Ltd., Pharmaceutical Division, Hillcrest Research Station, Belton, *Loughborough, Leicestershire* (UK)

Medical Primatology 1972. Proc. 3rd Conf. exp. Med. Surg. Primates, Lyon 1972, part III, pp. 73–79 (Karger, Basel 1972)

Chimpanzee Post-Streptococcal Nephritis Following Induced Group A Infection and M-1 Protein Injections[1]

D. H. KRUSHAK, R. A. ZIMMERMAN and J. D. KNOSTMAN

Disease Investigations Section, Phoenix Laboratories, CDC, Phoenix, Ariz. and Streptococcal Disease Section, Fort Collins Laboratories, CDC, Fort Collins, Col.

Several authors have described the clinical signs of group-A β-hemolytic streptococcal infection in chimpanzees [4, 6] and the similarity of these signs to those found in man [17].

Epidemiological and serological observations have shown antecedent streptococcal infection to be related to acute glomerulonephritis (AGN) [9, 10]. The disposition of immunoglobulins, complement, and streptococcal antigen and antibodies along the glomerular membrane, as shown by electro-immunofluorescent microscopy support an immune mechanism similar to that seen experimentally in serum sickness, where circulating antigen-antibody complexes induce glomerular damage [1, 2, 3, 7]. In humans, the study of AGN pathology has usually been limited to specimens obtained after the disease is clinically apparent, when perhaps the initiating factors are in complex or have disappeared.

The use of animal models has been limited by (1) phylogenic differences, (2) the artificial methods used to introduce the streptococci or streptococcal products, and (3) the somewhat dissimilar clinical and pathological findings when compared to the human disease [13].

This report presents our findings of kidney pathology following sequential induced streptococcal pharyngitis and injections of semipurified M-1 protein which produced high serum levels of antigen and antibody.

Material and Methods

Four three-year-old chimpanzees, weighing approximately 18 kg, without prior streptococcal experience were used in these studies. Three chimpanzees were inoculated; one chimpanzee (a control) was not inoculated with any antigenic agent.

Group A streptococci, serotype M-1, isolated during a human study were used to induce infection and prepare M-1 protein. Immunoglobulin G (IgG) was obtained from M-1 hyperimmune serum from another chimpanzee. The IgG was tagged with a ferritin tracer [12].

The three phases of the study were;

(1) antibody production, (2) challenge, and (3) convalescence, as presented in table I. M-1 TSA were produced in response to pharyngeal infection and i.m., or intradermal, injections of semipurified M-1 protein. On challenge day 0, the three chimpanzees received an i.m. injection of M-1 antigen or an intranasal inoculation of group-A, M-1, streptococci

Table I. Protocol for induction of poststreptococcal acute glomerulonephritis in chimpanzees

Animal	Pre-experiment day	Antibody formation, day		Challenge, day		Recovery, day		
	–115	–90	–59	0	3	4	33	124
Faye	B	1 ml 4-hour M-1 culture in nares	0.6 mg MAg i.m.	1.5 mg MAg i.m.	35 mg FE-M-1 Ab + 0.8 mg MAg i.v.	B	B	B
Gaby	B	0.6 mg MAg with adj. i.m.	0.3 mg MAg i.d.	1.4 mg MAg i.m.	35 mg FE-M-1 Ab + 0.8 mg M-1 Ag i.v.	B	B	B
Hy	B	0.6 mg MAg with adj. i.m.	0.3 mg MAg i.d.	2 ml 4-hour M-1 culture in nares	35 mg FE-M-1 Ab + 0.8 mg MAg i.v.	B	B	B

B = percutaneous needle biopsy; MAg = semipurified type 1 M-protein; M-1 Ab = hyperimmune type 1 IgG; adj. = Freund's incomplete adjuvant; i.d. = intradermal; FE = ferritin.

culture. On challenge day 3, the three chimpanzees received i.v. injections of antigen and tagged IgG. The fourth uninoculated chimpanzee received ferritin tagged IgG only.

Throughout the experiment the chimpanzees were monitored three times a week for changes in temperature, white blood cell count, blood pressure, and proteinuria and hematuria; blood was obtained to determine M-1 TSA and B_1C globulin levels. Indirect hemagglutination [18] and immunodiffusion techniques [16] were used to detect TSA. Percutaneous kidney biopsies were performed prior to the study and on the days listed in table I. Kidney tissue was 10% formalin fixed for light microscopy and a portion was fixed with osmium tetroxide and mounted in Epon 9 for electron microscopy.

Results

During the antibody formation period, M-1 TSA developed in all chimpanzees. Faye, the chimpanzee who received the intranasal inoculation of live streptococci developed pharyngitis. No urine abnormalities were noted in any animal.

The clinical response during the challenge and recovery periods is summarized in table II. Following the i.m. injection of Gaby and Faye on day 0 with M-1 antigen there were no urine, blood pressure, or B_1C globulin level changes. Hy, who received the intranasal inoculation, colonized and developed clinical pharyngitis. On day 3, following the i.v. administration of antigen and tagged antibody, hematuria and hypertension developed in all three chimpanzees accompanied by a low-grade fever and leukocytosis. The hypertension appeared most severe in Gaby, who subsequently was shown to have the greatest histopathology. Faye and Hy had mild hypertension and slowly returned to normal.

Urinary Findings

After the injection of antigen and antibody, moderate hematuria persisted intermittently for 12 days. Microscopic examination of the urine sediment revealed numerous red cells but no casts or WBC. Proteinuria was intermittent and mild (less than 30 mg %).

Serological Findings

Hemagglutinating and precipitating type specific antibody levels increased from moderate titers seen in the antibody formation period to extre-

Table II. Chimpanzee serological and clinical response to sequential streptococcal infection and sermipurified M-1 protein injections

Phase	I	II¹			II²	*									III*
Day	−1	0	1	2	3	4	5	6	7	8	9	10	11	12	33
Gaby															
HA (M-1) titer	2^7	2^8		2^7	2^7	2^8			2^{14}		2^{18}				2^9
ID (M-1) titer	1+	2+		2+	2+	2+			4+		4+				4+
Hematuria	−	−	−	−	+	−	+	+	−	+	−	−	−	+	+
Proteinuria	−	−	−	T	−	+	−	−	−	−	−	−	−	−	−
Blood pressure	120/82	128/82		134/80	152/110	212/130			180/134				192/138		162/80
Faye															
HA (M-1) titer	2^5	2^7		2^5	2^5	2^8			2^{16}		2^{15}				2^8
ID (M-1) titer	3+	3+		3+	3+	4+			4+		4+				
Hematuria	−	−	−	−	+	+	+	2+	−	+	+	−	−	+	−
Proteinuria	−	−	−	−	−	−	−	−	−	−	−	−	−	−	−
Blood pressure	138/66	140/64		142/82	142/90	132/62			150/108				140/90		130/82
Hy															
HA (M-1) titer	2^9	2^8		2^7	2^9	2^9			2^9		2^{14}				2^{11}
ID (M-1) titer	1+	2+		2+	1+	1+			2+		3+				
Hematuria	−	−	−	−	+	−	+	+	−	−	+	−	+	2+	−
Proteinuria	−	−	−	−	−	+	T	−	−	−	−	−	−	−	−
Blood pressure	106/72	120/78		136/44	140/88	142/98			138/78				138/82		142/104

* = Day of kidney biopsy; HA = hemagglutination test; ID = immunodiffusion test. Phase II¹ = antigen inoculation; phase II² = antigen-antibody i.v. injections.

mely high levels after the challenge dose of antigen. Unlike the usual slow decay of natural antibody levels observed in previous experiments, the high titers returned to near prechallenge levels within 30 days. B_1C globulin levels remained within normal limits or slightly elevated throughout the experiment.

Histologic Findings

The interpretations of the light microscopic sections read by three pathologists were similar; normal findings were noted in all pre-experimental biopsy tissue. In postchallenge tissue, changes of variable severity were limited to the glomeruli. The degree of histopathology in sequential biopsies correlated directly with the clinical response, being most marked in Gaby and minimal in Hy. The 24-hour postchallenge biopsies revealed slight hypercellularity and increased matrix in mesangial areas. There were no exudates or basement membrane changes. On day 33, Hy's kidney tissue was normal; in contrast, Faye and Gaby showed an increase in mesangial matrix with focal areas of hypercellularity. The renal pathology was limited to the glomerular apparatus. Four month follow-up biopsies on Hy and Faye were interpreted as normal and a six month biopsy on Gaby showed a persistence of a diffuse mesangial sclerosis.

Electron micrographs of the 24-hour kidney tissue specimen revealed electron dense material identifying the ferritin tagged antibody distributed throughout the basement membrane, primarily in the lamina densa. The concentration of antigen-antibody aggregates correlated with the light microscopy findings and clinical response. Small quantities of ferritin were detected in the capillary lumen, endothelial and epithelial cells, and mesangial areas. Other changes were focal areas of swelling or contraction of the visceral epithelial foot processes and obliteration of the lamina rara interna. On day 33, only a few ferritin particles were observed in Hy's kidney tissue; in Gaby's tissue, aggregates were located in the lamina densa, the lamina rara externa, and in the epithelial foot processes. Ferritin was not detected in the four and six-month biopsy specimens.

The control chimpanzee who received only ferritin tagged antibody showed no apparent urine changes or kidney pathology. In the 24-hour postinoculation tissue, examined by electron microscopy, ferritin molecules were detected in the capillary lumen and epithelial cell cytoplasm. The 33 day kidney tissue was normal.

Discussion

Chimpanzees were used in this study because of their phylogenic relationship with humans and similar clinical response to group-A streptococcal infection. M-protein was used as the antigen because (1) M-protein given i.v. is deposited in the renal glomeruli [5, 8]; (2) M-protein antigen and anti-M-protein globulins have been detected in the glomeruli in rare human cases [11] and in experimental animals [15].

In this study, chimpanzee hematuria, hypertension, and slight proteinuria developed after sequential natural and parenteral challenge with M-1 antigen, these signs have been associated with human AGN. The kidney pathology was not considered to be a toxic reaction, because only glomerular changes were detected and no tubular pathology were observed [14], furthermore, the control animal who received only tagged globulin had no renal changes. The glomerular changes in chimpanzee kidney tissue were primarily mesangial, which in part differed from most human poststreptococcal AGN histopathology. Complement levels did not decrease as is seen in human cases; therefore, the involvement of complement has yet to be studied. It appears that injury and permanent scarring resulted from the presence of induced streptococcal antigen-antibody aggregates in the chimpanzee glomerular apparatus.

Although the chimpanzees were not completely challenged in a natural manner, and the renal pathology was in some ways dissimilar to that observed in human AGN, we believe that these primates will be useful in the elucidation of the pathogenesis of poststreptococcal AGN.

References

1 ANDRES, G.A.; ACCINI, L.; HSU, K.C.; ZABRISKIE, J.B., and SEEGAL, B.C.: Electron microscopic studies of human glomerulonephritis with ferritin-conjugated antibody. J.exp.Med. *123:* 399–412 (1966).

2 DIXON, F.J.; FELDMAN, J.D., and VASQUEZ, J.J.: Experimental glomerulonephritis. The pathogenesis of a laboratory model resembling the spectrum of human glomerulonephritis. J.exp.Med. *113:* 899–920 (1961).

3 FELDMAN, J.D.; MARDINEY, M.K., and SHULER, S.E.: Immunology and morphology of acute post-streptococcal glomerulonephritis. Lab.Invest. *15:* 283–301 (1966).

4 FRIOU, J.F.: Experimental infection of the upper respiratory tract of young chimpanzees with group A hemolytic streptococci. J.infect.Dis. *86:* 264–274 (1950).

5 KAPLAN, M.H.: Localization of streptococcal antigens in tissues. I. Histologic distribution and persistence of M-proteins, type 1, 5, 12 and 19 in the mouse. J.exp.Med. *107:* 341–352 (1958).

6 KRUSHAK, D.H.; ZIMMERMAN, R.A., and MURPHY, B.L.: Induced group A beta hemolytic streptococci infection in chimpanzees. J.amer.vet.med.Ass. *157:* 742–744 (1970).

7 MICHAEL, A.F.; DRUMMOND, K.N.; GOOD, R.A., and VERNIER, R.L.: Acute poststreptococcal glomerulonephritis. Immune deposit disease. J.clin.Invest. *45:* 237–248 (1966).

8 MILLER, F.: Renal localization and persistence of type 12 streptococcal M-protein. Proc.Soc.exp.Biol.Med. *108:* 539–543 (1961).

9 RAMMELKAMP, C.H., jr.: Acute hemorrhagic glomerulonephritis; in MCCARTY Streptococcal infections, pp.197–207 (Columbia University Press, New York 1954).

10 RAMMELKAMP, C.H., jr.: Concepts of pathogenesis of glomerulonephritis derived from studies in man; in UHR The streptococcus, rheumatic fever and glomerulonephritis, pp.289–300 (Williams & Wilkins, Baltimore 1964).

11 Seegal, B.C.; Andres, G.A.; Hsu, K.C., and Zabriskie, J.B.: Studies on the pathogenesis of acute and progressive glomerulonephritis in man by immunofluorescein and immunoferritin techniques. Fed.Proc. *24:* 100–108 (1965).
12 Sri Ram, J.; Tawde, S.S.; Pierce, G.B., jr., and Midgley, A.R.: Preparation of antibody-ferritin conjugates for immuno-electron microscopy. J.Cell Biol. *17:* 673–675 (1963).
13 Tan, E.M.: Experimental renal disease induced by streptococci; in Uhr The streptococcus, rheumatic fever and glomerulonephritis, pp.238–247 (Williams & Wilkins, Baltimore 1964).
14 Tan, E.M. and Kaplan, M.H.: Renal tubular lesions in mice produced by streptococci in intraperitoneal diffussion chambers. Role of streptolysin S. J.infect.Dis. *110:* 55–62 (1962).
15 Vosti, K.L.; Lindberg, L.H.; Kosek, J.C., and Raffel, S.: Experimental streptococcal glomerulonephritis. Longitudinal study of a laboratory model resembling human acute poststreptococcal glomerulonephritis. J.infect.Dis. *122:* 249–259 (1970).
16 Zimmerman, R.A.; Auernheimer, A.H., and Taranta, A.: Precipitating antibody to group A streptococcal polysaccharide in humans. J.Immunol. *107:* 832–841 (1971).
17 Zimmerman, R.A.; Krushak, D.H.; Wilson, E., and Douglas, J.: Human streptococcal disease syndrome compared with observations in chimpanzees. II. Immunologic responses to induced pharyngitis and the effect of treatment. J.infect.Dis. *122:* 280–289 (1970).
18 Zimmerman, R.A.; Mathews, J., and Wilson, E.: Microtiter indirect hemagglutination procedure for identification of streptococcal M-protein antibodies. Appl. Microbiol. *16:* 1640–1645 (1968).

Authors' address: Dr. D.H. Krushak, Dr. R.A. Zimmerman and Dr. J.D. Knostman, Disease Investigations Section, Phoenix Laboratories, CDC, 4402 No.7th 5 T., *Phoenix, AZ* (USA)

Medical Primatology 1972. Proc. 3rd Conf. exp. Med. Surg. Primates, Lyon 1972, part III, pp. 80–87 (Karger, Basel 1972)

The Chimpanzee in Venereal Disease Research

U.S.G. KUHN, III

Venereal Disease Research Unit, Laboratory Division, Center for Disease Control, USPHS, Atlanta, Ga.

One of the most challenging disease control problems facing the world today is venereal disease. Gonorrhea is increasing at an alarming rate in most countries of the world. Syphilis, too, despite the availability of excellent diagnostic tests, therapeutic agents and elaborate administrative control programs, has recently shown an upward trend.

Research needs in meeting the challenge are broad. These include a serologic test with which to detect gonorrhea in asymptomatic carriers, a most important reservoir of human infection. Another diagnostic test which would greatly facilitate venereal disease control measures is a serologic test for incubating syphilis, one which would detect the presence of disease prior to the time of communicability. Along with these there is a strong feeling in some quarters that vaccines against both syphilis and gonorrhea will be required to achieve the ultimate goal of eradication of these diseases. As the biomedical research community responds to these needs, consideration of an experimental animal model is inevitable. During the past six years we have found the chimpanzee ideally suited to this role in treponemal research. More recently gonorrhea has been successfully established in the chimpanzee allowing for the first time its characterization in an animal model. This summarization of recent research on venereal disease is intended to illustrate the suitability and usefulness of chimpanzees as animal models for the study of experimental syphilis and gonorrhea.

Syphilis is the most important of a group of diseases of man caused by bacteria of the genus *Treponema.* All pathogenic treponemas are capable of causing infection in the chimpanzee. These include: *Treponema pallidum, Treponema pertenue* and *Treponema carateum,* the causative organisms, respectively, of syphilis, yaws, and pinta in humans, and *Treponema cuniculi,* the causative organism of venereal spirochetosis of rabbits. Previous reports have detailed some of the historical and current aspects of such studies [7, 8].

The intracutaneous inoculation of pathogenic *T.pallidum* in the chimpanzee results within two to three weeks in the development of a papule, approximately 3–4 mm in diameter, which, as it enlarges becomes ulcerated on the surface and assumes the configuration of the typical chancre, the indurated, painless primary syphilitic lesions seen in infected humans. At or about the time of appearance of the chancre, specific treponemal antibody is detectable in the blood serum by both the fluorescent treponemal antibody-absorption (FTA-ABS) test [17] and by the automated hemagglutination – *Treponema pallidum* (AMHA-TP) test [4]. We have found the initial serologic reactivity in infected chimpanzees to reside in the IgM fraction or in both the IgM and IgG fractions of the immune globulin. Reagenic antibody reactions to the cardiolipin antigen serologic tests for syphilis (VDRL) [17] appear usually within a week following. The immobilizing antibody, another specific treponemal antibody, is detectable by the *Treponema pallidum* immobilization-200 (TPI-200) test [18] around five to six weeks after infection.

Treponemes are abundant in the primary lesion and may be readily demonstrated by dark-field microscopic examination of lesion fluid until it has completely regressed, a period of three to four weeks. Interestingly, a tissue immunity develops early in the course of the chancre development. During the first week or so of its existence it is possible to induce additional lesions on the same animals by transfer of the lesion fluid to additional skin sites. Indeed, spontaneous development of additional lesions have been observed when the primary lesion is located where it comes into contact with normal skin. However, within a week or so after the appearance of the primary lesion, this susceptibility disappears and additional lesions cannot be induced anywhere on the animal's body.

Coinciding with the disappearance of the primary skin lesion specific treponemal antibody may be detected in the cerebrospinal fluid (CSF) by an FTA technique [5]. Reagin appears in the CSF some two to four weeks afterward.

Secondary lesions of syphilis, as evidenced by a dark-field positive macular rash has only been observed in one of 25 chimpanzees infected with syphilis in our series of experiments. Nor have late manifestations such as those seen in symptomatic neurosyphilis of man been observed in chimpanzees infected up to six years, albeit the presence of CSF antibody, polycytosis, and increased spinal fluid protein. The latter set of circumstances would place the infected chimpanzees in a category af asymptomatic neurosyphilis in comparison to the usual experience with the natural host, man.

Venereal syphilis of man is, of course, transmitted from one individual to another by intimate, usually sexual, contact, There is, however, another type of human syphilitic infection, endemic syphilis, which exists in several underdeveloped arid regions of the world and which is transmitted by intimate contact alone, as that between a mother and child, or between small children. We have observed a similar degree of communicability in the natural transmission of syphilis from one experimentally-infected chimpanzee to his male cage partner. In this single instance a primary lesion was not observed on the passively-infected animal, possibly overlooked on a mucous membrane or other hidden location.

One intriguing aspect of recent clinical research in syphilis has been the reported presence of treponemal forms in the body fluids of humans presumably adequately treated with penicillin [3, 14]. Questions surrounding the significance of these findings are further compounded by reports of progression of disease in neurological manifestations of late syphilis in spite of adequate therapy [13, 19].

A systematic study of body fluids of chimpanzees infected with syphilis and untreated for as long as six years revealed treponemal forms in both or either aqueous humor and CSF in three of 294 samples [6]. The treponemal forms were detected by direct fluorescent antibody stain techniques. In no instance were similar forms detected by direct dark-field microscopy. However, one CSF sample proved infectious when injected into susceptible rabbits.

The question of immunity following syphilitic infection is of course of primary interest in our work. Chimpanzees infected with syphilis for periods of over six months do not develop typical primary lesions after challenge with virulent organisms. Instead, a transitory dark-field negative wheal similar to a delayed hypersensitivity reaction has been observed in those animals so treated. Some chimpanzees carry treponemal antibody when imported from the wild. Infectivity experiments with such animals suggests that so-called skin immunity, or failure to develop a typical primary lesion upon inoculation of virulent *T.pallidum,* may be related to sex. Three naturally reactive females failed to develop lesions following challenge, whereas three male chimpanzees did. All of the animals became infected (superinfected) as evidenced by recovery of virulent organisms from lymph nodes.

The quest for a means of inducing immunity to syphilis led to experiments involving pinta infections in chimpanzees. Immunity against syphilis in humans with naturally-acquired or experimental infection with *T. carateum* has been suggested by the work of MEDINA [12]. To test this hypothesis under controlled laboratory conditions, six chimpanzees were inoculated with lesion material from humans with naturally-acquired pinta [9, 10]. The resultant primary lesion in the chimpanzee was first observed as a small (3 mm) erythematous dark-field positive papule which progressed over the following months to large desquamative plaques, up to 70 mm in diameter. Regression of the lesions was accompanied by hyper- or reversible hypopigmentive changes. No secondary lesions, i.e. pintids, were observed in the experimentally-infected chimpanzees, but new lesions could be induced repeatedly by transfer of material from active lesions to additional skin sites on the same or other animals. The pattern of humoral antibody development was sequentially analogous to that of the syphilis-infected animals, but the time period over which it occurred was protracted in the order of four times. For instance, whereas specific treponemal antibody was detectable within two to three weeks after infection with *T. pallidum,* the chimpanzees inoculated with *T. carateum* demonstrated the same antibody, on the average, at three months after infection. Histologically, the chimpanzee pinta lesions were, in most respects, identical to those seen in human subjects [2]. Parakeratosis, acanthosis and inflammatory infiltration of the upper dermis were notable features. However, *T. carateum* could be demonstrated in the upper dermis, in a location rarely or never observed in human lesions. Also, the presence of dermal melanotic melanocytes in the chimpanzee skin may have been associated with the usual reversibility of the hypopigmentive changes observed in chimpanzees in contrast to the permanent hypopigmentation observed to follow in the wake of *T. carateum* infection in human skin.

Three years after infection with *T. carateum,* four chimpanzees were challenged with 10^6 virulent *T. pallidum.* All of the animals became infected, developing typical dark-field positive chancres. Their regional lymph nodes also contained viable *T. pallidum,* as evidenced by rabbit infectivity tests. The syphilis lesion in all cases appeared larger, more active and longer lasting than that seen in ordinarily susceptible animals, suggesting the association of a delayed hypersensitivity reaction with the challenge inoculation. Curiously, in one animal a pinta lesion persisted for approximately a year after the *T. pallidum* challenge. Motile spirochetes transferred on repeated occasions from the lesion to susceptible rabbits failed to induce infection, suggesting that the organisms remaining in the pinta lesion were indeed *T. carateum.*

A second generation of pinta-infected chimpanzees is now being studied and may possibly serve to answer some of the questions posed by the initial experiment, such as the effect of the size of the syphilis challenge inoculation in relation to the levels of immunity extant in the chimpanzee with pinta infection.

The expense of maintaining chimpanzees for experimental use precludes following some of the intriguing possibilities of cross-immunity in treponemal infections such as that implied in the relative occurrence of syphilis in human populations in which yaws is endemic. However, the existence of *T. cuniculi* infections in rabbits throughout the temperate zones of the world begs for answer to what degree of cross-immunity this virulent treponema, diverted to one species of lower animals early in the course of evolution, could confer against human syphilis. Rabbits infected with *T. cuniculi* have been shown to possess a substantial degree of cross-immunity to syphilis [16]. TURNER and HOLLANDER [15], in their careful and classical studies on experimental treponemal infections in animals, described *T. cuniculi* infection of the rhesus monkey and postulated the possibility of human infection with the organism. In our laboratory we have been successful in infecting a chimpanzee.[1] A superficial dark-field positive encrusted lesion developed within three weeks after intradermal inoculation with infected rabbit preputial washings and regressed completely over the following two weeks. A humoral antibody was first evident in the results of the AMHA-TP test at the time coinciding with the lesion appearance. The FTA-ABS test became positive six weeks after inoculation, and the reagin antibodies were seen at eight weeks. Notable changes did not occur in the CSF throughout one year postinfection. At this time the animal was challenged by an intracutaneous inoculation of 10^6 *T. pallidum*. The resultant lesion three weeks postchallenge was so inconsequential that it nearly escaped dark-field examination. However, when a small amount of serum was expressed from the inoculation site, it was found to contain abundant and vigorously motile treponemes, and the same material produced typical syphilitic lesions when inoculated into susceptible rabbits. Additional studies seem warranted, especially in regard to the development of a practical or useful degree of immunity.

A new and fascinating chapter in venereal disease research has been opened by the successful infection of chimpanzees with *Neisseria gonorrhea*. For decades gonorrhea research has been limited by the lack of an experimental animal model in which to study the biology of the organism and details of the host response. Recently, however, scientists at our laboratory were able to induce gonorrhea in chimpanzees by the intraurethral inoculation of human infectious material [11]. In the initial trials a pool of gonococcal exu-

1 KUHN, U.S.G. and CLARK, W.J.: Unpubl. data from studies in progress.

date from five male patients was inoculated into the urethrae of four male chimpanzees. All animals became culture positive within four days. The cultures reverted to negative from the 9th to the 30th week postinfection. A small amount of exudate could be stripped from the chimpanzee urethra on the 4th day of infection, and one animal exhibited subjective signs of discomfort early in this period. In the other animals the urethral exudate became prominent from the 7th to the 14th day and then diminished over the next two weeks. One chimpanzee developed a unilateral conjunctivitis which yielded *N. gonorrhea* on culture. This particular animal was treated with penicillin and subsequently reinfected some 14 weeks later with essentially the same pattern of results. A female cagemate of an infected male was found to harbor *N. gonorrhea* by culture of her cervical mucosa after 16 weeks of exposure, suggesting natural venereal transmission of the infection in the chimpanzee.

Following the experiments with human exudate, an attempt was made to infect animals with organisms from pure culture [1]. *Neisseria gonorrhea* was obtained from an infected human female and subjected to six selective transfers on a solid medium. The final culture colonies were removed into trypticase-soy broth and inoculated into the urethra of a male chimpanzee. The animal became culture positive within three days and remained so through the following 46 days. He presented evidence of an urethritis from the 10th to the 15th day, the exudate containing gram-negative intracellular diplococci. From the time of inoculation, this male was caged with a sexually mature female. A cervical culture of the female yielded *N. gonorrhea* from the 5th through the 39th day. She had an estral discharge at the time of exposure, but no evidence of an inflammatory discharge was noted subsequent to her infection.

Sequential blood serum samples of all of the chimpanzees infected with human gonococcal exudate or cultured *N. gonorrhea* were subjected to several serologic procedures.[2] These revealed complement-fixing antibody in all of the male chimpanzees appearing between the 2nd and 3rd week following infection. Antibody detectable by an indirect fluorescent antibody technique was found in four males and one female between the 3rd and 4th week post-inoculation. The complement-fixing antibody persisted for varying lengths of time up to 35 weeks; the fluorescent antibody technique was reactive throughout a period of more than 40 weeks.

As a corollary to the presumed autoinoculation of virulent *N. gonorrhea* from the urethra to the eye of one chimpanzee, in another the situation was

2 Brown, W.J. and Lucas, C.T.: Unpubl. data from studies in progress.

somewhat reversed. On this occasion *N.meningiditis* was isolated from the urethra of an animal known to be a chronic nasopharyngeal carrier of the meningococcus. He was also observed to frequently engage in self oral-genital contact.[3]

At the present time a second generation of gonorrhea studies utilizing the chimpanzee model has begun.[4] A single strain of *N.gonorrhea* was isolated from a primary human case of acute gonorrhea, grown in one large scale single passage and stored frozen for use in all phases of the study. The first question to be answered is the minimal number of organisms required to infect the chimpanzee by intraurethral inoculation. Following this, the kinetics and the degree of the immune response will be characterized. Studies of cell-mediated immunity, by means of lymphocyte transformation of the chimpanzee cells, are proceeding concurrently. Regularly taken sequential serum samples are being banked to serve as reference material in the development and comparison of serologic tests for gonorrhea. Following the natural course of any resultant infection there will be an opportunity to assess any possible immunity to reinfection with homologous or heterologous strains of the gonococcus.

As serologic test development for both syphilis and gonorrhea proceed, the chimpanzee will offer the logical source of biological materials produced under controlled conditions necessary for evaluation preliminary to extended trials with human sera catagories. And, of course, when vaccines for either gonorrhea or syphilis are ready for trial, the chimpanzee should again be a logical candidate for the preliminary evaluation.

3 BROWN, W.J.; KRAUS, S.J., and ARKO, R.J.: Chimpanzee urethral meningococci subm. for publ. to New Engl.J.Med.).

4 KRAUS, S.J.; ARKO, R.J., and BROWN, W.J.: Unpubl. data from studies in progress.

References

1 BROWN, W.J.; LUCAS, C.T., and KUHN, U.S.G.: Gonorrhea in the chimpanzee. Infection with laboratory-passed gonococci and natural transmission (in press).

2 CHANDLER, F.W.; KAUFMANN, A.F., and KUHN, U.S.G.: The histopathology of experimental pinta in the chimpanzee. J.invest.Derm. *58:* 103 (1972).

3 COLLART, P.; BOREL, L.-J., and DUREL, P.: Significance of spiral organisms found after treatment in late human and experimental syphilis. Brit.J.vener.Dis. *40:* 81 (1964).

4 COX, P.M.; LOGAN, L.C., and NORINS, L.C.: Automated quantitative microhemagglutination assay for *Treponema pallidum* antibodies. Appl.Microbiol. *18:* 485 (1969).

5 Duncan, W.P. and Kuhn, U.S.G.: Reactivity of treponemal and nontreponemal tests with cerebrospinal fluid from syphilitic chimpanzees. J. infect. Dis. *125:* 61 (1972).

6 Elsas, F.J.; Cox, P.M.; Bullard, J.C.; Kuhn, U.S.G., and Chandler, F.W.: Treponeme like forms in chimpanzee aqueous humor and cerebrospinal fluid. Arch. Ophthal., Chicago *87:* 333 (1972).

7 Kuhn, U.S.G.: The treponematoses; in Bourne The chimpanzee, vol. 3, pp. 71–81 (Karger, Basel 1970).

8 Kuhn, U.S.G.: Humoral aspects of treponematoses of chimpanzees; in Goldsmith and Moor-Jankowski Medical primatology 1970, pp. 761–765 (Karger, Basel 1971).

9 Kuhn, U.S.G.; Medina, R.; Cohen, P.G., and Vegas, M.: Inoculation pinta in chimpanzees. Brit. J. vener. Dis. *46:* 311 (1970).

10 Kuhn, U.S.G.; Varela, G.; Chandler, F.W., and Osuna, G.G.: Experimental pinta in the chimpanzee. J. amer. med. Ass. *206:* 829 (1968).

11 Lucas, C.T.; Chandler, F.W.; Martin, J.E., and Schmale, J.D.: Transfer of gonococcal urethritis from man to chimpanzee. J. amer. med. Ass. *216:* 1612 (1971).

12 Medina, R.: El carate en Venezuela. Estudie de la enfermedad enel medio natural y resultado de los ensayos de inoculaction experimental. Sep. Rev. Derm. Venez. *3:*160 (1962).

13 Short, D.H.; Knox, J.M., and Glicksman, J.: Neurosyphilis, the search for adequate treatment. A review and report of a study using benzathine penicillin G. Arch. Derm., Chicago *93:* 87 (1966).

14 Smith, J.L. and Israel, C.W.: Spirochetes in the aqueous humor in seronegative ocular syphilis. Persistance after penicillin therapy. Arch. Ophthal., Chicago *77:* 474 (1967).

15 Turner, T.B. and Hollander, D.H.: Biology of the treponematoses (World Health Organization, Geneva 1957).

16 Turner, T.B. and McLeod, C.P.: Crossimmunity in experimental syphilis yaws and venereal spirochetosis of rabbits. Trans. Ass. amer. Physicians *57:* 265 (1942).

17 US Department of Health Education and Welfare. Manual of Tests for Syphilis. PHS Publication No. 411 (US Government Printing Office, Washington 1969).

18 US Department of Health, Education and Welfare. Serologic Tests for Syphilis. 1964 Manual. PHS Publication No. 411 (US Government Printing Office, Washington 1964).

19 Wilmer, E. and Brady, J.A.: Prognosis of general paresis after treatment. Lancet *ii:* 1370 (1968).

Author's address: U.S.G. Kuhn, III, Venereal Disease Research Unit, Laboratory Division, Center for Disease Control, USPHS, *Atlanta, GA.* (USA)

Medical Primatology 1972. Proc. 3rd Conf. exp. Med. Surg. Primates, Lyon 1972, part III, pp. 88–96 (Karger, Basel 1972)

Nonhuman Primates for Investigations of Parasite Oncology[1]

Robert E. Kuntz and Betty June Myers

Division of Microbiology and Infectious Diseases,
Southwest Foundation for Research and Education, San Antonio, Tex.

Introduction

Man is plagued by many parasite infections. However, parasitic diseases *per se,* except for a few (hookworm disease, the malarias, the schistosomiases, etc.) do not account for large numbers of deaths. As a consequence, priorities of basic parasitological research have been stifled, and simians less used as experimental models for parasitology than for studies of other diseases.

The overall parasitology of nonhuman primates and their role as models for investigations has been presented in reviews [18, 20, 29] and their potential for specialized studies in experimental schistosomiasis hematobia has been discussed by Kuntz *et al.* [30, 33].

Parasites as Carcinogens

The ability of parasites to serve as carcinogens has been discussed since the begining of this century. However, the field of parasite oncology is poorly developed, and the concept of parasite-cancer relationships has been downgraded in the absence of model systems for conclusive evidence, even though veterinary medicine includes records on cancer in association with parasite diseases.

Although there are instances suggesting a possible association of proto-

1 Supported by the United States-Japan Co-operative Medical Science Program administered by USPHS, NIH, NIAID, grant AI 08207, NCI grant CA 13208, and NIH grants RR 05519, RR 00278, and RR 00451.

zoa and cancer, the literature compiled by us leans heavily on the helminths, especially those which are tissue invaders, or those intimately associated with host tissues. For man, a good proportion of available records is concerned with schistosomiasis or a combination of schistosome infection and other parasites in association with cancer. Different theories (trauma, physical or chemical irritation, influence of metabolic products on irritated tissues, etc.) have been proposed to explain the carcinogenic features of parasite infection. Even in early writings [17] there was a surmise that a virus accompanying the parasite may have been involved. However, many past reports are far from satisfactory. Apparently, misjudgements have been made in the evaluation of macroscopic lesions, some designated as 'cancerous-like', on one hand, while on the other, it seems likely that malignancies in parasite infections may have been overlooked. This was due in part to lack of communication between the parasitologist and the pathologist. Thus, while a review of the literature reveals many references which suggest malignancy due to parasite infections, a more critical evaluation points to considerable uncertainty or nondocumented pathology. Several reviews [2, 3, 43, 49] concerned with cancer, neoplasia, and pertinent pathology as related to cancer, describe the works of many authors who have touched upon the subject of cancer associated with or induced by parasites.

It is difficult to pinpoint the time at which cancer or tumors were first observed. However, ancient Egyptian records include descriptions presumably in reference to tumors, and it seems probable that it may have been related to schistosomiasis [35].

There is little point in an extensive listing of known or suggested cases of parasite-cancer associations. However, parasites of greatest concern are *Gongylonema, Hydatigera taeniaeformis (Cysticercus fasciolaris), Spirocerca, Clonorchis* and *Schistosoma*. Even though there have been questions and disclaimers regarding the malignancy of the gastric 'cancers' described for *Gongylonema neoplasticum* in rats by FIBIGER [15, 16] his work stimulated interest in the possibility of a parasite-cancer relationship. At the time it was assumed that a laboratory model for cancer research had been realized. Another situation which evoked interest was based upon the causal association of *Cysticercus fasciolaris,* a larval cestode in rats, and liver sarcoma [5]. Although the precise factors for neoplasia were not demonstrated, later investigations [9] showed an active agent in larvae which produced peritoneal sarcoma when injected peritoneally. Research on esophageal sarcoma induced by *Spirocerca lupi* have been well described by BAILEY [2, 3]. *Clonorchis sinensis,* the Oriental liver fluke, has received less attention, but HOU [21–23] has described carcinoma in the bile ducts of man as well as in experimentally-infected cats and dogs. Pros and cons on this pathology have been reviewed by YAMAGATA and YAEGASHI [52]. Varied pathology and malignancy associated with the schistosomiases covers a period of 75 years and will be discussed later in more detail.

Other studies on parasites have cast an entirely different light upon the field of parasite oncology. In one instance it has been intimated that heat-killed or lyophilized trypanosomes *(T. cruzi)* have an antineoplastic action on epithelial cancer cells [51]. In another, it was demonstrated that growth of Walker sarcoma could be entirely suppressed or enhanced in *Nippostrongylis brasiliensis* infected rats, depending on the time of tumor cell inoculation in relation to status of parasite infection [28].

Nonhuman Primates as Models for Parasite Oncology

Schistosoma haematobium and Cancer of the Urinary Bladder

Schistosomiasis, including the three principal species found in man, is recognized as the most important parasite disease, affecting the health of extensive populations. It is a debilitating infection that results from a varied and serious pathology which may affect any organ of the body. The most severe pathology involves the intestinal tract, the urogenital system and other abdominal viscera. All three of the schistosomes *(S. japonicum, S. haematobium,* and *S. mansoni)* of man but mainly *S. haematobium* have been incriminated as agents with causal relationships to cancer (table I).

Man has hosted *S. haematobium* for several millenia and descriptions of hematuria in the texts of the early papyri of Egypt, along with the finding of *S. haematobium* eggs in mummy remains leave little doubt that schistosomiasis hematobia has been endemic along the Nile for a long time. It was not unexpected that the first incrimination of this parasite as a possible cause of cancer should be reported from Cairo. In 1911, FERGUSON [14], after six years of observations on schistosomiasis hematobia in Egyptians, reported on 40 cases of infection and associated this disease with malignancy of the urinary bladder. HUEPER [24], in reviewing carcinoma of the bladder, stated that in all probability vesical schistosomiasis is the oldest occupational disease with neoplastic potentialities. At a later date, he [25] again reviewed the *S. haematobium*-carcinoma situation and presented pertinent statistics for a causal relationship between the parasite and bladder cancer. Additional evidence

Table I. Varied pathology recorded in schistosome infections

Schistosoma haematobium		
cancer, urinary bladder	human	Ferguson [14]
cancer, urinary bladder	human	El-Gazayerli and Koraitum [11]
cancer, bladder, liver, prostate, etc.	human	Shamma [44]
malignant growth, bladder wall	*Papio anubis*	Edwards and McCullough [10]
papillomata, urinary bladder	*Cercopithecus*	Fairley [13]
transitional cell papillomata, bladder	opossum	Kuntz *et al.* [33]
transitional cell carcinoma, bladder	*Cebus, Cercopithecus*	Kuntz *et al.* [30]
cancer, urinary bladder	human	Mustacchi and Shimkin [37]
carcinoma, urinary bladder	human	Talib [47]
hyperplastic and metaplastic changes, urinary bladder	albino mice	Hashem and Boutros [19]
Schistosoma japonicum		
carcinoma, colon and rectum	human	Ch'en *et al.* [6]
carcinoma, liver	human	Suzuki, T. [46]
carcinoma, parotid gland	human	Tangchai and Poshayalakshana [48]
Schistosoma mansoni		
carcinoma, stomach, hepatoma	wild rat	Oettlé *et al.* [41]
hepatoma, liver (w/chemical carcinogen)	white mice	Domingo *et al.* [8]
adenocarcinoma, pancreas	human	Ishak [26]
adenocarcinoma, large intestine	human	Dimmette *et al.* [7]
cancer, large intestine	human	Barsoum [4]

for and against this thesis has been published over the past few decades [36, 47].

As a rule such controversy would elicit the interests of the experimentalists and initiate research to prove or refute the points in concern. Basic research on the topic, however, was hampered by the fact that *S. haematobium* infection in lower vertebrates does not present the clinical manifestations found in man and, in general, there is little or no involvement of the urogenital system. A possible exception is the occurrence of transitional cell papillomata of the bladder accompanying *S. haematobium* infection in the American opossum [32]. Attempts to circumvent the use of infected animals for studies in schistosome carcinogenesis by injecting mice s.c. with living worms and lyophilized cercariae and eggs were unsuccessful [45]. At a later date, AL-HUSSAINI and MCDONALD [1] made an unsuccessful attempt to elicit tumors in the bladder of mice given intravesical applications of lyophilized *S. haematobium* eggs in mineral oil. EL-GHAFFAR [12], likewise, failed to initiate bladder tumors by surgically implanting paraffin pellets with lyophilized urine from patients with schistosomiasis hematobia.

The situation in nonhuman primates has been somewhat different and much more encouraging. A fairly formidable list of species which have been exposed to *S. haematobium* from different geographic areas with resulting urinary bladder pathology includes *Cebus apella* [34], *Cercopithecus aethiops* [13, 40], *Cercopithecus talapoin* [38], *Pan* [43, 50], *Pan* and *Cercocebus* [50] *Papio anubis* [10, 27], *Papio hamadryas* [31] and *Presbytis cristatus* [39].

In a most recent report [30] causal relationship was demonstrated between experimental schistosomiasis hematobia in lower primates and carcinoma of the bladder. Lesions with features of papillary transitional cell carcinoma were described in the bladder of a talapoin *(Cercopithecus talapoin)* and a capuchin monkey *(Cebus apella)* exposed to 1,000 and 2,000 parasites, respectively. The inner surface of the bladder of the talapoin was covered by prominent cauliflower-like projections (up to 3.5 mm in diameter) some of which were intimately associated with the eggs of *S. haematobium*. There were numerous independent tumors several millimeters away from the principal lesions. A KOH (potassium hydroxide) digest indicated approximately 9,500 schistosome eggs/gram of tissue. In the capuchin monkey, the mucosal surface of the bladder was covered with soft, dirty yellow mucosal plaques. The most prominent lesion consisted of a large (1.7 × 0.5 cm) cone-shaped projection into the urethra, and there were marked epithelial proliferations some distance away. Microscopically, there were well-differentiated nests of transitional cells in the lamina propria and at some sites between muscle bundles. Small areas of squamous metaplasia occurred in the proximity of eggs deposited in the submucosa. KOH digest indicated approximately 70,000 eggs/gram of tissue.

An African baboon *(Papio cynocephalus)*, exposed to 1,000 cercariae of *S. haematobium* and examined 52 weeks later, presented a tumor (grade I papillary carcinoma) in the ureter near the bladder. Significant bladder lesions occurred also in two squirrel monkeys *(Saimiri sciureus)* which demonstrated large polypoid projections caused by marked granulomatous inflammation or edema of the submucosa and proliferation of the epithelium. This pathology was classed as epithelial hyperplasia with squamous metaplasia.

The nature of malignancy and the relatively small number of hosts at risk, i.e. cancer in one of two talapoins, one of seven capuchin monkeys, and in one of 14 baboons, indicates the need for continued research on the association of *S. haematobium,* cancer of the urinary bladder and helminth oncogenesis.

Knowledge of the basic phenomena involved in cancer is far from satisfactory with need for models for more sophisticated investigations. At present, the cause, mechanisms at play (single or combination of factors) and the reproducibility of pathology in schistosome oncogenesis is unknown. Potentials for development of a model system have been demonstrated. In the future, it will be necessary to determine more precisely the role in parasite oncogenesis of basic host-parasite relationships such as intensity of infection with schistosomes, duration of infection; effects of mixed, super- and supra-infections upon bladder pathology, age of hosts at time of introduction of parasites, status of infection in relation to introduced endogenous and exogenous factors, stress in captivity, diet and other influencing conditions.

References

1 Al-Hussaini, M. and McDonald, D.F.: Lack of urothelial topical tumorigenicity and cotumorigenicity of schistosome ova in mice. Cancer Res. *27:* 228–229 (1967).

2 Bailey, W.S.: Parasites and cancer. Ann.N.Y.Acad.Sci. *108:* 890–923 (1963).

3 Bailey, W.S.: *Spirocerca lupi:* a continuing inquiry. J.Parasit. *58:* 3–22 (1972).

4 Barsoum, H.: Cancer in Egypt. Its incidence and clinical forms. Acta Un.int.Cancr. *9:* 241–250 (1953).

5 Bullock, F.D. and Curtis, M.R.: Spontaneous tumors of the rat. J.Cancer Res. *14:* 1–115 (1930).

6 Ch'en, M.C.; Hu, J.C.; Chang, P.Y.; Chuang, C.Y.; Ts'ao, P.F.; Chang, S.H.; Wang, F.P.; Ch'en, T.L., and Chou, S.C.: Pathogenesis of carcinoma of the colon and rectum in schistosomiasis japonica. A study of 90 cases. Chin.med.J. *84:* 513–525 (1965).

7 Dimmette, R.M.; Elwi, A.M., and Sproat, H.F.: Relationship of schistosomiasis to polyposis and adenocarcinoma of large intestine. Amer.J.clin.Path. *26:* 266–276 (1956).

8 Domingo, E.O.; Warren, K.S., and Stenger, R.J.: Increased incidence of hepatoma in mice with chronic schistosomiasis mansoni treated with a carcinogen. Amer.J.Path. *51:* 307–321 (1967).

9 Dunning, W.F. and Curtis, M.R.: Multiple peritoneal sarcoma in rats from intraperitoneal injection of washed, ground *Taenia* larvae. Cancer Res. *6:* 668–670 (1946).

10 Edwards, E.E. and McCullough, F.S.: Studies on the life-cycles of *Schistosoma haematobium* and *S. mansoni* in the Gold Coast. Ann.trop.Med.Parasit. *48:* 164–177 (1954).

11 EL-GAZAYERLI, M. and KORAITUM, M.: The role of bilharziasis in the pathogenesis of bladder cancer; in MOSTOFI Bilharziasis. Int. Acad. Path. Special Monogr., pp. 84–85 (Springer, New York 1967).

12 EL-GHAFFAR, Y.A.: Failure to induce bladder cancer in mice. Bladder implantation with paraffin wax pellets of lyophilized urine from bilharzial patients. Cancer, Philad. *19:* 1225–1230 (1966).

13 FAIRLEY, N.H.: A comparative study of experimental bilharziasis in monkeys contrasted with the hitherto described lesions in man. J. Path. Bact. *23:* 289–314 (1920).

14 FERGUSON, A.R.: Associated bilharziosis and primary malignant disease of the urinary bladder, with observations on a series of forty cases. J. Path. Bact. *16:* 76–94 (1911).

15 FIBIGER, J.A.G.: Untersuchungen über eine Nematode (*Spiroptera* sp.n.) und deren Fähigkeit, papillomatöse und carcinomatöse Geschwulstbildungen im Magen der Ratte hervorzurufen. Z. Krebsforsch. *13:* 217–280 (1913).

16 FIBIGER, J.A.G.: On *Spiroptera* carcinomata and their relation to true malignant tumours. With some remarks on cancer age. J. Cancer Res. *4:* 367–387 (1919).

17 FIBIGER, J.A.G.: Helminths in cancer (editorial). Brit. med. J. *i:* 777–778 (1920).

18 FIENNES, R.: Zoonoses of primates. The epidemiology and ecology of simian diseases in relation to man (Cornell University Press, Ithaca 1967).

19 HASHEM, M. and BOUTROS, K.: The influence of bilharzial infection on the carcino-genesis of the mouse bladder. An experimental study. J. Egypt. Med. Ass. *44:* 598–606 (1961).

20 HOEPPLI, R.J.C.: Parasites and tumour growth. Chin. med. J. *47:* 1075–1111 (1933).

21 HOU, P.C.: The relationship between primary carcinoma of the liver and infestation with *Clonorchis sinensis*. J. Path. Bact. *72:* 239–246 (1956).

22 HOU, P.C.: Hepatic clonorchiasis and carcinoma of the bile duct in a dog. J. Path. Bact. *89:* 365–367 (1965).

23 HOU, P.C.: Pathological changes in the intrahepatic bile ducts of cats *(Felis catus)* infested with *Clonorchis sinensis*. J. Path. Bact. *89:* 357–364 (1965).

24 HUEPER, W.C.: Occupational tumors and allied diseases (Thomas, Springfield 1942).

25 HUEPER, W.C.: Occupational and environmental cancer of the urinary system (Yale University Press, New Haven 1969).

26 ISHAK, KG.: Adenocarcinoma of the head of the pancreas associated with *S. mansoni* infestation. Report of a case. J. Egypt. med. Ass. *40:* 59–63 (1957).

27 JORDAN, P.; LICHTENBERG, F. VON, and GOATLY, K.D.: Experimental schistosomiasis in primates in Tanzania. Preliminary observations on the susceptibility of the baboon *Papio anubis* to *Schistosoma haematobium* and *Schistosoma mansoni*. Bull. Wld Hlth Org. *37:* 393–403 (1967).

28 KELLER, R.; OGILVIE, B.M., and SIMPSON, E.: Tumour growth in nematode-infected animals. Lancet *i:* 678–680 (1971).

29 KUNTZ, R.E.: Models for investigations in parasitology; in BOURNE Nonhuman primates in biomedical research (Academic Press, New York, in press).

30 KUNTZ, R.E.; CHEEVER, A.W., and MYERS, B.J.: Proliferative epithelial lesions of the urinary bladder of nonhuman primates infected with *Schistosoma haematobium*. J. nat. Cancer Inst. *48:* 223–235 (1972).

31 KUNTZ, R.E. and MALAKATIS, G.M.: Susceptibility studies in schistosomiasis. III. Infections of various experimental hosts with *Schistosoma haematobium* in Egypt. Amer. J. trop. Med. Hyg. *4:* 75–89 (1955).

32 Kuntz, R.E.; Myers, B.J., and Cheever, A.W.: *Schistosoma haematobium* infection in the oppossum *(Didelphis marsupialis)*. Involvement of the urogenital system. Bull. Wld Hlth Org. *45:* 21–25 (1971).

33 Kuntz, R.E.; Myers, B.J.; Huang, T.C., and Moore, J.A.: Use of nonhuman primates in experimental schistosomiasis haematobia; in Biegert and Leutenegger Proc. 3rd Int. Congr. Primatology, vol. 2, pp. 162–172 (Karger, Basel 1971).

34 Kuntz, R.E.; Myers, B.J.; Moore, J.A., and Huang, T.C.: *Schistosoma haematobium*. Experimental infection in capuchin monkey, *Cebus apella*. Exp. Parasit. *29:* 33–41 (1971).

35 Magahed, M.S.; Schlagenhauff, R.E., and Wagshul, A.: Cerebral schistosomiasis. J. Med. *1:* 201–212 (1970).

36 Mostofi, F.K. (ed.): Bilharziasis. Int. Acad. Path., Special Monogr. (Springer, New York 1967).

37 Mustacchi, P.O. and Shimkin, M.B.: Cancer of the bladder and infestation with *Schistosoma hematobium*. J. nat. Cancer Inst. *20:* 825–842 (1958).

38 Myers, B.J.; Kuntz, R.E.; Huang, T.C., and Moore, J.A.: Urinary bladder involvement in the talapoin (*Cercopithecus talapoin* Schreber) due to infection with *Schistosoma haematobium* (Bilharz, 1852) Weinland, 1858. Lab. Anim. Care *20:* 1004–1006 (1970).

39 Myers, B.J.; Kuntz, R.E.; Huang, T.C., and Moore, J.A.: Urinary bladder involvement in the langur *(Presbytis)* infected with *Schistosoma haematobium* (Bilharz, 1852) Weinland, 1858. Proc. helminth. Soc. Wash. *37:* 189–192 (1970).

40 Obuyu, C.K.: Preliminary communication on gross pathological lesions in the genital-urinary systems of vervet monkeys *(Cercopithecus aethiops)* experimentally infected with *Schistosoma haematobium*. Ann. trop. Med. Parasit. *64:* 395–398 (1970).

41 Oettlé, A.G.; Meillon, B. de, and Lazer, B.: Carcinomas of the glandular stomach and hepatomas in *Rattus (Mastomys) natalensis* infected with *Bilharzia mansoni*. Acta Un. int. Cancr. *15:* 200–202 (1959).

42 Sadun, E.H.; Lichtenberg, F. von; Cheever, A.W.; Erickson, D.G., and Hickman, R.L.: Experimental infection with *Schistosoma haematobium* in chimpanzees. Amer. J. trop. Med. Hyg. *19:* 427–458 (1970).

43 Schwabe, C.W.: Helminth parasites and neoplasia. Amer. J. vet. Res. *16:* 485–488 (1955).

44 Shamma, A.H.: Schistosomiasis and cancer in Iraq. Amer. J. clin. Path. *25:* 1283–1284 (1955).

45 Shimkin, M.B.; Mustacchi, P.O.; Cram, E.B., and Wright, W.H.: Lack of carcinogenicity of lyophilized *Schistosoma* in mice. J. nat. Cancer Inst. *16:* 471–474 (1955).

46 Suzuki, T.: A case of the cancer originated from the liver containing eggs of *Schistosoma japonicum*. Zyuzenkai Zassi *45:* 948–961 (1940).

47 Talib, H.: The problem of carcinoma of bilharzial bladder in Iraq. Critical review. Brit. J. Urol. *42:* 571–579 (1970).

48 Tangchai, P. and Poshayalakshana, P.: Schistosomal granuloma with muco-epidermoid carcinoma of parotid gland. J. trop. med. Hyg. *71:* 134–136 (1968).

49 Unio Internationalis Contra Cancrum Acta *18:* 517–688 (1962).

50 Vogel, H.: Experimentelle Infektionen mit *Schistosoma haematobium* an Mangaben und Schimpansen. Ann. Soc. belge Méd. trop. *47:* 107–116 (1967).

51 Wery, Ph.: Trypanosomiase et cancer. Rev. Path. gén. *63:* 229–235 (1963).
52 Yamagata, S. and Yaegashi, A.: Clinical problems of clonorchiasis; in Morishita *et al.* Progress of medical parasitology in Japan, vol. 1, pp. 663–721 (Meguro Parasit. Museum, Tokyo 1964).

Authors' address: Drs. Robert E. Kuntz and Betty June Myers, Department of Parasitology, Division of Microbiology and Infectious Diseases, Southwest Foundation for Research and Education, *San Antonio, TX 78284* (USA)

Medical Primatology 1972. Proc. 3rd Conf. exp. Med. Surg. Primates, Lyon 1972, part III, pp. 97–109 (Karger, Basel 1972)

Use of Chimpanzees as a Model for the Study of Hepatitis B Virus Infections[1]

A. M. PRINCE

Laboratory of Virology, New York Blood Center and Department of Pathology, New York Hospital, Cornell Medical Center, New York, N.Y.

Introduction

Until recently man was the only available model for the study of human hepatitis infection. Demonstration of the specificity of an antigen, now termed the hepatitis B antigen (HB ag, HAA, SH, Australia antigen) for infections with hepatitis B (serum hepatitis) virus [15] and the demonstration that this antigen may be found in the serum of some primates [3, 4, 10] suggested that animal models for hepatitis B infections would become available. The present report presents additional confirmation of this expectation. We shall show that chimpanzees are susceptible to infections with hepatitis B virus and that they may develop both transient and persistent types of infections. In addition, we will indicate the usefulness of this species for the study of the chronic virus carrier state; and for the production of high titer hepatitis B antibody which may be useful for immunoprophylaxis in man.

Materials and Methods

All serum specimens were tested for SGPT by the kinetic spectrophotometric method routinely employed in our laboratory [18]. We routinely employ frozen serum controls to insure accuracy and reproducibility. The upper limit of normal in our laboratory (95 % of volunteer blood donors) is 30 Karmen units. Our experience with serial blood sample col-

1 These studies were aided by grants No. HE-09011 and AI-09516 from the National Institutes of Health, contract No. 70-2236, from the National Heart and Lung Institute, and grants in aid from the Kresge Foundation and from the Strasburger Foundation. Dr. PRINCE is a Career Scientist of the Health Research Council of the City of New York under contract No. 1-533.

lections from approximately 35 chimpanzees during the past three years indicates that these animals do not differ significantly from man in normal mean SGPT levels.

Sera were also tested for HB ag and HB ab by agar gel diffusion [9], IEOP [14], passive hemagglutination (HA), and hemagglutination inhibition (HAI) [17], and more recently by the direct radioimmunoassay (RIA) of Ling and Overby, utilizing AUSRIA™ kits supplied by Abbott Laboratories.

Results

'Spontaneous' Development of HB Antigen in Chimpanzees Held in Captivity

HB antigen was detected in the serum of eight of 138 chimpanzees tested [10]. In each case antigen was present in the first of the serial sera examined. It was, thus, not possible to determine whether the antigenemia had originated in Africa or in the United States. This is an important question for two reasons: first, it is likely that if infection occurs in captivity at least some newly-imported chimpanzees should be susceptible to infection with hepatitis B virus; and second, if the prevalence of the antigen carrier state in chimpanzees in the wild approximates the high rate found in native populations in the areas from which the chimpanzees originate [2, 11] this would have important implications for an understanding of the natural route of transmission of hepatitis B virus in tropical regions.

Fortuitously, Dr. K. F. SOIKE had stored earlier sera samples from seven of the animals in whom antigen was detected and had available serial samples from one additional animal. These additional serum specimens were tested by the agar gel diffusion test and, in some cases, also by the more sensitive immunoelectroosmophoresis (IEOP) test. In four animals antigen was detected in the earliest of the available serum specimens. However, as shown in table I, three of the original series of positive animals and the additional animal examined had previously been negative for HB antigen but acquired the antigen following importation into the United States. Minimal intervals prior to appearance of the antigen varied from four months to five years. It is likely that at least animals 178, 466 and 505 acquired their infections during captivity.

It is unlikely that the absence of detectable antigen in the early sera is due to inactivation during storage as this antigen is extremely stable in the frozen state. It has been readily detected in specimens stored for more than 15 years at –20 °C [3].

Table I. Development of hepatitis B antigen in chimpanzees held in captivity

Animal No.	Date received from importer	Date of serum specimen	Detection of Hb ag		Minimum interval prior to appearance of antigen
			Ouchter-lony test	IEOP test	
178	7/29/62	3/64	–	ND	5 years
		10/64	–	–	
		6/67	–	–	
		9/67	+	+	
		10/67	+	ND	
		8/68	–	–	
466	4/22/66	5/66	–	–	10 months
		2/67	–	–	
		8/68	+	ND	
		3/69	+	ND	
		2/70	–	ND	
705	10/31/68	1/27/69	–	–	4 months
		2/3/69	–	–	
		3/10/69	+	+	
		3/17/69	+	ND	
505	7/19/66	1/67	–	–	8 months
		3/67	–	–	
		6/67	+	+	
		6/68	+	ND	
		4/69	+	ND	
		10/69	+	ND	

ND = not done.

The source of these infections cannot be definitely established. It may be significant that chimpanzee 178 received injections of human blood on several occasions between January, 1966, and April, 1969. However, the remaining animals did not receive injections of human or chimpanzee origin. These animals may, therefore, be presumed to have been infected by a nonparenteral route, as has been postulated to explain antigen-positive cases of hepatitis which occur among urban adults lacking a history of parenteral exposure [15].

The fact that chimpanzees may acquire HB antigenemia in captivity suggests that some of these animals may be susceptible to challenge infection with serum hepatitis virus shortly after importation. Whether some animals contain the antigen in the wild state prior to capture remains to be determined.

Susceptibility of Chimpanzees to Intentional Challenge Infection

The high prevalence of HB ag in the chimpanzees examined [10] suggested widespread past exposure in this species. It has been found that human beings with serologic evidence of past hepatitis B infection (i.e. anamnestic antibody responses detectable by passive hemagglutination assay) may, nevertheless, develop hepatitis if exposed to large doses of virus by blood transfusion [13]. We, therefore, chose to expose chimpanzees to infection in a comparable manner. On August 13, 1970, chimpanzees ranging in age from 32 to 60 months were challenged with 70–100 ml of plasma obtained from chimpanzee 20, a chronic HB ag carrier, whom we have studied since 1969. In each case, one unit of blood was withdrawn from the chimpanzee to be challenged, the red cells were resuspended in the antigenemic plasma from chimpanzee 20 and reinfused. Serum samples were then obtained at weekly intervals for eight months and again 18 months after challenge.

The results of these experiments are summarized in figures 1–6, and table II. When the passive hemagglutination assay became available, it became feasible to examine the preinoculation sera with a sensitive test for HB ag. This revealed that all except two animals had pre-existing levels of this antibody and had, therefore, in all probability, been previously exposed to infection. It was of interest that the inoculated antigen disappeared at

Table II. Results of challenge of six chimpanzees with 70–100 ml chimpanzee 20 (ad) plasma

Chimpanzee No.	Age when challenged months	Weight when challenged kg	Preinoculation HA titer (reciprocal)	Duration of antigenemia weeks		SGPT rise			Antibody response	
				HAI	RIA	incubation period weeks	peak	weeks	incubation period weeks	peak titer first eight months
23	34	13	32	5	11	14	150	16	–	64
25	32	11	<2	4	4	4	84	9	5	2,048
27	46	16	8	2	3	6	51	7	4	1,024
29	60	18	64	<1	9	16	141	17	4	4,096
31	46	15	<2	8	∞[1]	16	89	20	8	256
38	34	13	4	1	1	12	76	13	7	128

1 Induction of chronic carrier state.

differing rates, becoming nondetectable by HAI after an interval varying from less than one to eight weeks. There was no apparent correlation between prior HB ab levels and rate of disappearance of antigen. All animals revealed transaminase elevations between four and 16 weeks after challenge. The elevations were mild to moderate, peak SGPT varying between 51 and 150 Karmen units. Distinct seroconversion (i.e. a fourfold or greater rise in HB ab titer detectable by passive hemagglutination) was seen in all except one animal (chimpanzee 23). The initially seronegative animals, No. 25 and 31 and chimpanzee 38 who had a preinoculation titer of 1:4 showed antibody rises occurring between five and eight weeks after exposure, i.e. typical primary antibody response [13].

The above results were strongly suggestive but did not prove infection. Through the kindness of Drs. LING and OVERBY of Abbott Laboratories, we have been able to examine the sera from this experiment by their direct radioimmunoassay technique. The most convincing results were those found when the sera of chimpanzee 31 were examined (fig. 5). It will be seen that by RIA technique, antigen never became nondetectable; indeed, beginning three to four months after exposure a chronic carrier state became apparent. During the period between three and nine months antigen remained at relatively low

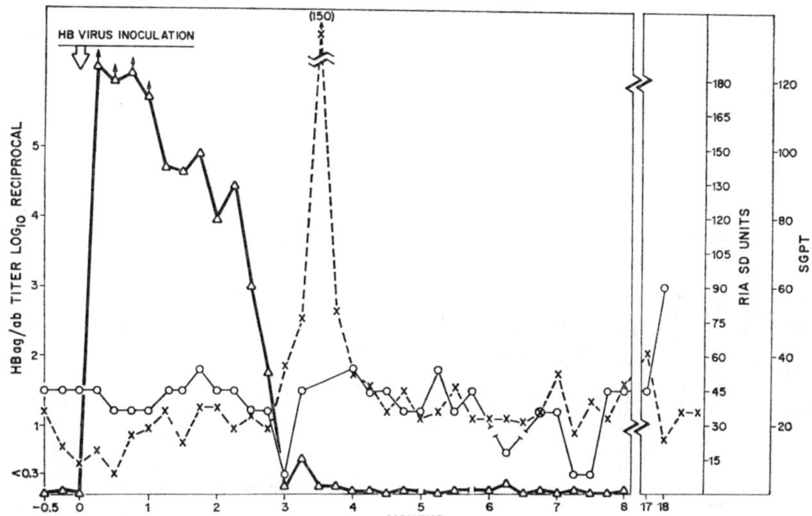

Fig. 1. Challenge experiment: inoculation of chimpanzee 23 with 100 ml chimpanzee 20 (HB ag, +) plasma. △ = RIA SD units; × = SGPT; ○ = HB ab – HA test.

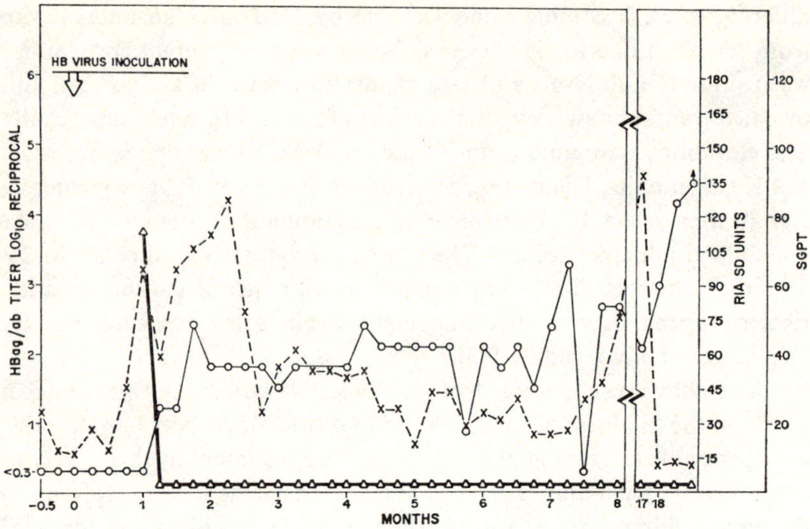

Fig. 2. Challenge experiment: inoculation of chimpanzee 25 with 100 ml chimpanzee 20 (HB ag, +) plasma. △ = RIA SD units; × = SGPT; ○ = HB ab – HA test.

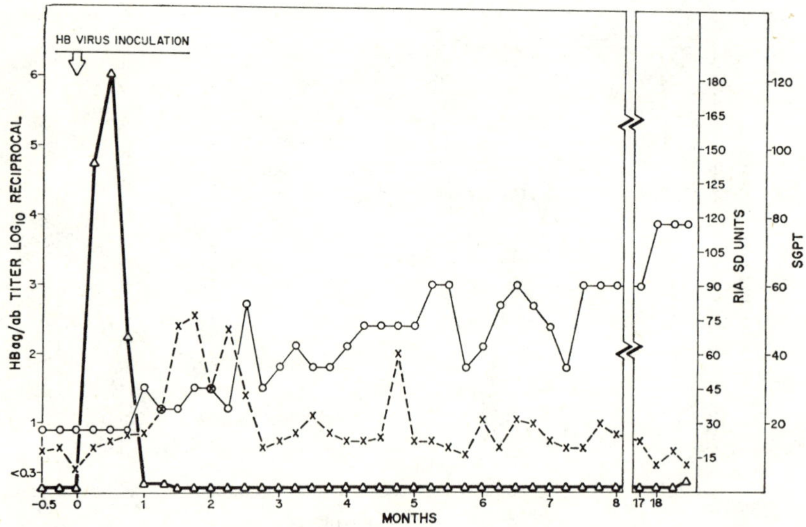

Fig. 3. Challenge experiment: inoculation of chimpanzee 27 with 100 ml chimpanzee 20 (HB ag, +) plasma. △ = RIA SD units; × = SGPT; ○ = HB ab – HA test.

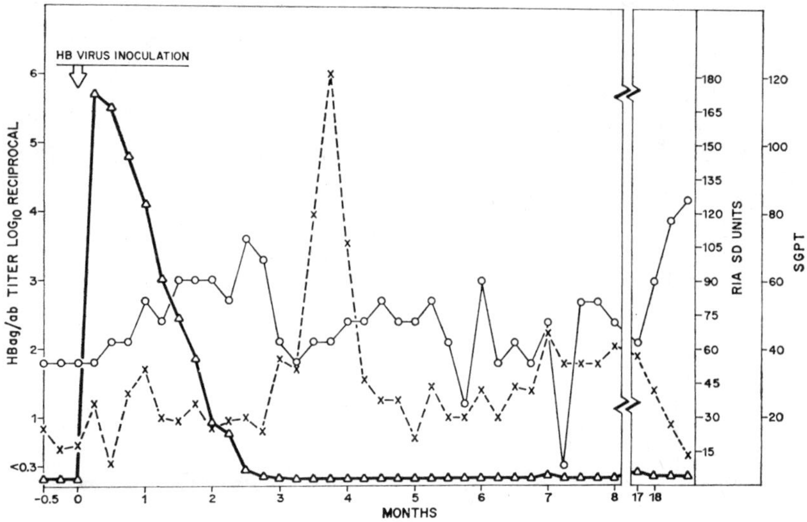

Fig. 4. Challenge experiment: inoculation of chimpanzee 29 with 70 ml chimpanzee 20 (HB ag, +) plasma. △ = RIA SD units; × = SGPT; ○ = HB ag – HA test.

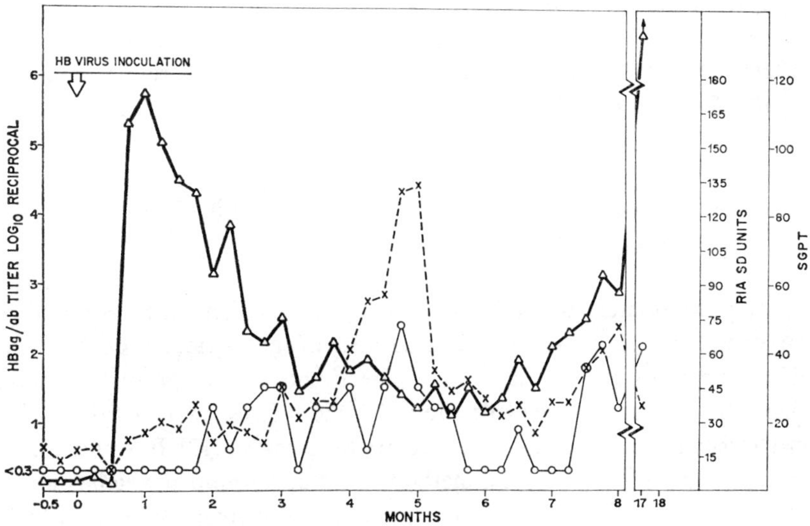

Fig. 5. Challenge experiment: inoculation of chimpanzee 31 with 85 ml chimpanzee 20 (HB ag, +) plasma. △ = RIA SD units; × = SGPT; ○ = HB ag – HA test.

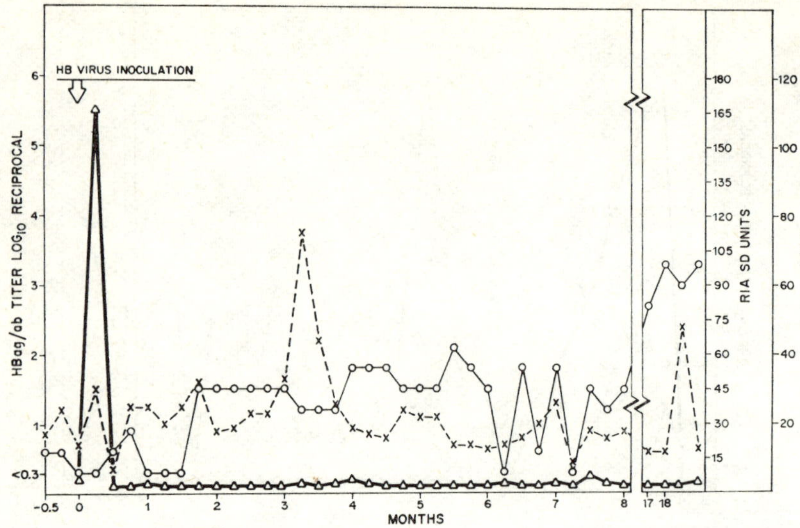

Fig. 6. Challenge experiment: inoculation of chimpanzee 38 with 100 ml chimpanzee 20 (HB ag, +) plasma. Δ = RIA SD units; × = SGPT; ○ = HB ag – HA test.

levels detectable only by radioimmunoassay. The quantity of circulating antigen began to rise at about six months, reaching levels corresponding to about 90 standard deviation units. A follow-up specimen taken 17 months after exposure revealed antigen to be detectable by radioimmunoassay, hemagglutination inhibition, and now even by agar gel diffusion and IEOP.

Chimpanzees as a Model for the Chronic Hepatitis B Virus Carrier State

Approximately one million residents of the United States, and much larger numbers of people in the remainder of the world, are chronic carriers of the hepatitis B antigen. It may be estimated that approximately 5% of these chronic carriers will develop chronic aggressive hepatitis leading to cirrhosis and, in some cases, to primary liver cancer [12]. It would, therefore, be of the greatest interest if a method could be developed which could result in termination of the chronic infection. As all of the approaches which can be contemplated at the present time are potentially hazardous, the availability of an animal model for this chronic carrier state is of the greatest importance.

We have investigated a number of approaches to this problem and will illustrate just one of these. Figure 7 summarizes administration of HB ab to two chronic HB ag carriers: (1) Chimpanzee 20, who was given 4×10^8 leucocytes from chimpanzee 12 (who had been hyperimmunized with serum from chimpanzee 20 suspended in Freund's adjuvant). The latter animal had an HB ab titer of 1:128 by IEOP at the time of plasmapheresis. The leucocytes were suspended in 20 ml of autologous plasma, and were injected by slow i.v. injection using gravity flow from a plastic bag. After several minutes blood pressure and pulse became undetectable, probably as a result of ventricular fibrilation and cardiac arrest. Cardiac massage was immediately instituted. Atropine and epinephrine were administered: Cardiac function returned to normal over a 30-min period. The above reaction may well have represented passive 'systemic' anaphylaxsis. Cardiac arrest has also been observed during administration of HB ab plasma i.v. to one patient with fulminant hepatitis whose serum contained detectable HB ag [SCHAFFNER, personal commun.].

These observations suggest that HB ab-containing materials should be administered, whenever possible, only to subjects demonstrably free of HB ag. If it is thought desirable to administer such materials on an emergency

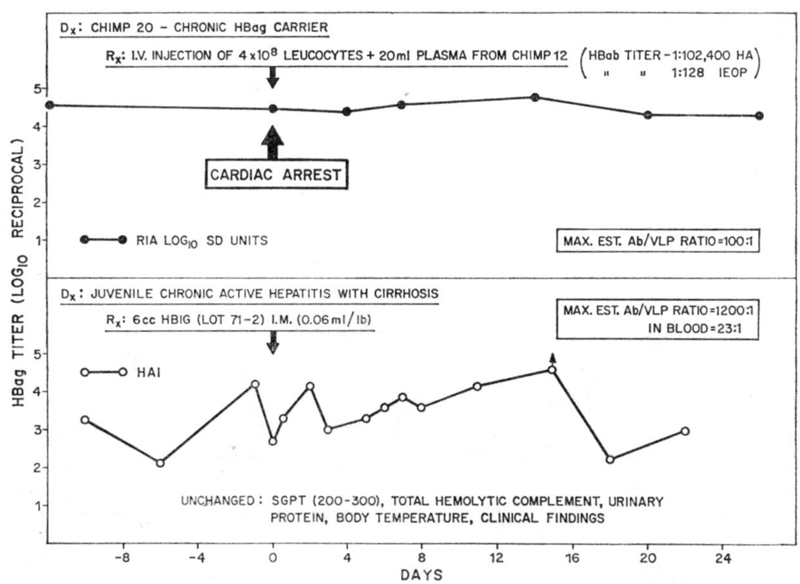

Fig. 7. Effect of HB ab on chronic HB ag carriers.

basis, where HB ag screening cannot be carried out, it would be desirable to carry out a skin test with HB ab-containing material prior to administration, and then to administer HB ab slowly and cautiously under conditions where resuscitative measures are immediately available.

Figure 7 summarizes administration of a high titer hepatitis B immune globulin (HBIG) [16] by the i.m. route to a patient with juvenile chronic active hepatitis and probable cirrhosis. No adverse effects were noted; however, it should also be pointed out that no benefit accrued.

We have also failed to influence the chronic carrier state by administration of exogenous human interferon.

Preparation of Hyperimmune Hepatitis B Immune Globulin in Chimpanzees

The use of chimpanzee plasma as an alternate source for HBIG is under consideration in our laboratory. Precipitating quantities of hepatitis B antibody have been observed in unimmunized chimpanzees [10] and have been induced by immunization [5] in these animals. Immunization with highly-

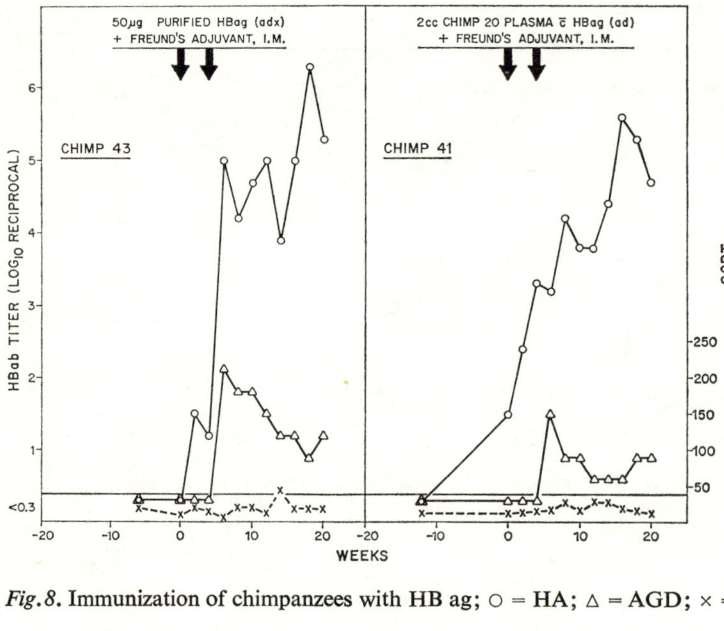

Fig. 8. Immunization of chimpanzees with HB ag; ○ = HA; △ = AGD; × = SGPT.

purified antigen results in the appearance of monospecific high titer antibody within two weeks after a booster injection of purified antigen suspended in Freund's adjuvant (fig. 8). The results presented are typical of those observed in 20 chimpanzees whom we have immunized during the past year; thus, large volumes of hyperimmune plasma can be obtained by plasmapheresis. If γ-globulin of chimpanzee origin can be shown to be no more immunogenic in man than pooled γ-globulin of human origin, as may be expected, chimpanzee γ-globulin could represent a logical source for protective antibody for human use.

It is noteworthy that none of the animals which have been immunized with purified antigen in Freund's adjuvant have developed significant transaminase elevations, suggesting that these preparation may be noninfectious under these conditions.

It was of interest that the precipitating antibody titers tended to fall subsequent to the second booster immunization at a time when hemagglutinating antibody was continuing to rise in titer. The mechanism of this phenomenon requires further investigation.

Discussion

The results presented in this report provide further indication that the chimpanzee represents a uniquely useful model for the study of hepatitis type B infections. It has been well established that the hepatitis B antigen and its associated particles are immunologically and morphologically very similar to those present in man [4, 8, 10]. The work presented in this report, as well as parallel studies in other laboratories, [1, 7] indicates clearly that chimpanzees may be experimentally infected with this virus. Indeed, recent evidence suggests that the rhesus monkey is also susceptible to this infection [6].

The disease induced in chimpanzees is clinically analogous to anicteric posttransfusion hepatitis. Replication of hepatitis B antigen was clearly demonstrated in one animal. It was found, as might be expected on the basis of posttransfusion follow-up studies in man [13] that past immunity did not protect against the development of at least mild forms of hepatitis.

The existence of animal models for this important human disease indicates that future studies of immunoprophylaxis and immunotherapy of hepatitis B infections should be based on prior exploration of possible risks and benefits in these animal models prior to further exploration of these approaches in man.

Acknowledgements

We are grateful for the technical assistance of B. CLINKSCALE, EDWINA ECHENROTH, ANNIE MAY MOFFATT, D. JOSS, and especially Mr. W. JOHNSON, Mr. B. TYRELL, and their co-workers at the Laboratory for Experimental Medicine and Surgery in Primates, Sterling Forest, N.Y. Dr. K. F. SOIKE kindly supplied stored serum samples from chimpanzees.

References

1 BARKER, L. F.; DALGARD, D.; MCGRATH, P. P.; CHISARI, F. V.; KIRCHSTEIN, R. L.; SHARP, D. G., and PETERSON, M. R.: Transmission of viral hepatitis to chimpanzees. Fed. Proc. *31:* 759 (1972).

2 BLUMBERG, B. S.; MELARTIN, L.; QUINTO, R. A., and WERNER, B.: Family studies of a human serum isoantigen system. Amer. J. hum. Genet. *18:* 594–608 (1966).

3 BLUMBERG, B. S.; SUTNICK, A. I., and LONDON, W. T.: Hepatitis and leukemia. Their relation to Australia antigen. Bull. N.Y. Acad. Med. *44:* 1566–1586 (1968).

4 HIRSCHMAN, R. J.; SHULMAN, N. R.; BARKER, L. F., and SMITH, K. O.: Virus-like particles in sera of patients with infectious and serum hepatitis. J. amer. med. Ass. *208:* 1667–1670 (1969).

5 LICHTER, E. A.: Chimpanzee antibodies to Australia antigen. Nature, Lond. *224:* 810–811 (1969).

6 LONDON, W. T.; ALTER, H. J.; LANDER, J., and PURCELL, R. H.: Serial transmission in rhesus monkeys of an agent related to hepatitis associated antigen. J. infect. Dis. *125:* 382–389 (1972).

7 MAYNARD, J. G.; BERQUIST, K. R., and DRUSHAK, D. H.: Studies of hepatitis candidate agents in tissue cultures and in animal models. Proc. Symp. Viral Hepatitis and Blood Transfusions, University of California, San Francisco 1972 (in press).

8 MAYNARD, J. G.; HARTWELL, W. V., and BERQUIST, K. R.: Hepatitis associated antigen in chimpanzees. J. infect. Dis. *123:* 660–664 (1971).

9 PRINCE, A. M.: An antigen detected in the blood during the incubation period of serum hepatitis. Proc. nat. Acad. Sci., Wash. *60:* 814–821 (1968).

10 PRINCE, A. M.: Hepatitis associated antigen: Long term persistence in chimpanzees; in GOLDSMITH and MOOR-JANKOWSKI Medical primatology 1970, pp. 731–739 (Karger, Basel 1971).

11 PRINCE, A. M.: Prevalence of serum-hepatitis-related antigen (SH) in different geographic regions. Amer. J. trop. Med. Hyg. *19:* 872–879 (1970).

12 PRINCE, A. M.: Role of serum hepatitis virus in chronic liver disease. Gastroenterology *60:* 913–921 (1971).

13 PRINCE, A. M.; BROTMAN, B., and CHERUBIN, C. E.: Immune response in patients who received blood containing serum hepatitis antigen. Studies with the passive hemagglutination technique. Amer. J. Dis. Child. *123:* 415–418 (1972).

14 PRINCE, A. M. and BURKE, K.: Serum hepatitis antigen (SH). Rapid detection by high voltage immunoelectroosmophoresis. Science *169:* 593–595 (1970).

15 PRINCE, A. M.; HARGROVE, R. L.; SZMUNESS, W.; CHERUBIN, C. E.; FONTANA, V. J.,

and JEFFRIES, G.H.: Immunologic distinction between infectious and serum hepatitis. New Engl. J. Med. *282:* 987–991 (1970).

16 PRINCE, A.M.; SZMUNESS, W.; BROTMAN, B.; IKRAM, H.; LIPPIN, A.; STRYKER, M.; EHRICH, B., and FINLAYSON, N.D.C.: Hepatitis B immune globulin. Availability, preparation, characterization and safety. Presented at Symp. Viral Hepatitis and Blood Transfusions, University of California, San Francisco 1972 (in press).

17 VYAS, G.N. and SHULMAN, N.R.: Hemagglutination assay for antigen and antibody associated with viral hepatitis. Science *170:* 332–333 (1970).

18 WROBLEWSKI, F. and LADUE, J.S.: Serum glutamic pyruvic transaminase in cardiac and hepatic disease. Proc. Soc. exp. Biol. Med. *91:* 569 (1956).

Author's address: Dr. ALFRED M. PRINCE, Laboratory of Virology, New York Blood Center, 310 East 67th Street, *New York, NY 10021* (USA)

Medical Primatology 1972. Proc. 3rd Conf. exp. Med. Surg. Primates, Lyon 1972, part III, pp. 110–115 (Karger, Basel 1972)

Pyelonephritis in the Nonhuman Primate[1]

J. A. ROBERTS

Tulane University Medical Center, Section of Urology and Delta Regional Primate Research Center, New Orleans and Covington, La.

Renal physiology [1] and natural disorders of the urinary tract such as hydronephrosis of pregnancy [8] in the nonhuman primate, are more representative of that in man than in other mammals. A recent evaluation of renal pathology in an autopsy series at the Delta Regional Primate Research Center shows that the incidence of chronic pyelonephritis in the nonhuman primate [7] of 0.65% compares closely to the incidence in man of 0.23 % recently determined by FARMER and HEPTINSTALL [2].

In order to allow correlation of bacteriuria with later autopsy findings in monkeys dying at the Center, percutaneous aspiration of bladder urine for culture is now being done. To date 240 primates have thus been studied and show an overall incidence of 3 % with bacteriuria. In the human population the incidence is from 2 to 5 % [6]. Only one bacteriuric animal came to autopsy and had normal kidneys. The low incidence of chronic pyelonephritis in comparison to that of bacteriuria would be expected, since cystitis is much more common than renal infection in the human population.

Vesicoureteral reflux, wherein bladder urine during voiding ascends the ureter, is abnormal in man. Progressive renal disease from nonobstructive bacterial infection infrequently occurs in the absence of such reflux of urine [4]. The frequency of reflux is high in animals such as the rat and rabbit, and has been evaluated in primates in combination with our studies of bacteriuria. At the time of percutaneous bladder puncture, the bladder is gravity filled with contrast material at a filling pressure of 40 cm of H_2O and an x-ray of the abdomen taken at the time of voiding. Table I shows the species thus evaluated and the percentage with vesicoureteral reflux. Note that the inci-

1 Supported by USPHS grants RR00164 and AM14681.

Table I. Vesicoureteral reflux and spontaneous urinary tract infection in the nonhuman primate

	Suprapubic bladder aspiration		
	number	% with reflux	% with bacteriuria
Old World monkeys			
Rhesus	118	6	1.8
Stump-tailed	42	0	4.7
Patas	20	0	5.0
Talapoin	10	0	10.0
Baboon	33	0	0
Chimpanzee	17	0	11.7
Total Old World	240	2.5	3.3
New World monkeys			
Squirrel	11	12.5	9.0
Callicebus	2	50.0	0
Total New World	13	20.0	7.6

dence is higher for New World monkeys as has been previously shown in the squirrel monkey [10]. The function of the ureterovesical junction of the Old World monkey is thus more similar to that in man than in other mammals (see fig. 1).

Reflux of urine occurs at a high frequency in the child with a urinary tract infection, but since the reflux often disappears following eradication of infection it has been suggested that vesicoureteral reflux is a change secondary to infection [5]. To test this theory, six stump-tailed monkeys without reflux had a chronic bladder infection produced by infecting the bladder in the presence of a foreign body. Although a proteus infection was maintained for 16 weeks by this technique, reflux was never seen on weekly voiding cystograms and no pyelonephritis was found at the time of autopsy.

The high incidence of reflux in children with urinary tract infections may only be due to a lack of maturation of the ureterovesical junction, since we have found in the infant rhesus monkey that the incidence of reflux is 30–50%, while by two years of age it has decreased to 2–5%. Recent studies [9] have shown a similar high incidence of reflux in normal children up to 3.5 years of age.

To evaluate whether ascending infection from the bladder will cause pyelonephritis, 200,000 *E. coli* were introduced by ureteral catheter into the

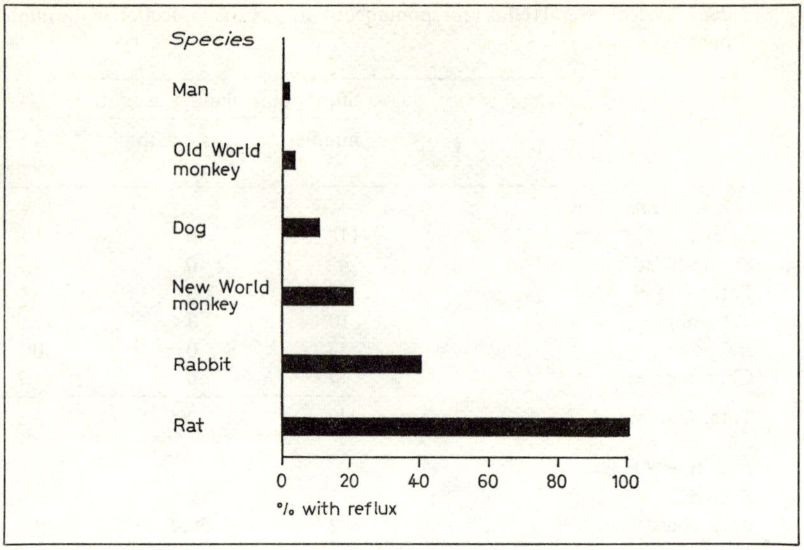

Fig. 1. A comparison of the incidence of vesicoureteral reflux in mammals.

renal pelvis in three animals. In only one was bacteriuria found for one week and this animal showed histologic changes of chronic pyelonephritis but no renal infection at the time of autopsy two months later. This points out the difficulty in producing a lasting renal infection, a problem common to all attempts to produce pyelonephritis experimentally. In the absence of renal trauma or obstruction, the inoculum necessary to produce hematogenous infection approaches the LD_{50} [3].

As we wish to evaluate possible changes in ureteral function secondary to infection itself, a nonsurgical technique was needed. It was found that feeding oxamide (the diamide of oxalic acid) would cause microtubular renal obstruction and that intravenous infection at the time of this obstruction would cause acute pyelonephritis as shown in table II. Upon cessation of the feeding of oxamide the crystalline aggregates were dissolved or washed away, leaving an unobstructed urinary tract. Bacteriuria in the stump-tailed monkeys thus studied often disappears within days after the acute pyelonephritis, and the length of time bacteriuria persists can be correlated with the severity of the renal disease (see fig. 2). In order to evaluate changes in ureteral function from the bacteria (presumably an effect of the endotoxin), both ureteral pressure studies for peristaltic activity, and renal scintiphoto studies were done. We have previously shown that partial ureteral obstruction causes

Table II. Acute hematogenous pyelonephritis

Monkey	WBC at 24 h	Urine culture at autopsy	Oxamide in papilla	Renal culture R	Renal culture L	Histology R	Histology L
1	26,600	4×10^5	+	+	+	–	+
2	29,900	3×10^5	+	+	+	+	–
3	10,400	1.7×10^4	+	+	+	+	–
4	17,900	3×10^7	+	+	+	+	+
5	20,800	1.3×10^6	+	+	+	–	+

Histologic change was present in all monkeys, however, animals marked + showed typical acute pyelonephritis and those marked – had minimal focal inflammation only.

delayed excretion of intravenous ^{131}I hippuran visualized by minute sequence polaroid exposures using the scintiphoto camera [11]. Such scintiphoto studies were thus done and correlated with the pathology found two months after infection. Figure 3 shows the difference between those with and without histologic change and suggests that a change in ureteral function occurred in monkeys with the final diagnosis of chronic pyelonephritis. In addition, ureteral pressure studies confirmed a change, as no peristaltic activity was seen in over half of the ureters draining kidneys with chronic pyelonephritis. However, none of the monkeys two months after infection continued to have bacteria in their kidneys, thus the change in ureteral function was not severe

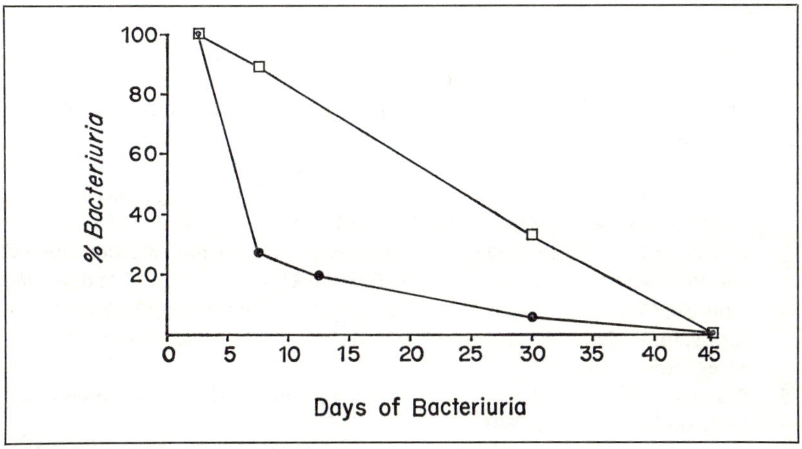

Fig. 2. Correlation bacteriuria (bladder urine) and final pathology. ● = Normal; □ = chronic pyelonephritis.

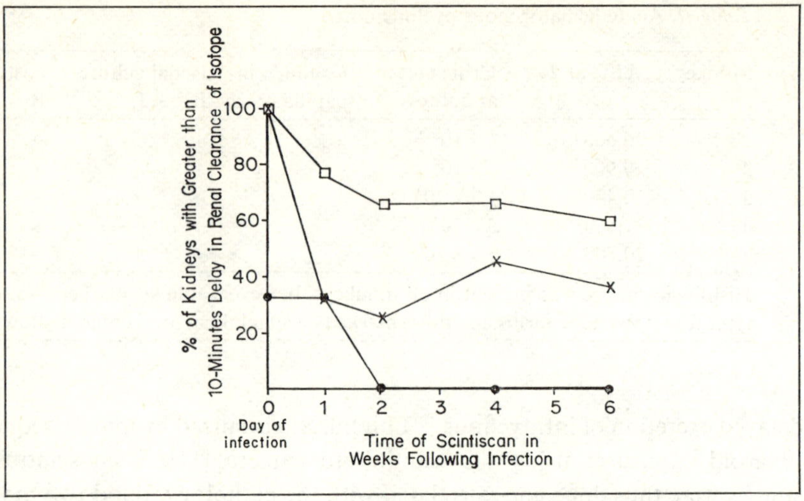

Fig. 3. Correlation of renal scintiphotos and final pathology. ● = No bacteriuria, normal histology; × = bacteriuria, normal histology; □ = bacteriuria, chronic pyelonephritis.

enough to maintain the infection. We are presently planning reinfection one month after the initial infection to determine whether monkeys with abnormal ureteral function are thus made more prone to a second hematogenous infection than those with normal ureters.

References

1 BENNETT, C.M.; BRENNER, B.M., and BERLINER, R.W.: Micropuncture study of nephron function in the rhesus monkey. J. clin. Invest. *47:* 203 (1968).

2 FARMER, E.R. and HEPTINSTALL, R.H.: Chronic non-obstructive pyelonephritis. A reappraisal; in Proc. Int. Symp. Pyelonephritis, Vesico-Ureteral Reflux and Renal Papillary Necrosis (Mercedes, Melbourne 1971).

3 GORRILL, R.H.: Susceptibility of the kidney to experimental infection; in O'GRADY and BRUMFITT Urinary tract infection (Oxford University Press, London 1968).

4 HODSON, C.J.: The mechanism of scar formation in chronic pyelonephritis; in Proc. Int. Symp. Pyelonephritis, Vesico-Ureteral Reflux and Renal Papillary Necrosis (Mercedes, Melbourne 1971).

5 HODSON, C.J. and EDWARDS, D.: Chronic pyelonephritis and vesico-ureteric reflux. Clin. Radiol. *11:* 219 (1960).

6 KUNIN, C.M.: The natural history of recurrent bacteriuria in school girls; in Proc. Int. Symp. Pyelonephritis, Vesico-Ureteral Reflux and Renal Papillary Necrosis (Mercedes, Melbourne 1971).

7 ROBERTS, J.A.; CLAYTON, J.D., and SEIBOLD, H.R.: The natural incidence of pyelonephritis in the nonhuman primate. Invest. Urol. *9:* 276 (1972).
8 ROBERTS, J.A. and WOLF, R.H.: Hydronephrosis of pregnancy. A naturally occurring disorder in non-human primates closely resembling that in man. Folia primat. *15:* 143 (1971).
9 SHOPFNER, C.E.: Vesicoureteral reflux. Radiology *95:* 637 (1970).
10 SINHA, D.P. and CLARKSON, T.B.: Ureteral reflux in the squirrel monkey *(Saimiri sciurius)*. Amer. J. vet. Res. *32:* 975 (1971).
11 WEXLER, N.S.; MCCLINTON, M.A.; CLAYTON, J.D., and ROBERTS, J.A.: Partial ureteral obstruction in the monkey. A comparison of hydrated *versus* dehydrated scintiphoto studies for evaluation. Invest. urol. (in press).

Author's address: Dr. JAMES A. ROBERTS, Delta Regional Primate Research Center, 3 Rivers Road, *Covington, LA 70433* (USA)

Medical Primatology 1972. Proc. 3rd Conf. exp. Med. Surg. Primates, Lyon 1972, part III, pp. 116–123 (Karger, Basel 1972)

Use of the Rhesus Monkey as a Model for Studies of Comparative Efficacy of Antibiotics in *Pseudomonas* Sepsis

S. Saslaw and H. N. Carlisle

Division of Infectious Diseases, Department of Medicine, Ohio State University College of Medicine, Columbus, Ohio

Pseudomonas aeruginosa infections represent a serious problem particularly in patients with chronic diseases or impaired defense mechanisms. In general, antibiotics that are active *in vitro* have been used in uncontrolled studies in man as far as comparative efficacy is concerned [3]. Lack of a suitable animal model simulating *Pseudomonas* sepsis in man has been a limit-

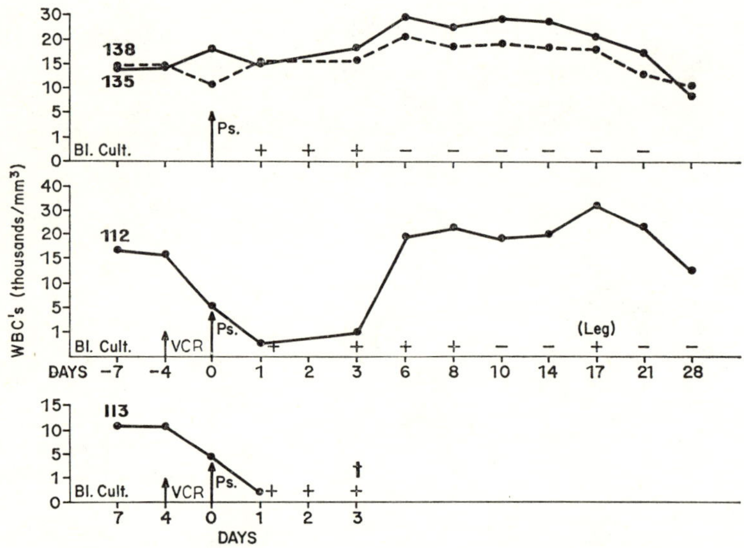

Fig. 1. Experiment 4. Effect of VCR (2.5 mg intratracheal) on *Pseudomonas* infections (4.2×10^{10} organisms i.v.).

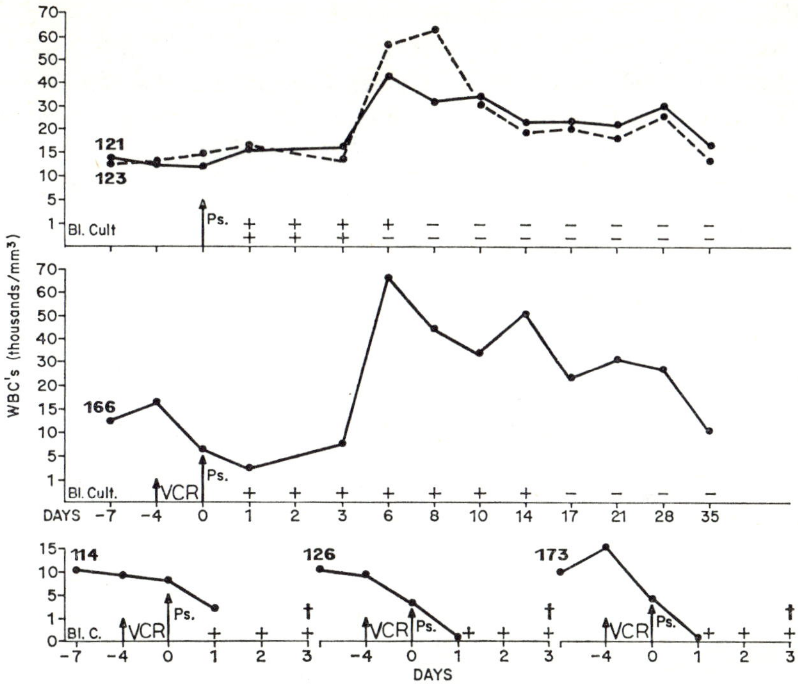

Fig. 2. Experiment 5. Effect of VCR (2.5 mg intratracheal) on *Pseudomonas* infections (6.8×10^{10} organisms i.v.).

ing factor. *Pseudomonas* septicemia has been a particular problem in patients with leukemia or agranulocytosis, and appears to be enhanced by antimetabolites [1, 2, 4].

Studies in this laboratory have been conducted to establish a biologic model for *Pseudomonas* sepsis to allow controlled studies of antibiotic therapy [8]. Preliminary studies showed that i.v. inoculation of $1\text{–}2 \times 10^{10}$ *Pseudomonas* organisms into rhesus monkeys caused acute illness for a four- to five-day duration with spontaneous recovery in 13 of 15; positive blood cultures were observed for three to 17 days, and all monkeys exhibited leukocytosis. Previous studies in this laboratory with different antineoplastic agents suggested that vincristine sulfate could be employed to induce granulocytopenia with lesser risk and toxicity in monkeys [6]. Subsequent studies demonstrated that i.v. or intratracheal administration of 2.0–2.5 mg of vincristine sulfate induced leukopenia by the fourth day. Intravenous challenge with $4.2\text{–}7.8 \times 10^{10}$ organisms during this leukopenic phase was followed by deaths in 11 of 14 monkeys while none of four receiving *Pseudomonas* alone died. Skin and visceral lesions were similar to those seen in human infections. Figures 1–3 indicate the effects of vincristine sulfate in *Pseudomonas* sepsis. It is the purpose of this report to describe the studies conducted to date on comparative efficacy of antibiotics on *Pseudomonas* sepsis.

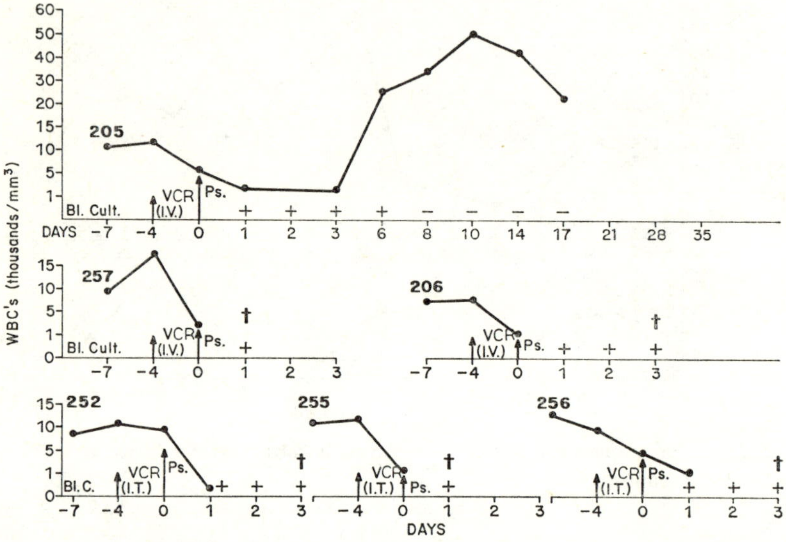

Fig. 3. Experiment 6. Effect of VCR (2.5 mg intratracheal [i.t.]) on *Pseudomonas* infections (7.8 × 10^{10} organisms i.v.).

Materials and Methods

Young adult fully-conditioned monkeys *(Macaca mulatta)* weighing 3.2–4.6 kg were used. Vincristine sulfate (Lilly) [5], hereinafter referred to as VCR, was used in these studies as was a pyocine type 6 strain of *Pseudomonas aeruginosa* (Bricker) as previously described [8]. Minimal inhibitory concentrations of tobramycin, gentamicin, colistin and carbenicillin for the *Pseudomonas* were 0.62, 2.5, 3.13 and 62.5 μg/ml, respectively.

Monkeys were challenged with 3.4 × 10^{10} to 8.7 × 10^{10} *Pseudomonas* cells four or five days after i.v. or intratracheal inoculation of 2.0 or 2.5 mg of VCR. Therapy with tobramycin, gentamicin, colistin and carbenicillin was instituted 16 h after challenge and continued for ten days. When two agents were given they were administered in separate syringes. The daily dose was divided equally and given i.m. at 8:00 a.m. and 5:00 p.m. Controls received normal saline at these time intervals.

Results

Comparison of Tobramycin, Gentamicin, Colistin and Carbenicillin

As can be seen in table I, comparable results were obtained in each therapy group. Four of 11, four of 11, three of ten and five of 12 monkeys treated with tobramycin, gentamicin, colistin and carbenicillin, respectively, died. Duration of illness in surviving monkeys was not significantly different in the four therapy groups. Monkeys treated with tobramycin, gentamicin, colistin and carbenicillin began to improve after two to seven days (mean 4.7), three to seven days (mean, 4.6), three to eight days (mean, 4.4) and two to six

Table I. Effect of therapy with tobramycin, gentamicin, colistin and carbenicillin on response of rhesus monkeys challenged i.v. with *Pseudomonas* four days after VCR administration

Antibiotic[1]	Experiment[2]	Mortality	Total	Day of death	Acute illness day	Mean	Total illness day	Mean
Tobramycin	1	2/3[3]	4/11	5, 11[4]	2	4.7	5	8.6
	2	1/4		2	3, 4, 7		6, 7, 8	
	3	1/4		12	5, 5, 7		6, 7, 21	
Gentamicin	1	1/3	4/11	3	4,7	4.6	8, 13	8.6
	2	2/4		3, 4	3, 6		7, 8	
	3	1/4		3	3, 4, 5		6, 6, 12	
Colistin	1	1/3	3/10	2	4, 4	4.4	6, 11	7.4
	2	2/3		2,2	4		5	
	3	0/4			3, 4, 4, 8		6, 7, 7, 10	
Carbenicillin	1	2/4	5/12	2, 2	2, 4	4.3	4, 12	7.0
	2	3/4		2, 3, 4	4		5	
	3	0/4			3, 5, 6, 6		6, 6, 8, 8	
Controls	1	3/3	8/9	1, 2, 3		9.0		26.0
	2	2/2		1, 3				
	3	3/4		1, 1, 2	9		26	

1 Five mg/kg/day of tobramycin, gentamicin, and colistin in all three experiments. Carbenicillin doses in experiments 1, 2, and 3 were 100, 200, and 400 mg/kg/day respectively.

2 Challenge doses in experiments 1, 2, and 3 were 3.4×10^{10}, 6.2×10^{10}, and 7.4×10^{10} *Pseudomonas* cells, respectively, given four days after 2.5, 2.0 and 2.0 mg of VCR i.v., i.v. and intratracheally, respectively.

3 Number that died over total number.

4 Concomitant *Proteus mirabilis* enteritis.

days (mean, 4.3), respectively. All but six of the 28 surviving monkeys appeared normal by day 9. All 28 surviving monkeys had positive blood cultures on day 3 and only four had positive blood cultures after this period: two in the gentamicin group, and one in each of the carbenicillin- and tobramycin-treated group. These data and other laboratory aspects will be discussed in detail elsewhere [7].

Comparison of Tobramycin and Gentamicin at High Dose Levels

When the two aminoglycosides were compared at higher dose levels comparable results were also observed. Twenty monkeys were given 2.0 mg VCR, intratracheally, and challenged four days later with 8.7×10^{10} *Pseudomonas* cells. Three of the four controls were dead by day 2 and the fourth animal was acutely ill for 11 days, and not completely recovered until day 25. *Pseudomonas* was recovered from the blood through day 10 in the surviving monkey, and from all major organs in the ones that died. No specific deaths were observed in two groups of four monkeys each treated with 20 mg/kg/day of tobramycin and gentamicin, respectively, for five days followed by 10 mg/kg/day for five days. Similarly no specific deaths were observed in two groups of four each receiving 10 mg/kg/day of the two antibiotics for five days followed by 5 mg/kg/day for five days. Two monkeys receiving the higher dose of gentamicin died on days 13 and 14. No organisms were recovered from the latter two monkeys and death was probably related in part to nephrotoxicity since both exhibited marked azotemia.

Comparison of Carbenicillin, Gentamicin and Carbenicillin-Gentamicin

Nineteen monkeys were inoculated, intratracheally, with 2.5 mg of VCR and challenged four days later with 6.0×10^{10} *Pseudomonas* cells. Two groups of four monkeys each were treated, i.m., with 50 and 2.5 mg/kg/day, respectively, of carbenicillin and gentamicin, respectively. Eight monkeys were treated with the same doses of both antibiotics in combination administered separately. Three monkeys served as untreated controls.

As shown in table II, the three controls died on days 1, 2 and 7, and *Pseudomonas* was isolated from all major organs and blood of all three monkeys. One of four monkeys treated with carbenicillin failed to survive and died on day 3. Similarly one of four treated with gentamicin died on day 3.

Table II. Comparison of carbenicillin, gentamicin and carbenicillin-gentamicin in *Pseudomonas* sepsis in rhesus monkeys

Antibiotic	Dose, mg/kg[1]	Mortality[2]	Day of Death[3]
Carbenicillin	50	1/4	3
Gentamicin	2.5	1/4	3
Carbenicillin plus gentamicin	50+2.5	2/8	2, 15
Controls	–	3/3	1, 2, 7

1 Daily dose divided equally and given at 8:00 a.m. and 5:00 p.m for ten days beginning 16 h after i.v. challenge with 6.0×10^{10} *Pseudomonas* cells.
2 Number dead over total number.
3 Day 0 = day of *Pseudomonas* challenge, or four days after intratracheal administration of 2.5 mg VCR.

On combined therapy two of eight monkeys receiving carbenicillin-gentamicin died on days 2 and 15, respectively. *Pseudomonas* was isolated at autopsy from the monkey dying on day 2. However, no *Pseudomonas* organisms were recovered from the monkey dying on day 15 who apparently suffered a late severe enteritis due to *Proteus mirabilis.*

Comparison of Carbenicillin, Colistin and Carbenicillin-Colistin

In one experiment 12 monkeys (table III) were inoculated with 6.2×10^{10} *Pseudomonas* organisms five days after intratracheal administration of 2.5 mg

Table III. Comparison of colistin, carbenicillin and colistin-carbenicillin in *Pseudomonas* sepsis in rhesus monkeys

Antibiotic	Dose, mg/kg[1]	Mortality[2]	Day of Death[3]	Dose, mg/kg	Mortality	Day of Death
Colistin	2.5	0/3		1.25	6/8	2, 2, 2, 3, 3, 3
Carbenicillin	50	0/3		25	3/7	3, 3, 5
Colistin plus Carbenicillin	2.5+50	1/3	20	1.25+25	4/9	2, 2, 2, 3
Controls	–	3/3	1, 1, 2	–	5/7	1, 1, 1, 2, 2

1 Daily dose divided equally and given at 8:00 a.m. and 5:00 p.m. for ten days beginning 16 h after i.v. challenge with 6.2×10^{10} *Pseudomonas* cells.
2 Number dead over total number.
3 Day 0 = day of *Pseudomonas* challenge, or five days after intratracheal administration of 2.5 mg VCR.

of VCR. All of three untreated controls died by the second day. All of three receiving either 2.5 mg/kg/day of colistin or 50 mg/kg/day of carbenicillin, survived. In three monkeys receiving both antibiotics at the same dose level, one of three failed to survive and died on day 20, but no *Pseudomonas* had been isolated after day 3 or at autopsy. Death was attributed to VCR toxicity.

In subsequent experiments (table III) using 1.25 mg/kg/day of colistin, 25 mg/kg/day of carbenicillin and both antibiotics at the same dosage, the following results were obtained: Deaths were observed in six of seven, three of seven, and four of nine in monkeys treated with colistin, carbenicillin, and colistin-carbenicillin combined respectively, while five of seven controls died.

Discussion

Although 115 monkeys were employed in these therapy studies, individual groups were too small to allow precise statistical evaluation. As in patients with *Pseudomonas* sepsis, many variables come into play including underlying disease, antecedent or concomitant therapy and blood picture. Although these monkeys were originally healthy animals, the prior administration of an antimetabolite enhanced their susceptibility to *Pseudomonas* infection. The decrease in leukocytes, particularly granulocytes, apparently served as a major factor in reference to increased susceptibility [6, 8] as has been observed in man [1, 2, 4]. Since there was variation in the effect of vincristine on leukocyte count in individual monkeys, one would have to consider that some were poorer risks than others. Analysis of this factor is too complex and beyond the purpose of this report and will be described in separate publications. The major purpose of this report is to demonstrate that a severe, fatal *Pseudomonas* sepsis can be induced in monkeys more regularly after administration of an antimetabolite like vincristine sulfate four to five days previously. Under the conditions of this study when therapy was instituted 16 h after i.v. inoculation of *Pseudomonas* organisms, tobramycin, gentamicin, colistin and carbenicillin yielded comparable results at the same dose levels usually employed in man. Combination therapy using gentamicin or colistin with carbenicillin did not show increased or decreased efficacy – i.e., there was no evidence of synergy or antagonism at the dose levels studied. Many more animals and different dose regimes would be required to further delineate if there are any significant differences in comparative efficacy of the antibiotics now being employed in the therapy of *Pseudomonas* sepsis.

References

1 Bodey, G.P.; Buckley, M.; Sathe, Y.S. *et al.:* Quantitative relationships between circulating leukocytes and infection in patients with acute leukemia. Ann.intern. Med. *64:* 328–340 (1966).

2 Bodey, G.P.; Rodriguez V., and Whitecar, J.P.: Severe infections in leukemic patients – an approach to antibiotic therapy; in Advances in the Management of *Pseudomonas* and *Proteus* infections, pp. 65–78 (Excerpta Medica Foundation, New York 1969).

3 Davis, S.D.; Iannetta, A., and Wedgwood, R.J.: Antibiotics for *Pseudomonas aeruginosa* sepsis. Inadequate proof of efficacy. J.infect. Dis. *124:* 104–106 (1971).

4 Hersh, E.M.; Bodey, G.P.; Nies, B.A. *et al.:* Causes of death in acute leukemia. A ten-year study of 414 patients from 1954–1963. J.amer.med.Ass. *193:* 105–109 (1965).

5 Johnson, I.S.; Armstrong, J.G.; Gorman, M., and Burnett, J.P., jr.: The vinca alkaloids. A new class of onocolytic agents. Cancer Res. *23:* 1390–1427 (1963).

6 Saslaw, S. and Carlisle, H.N.: Nonhuman primates in evaluation of hematotoxicity. Ann.N.Y.Acad.Sci. *162:* 646–658 (1969).

7 Saslaw, S.; Carlisle, H.N., and Moheimani, M.: Effect of vincristine sulfate on *Pseudomonas* infections in monkeys. Infect.Immunol. *6:* 277–282 (1972).

8 Schimpff, S.; Satterlee, W.; Young, V.M., and Serpick, A.: Empiric therapy with carbenicillin and gentamicin for febrile patients with cancer and granulocytopenia. New Engl.J.Med. *284:* 1061–1065 (1971).

Author's address: Samuel Saslaw, MD, PhD, Division of Infectious Diseases, Department of Medicine, Ohio State University College of Medicine, N-1148 University Hospital, 410 West 10th Avenue, *Columbus, OH 43210* (USA)

Medical Primatology 1972. Proc. 3rd Conf. exp. Med. Surg. Primates, Lyon 1972, part III, pp. 124–129 (Karger, Basel 1972)

Use of Nonhuman Primates for Vaccine Manufacture and Control as Related to Problems Posed by Infectious Processes

N. M. Tauraso

Department of Health, Education, and Welfare, Public Health Service, National Institutes of Health, Division of Biologics Standards, Laboratory of Virology and Rickettsiology, Bethesda, Md.

Introduction

Probably due to their close phylogenetic relationship, nonhuman primates and man are susceptible to many of the same or closely-related microbial agents. As a result, some nonhuman primates and their tissues have been useful for a long time both for the manufacture of viral vaccines and for vaccine control work. From the medical point of view, it becomes important that we consider the infectious diseases of these animals so that we can ensure not only the quality (i.e., purity and safety) of the biological products derived from simian tissues, but also the utmost safety of the personnel who must care for these nonhuman primates and process their tissues. The purposes of this paper are (1) to describe how nonhuman primates have been and are being employed for the manufacture and control of biologics products; (2) to describe some new developments in the field; and (3) to consider infectious diseases of nonhuman primates as they relate to these uses.

Vaccine Development and Manufacture

Nonhuman primates and their tissues have been used in the development of virus strains suitable for vaccine manufacture. After isolation in 1927, the pantropic Asibi yellow fever virus strain was maintained in the laboratory by 53 serial passages in rhesus monkeys *(Macaca mulatta)* and a single passage in *Cebus fatuellus* before cultivation in cultures of minced whole mouse embryos. Later, both virulent poliovirus strains used to manufacture inactivated (Salk) vaccine and attenuated strains employed in the live oral polio (Sabin) vaccine had numerous passages in the monkey by direct intraspinal inoculation and in primary cell cultures of kidneys from rhesus and cynomolgus monkeys *(Macaca fascicularis)*. Most recently, African green monkey *(Cercopithecus aethiops)* cell cultures were used in the attenuation of the HPV-77 rubella vaccine strain [12].

It should be noted that, during the period of developing attenuated virus strains suitable for vaccine manufacture, nonhuman primates were continuously required for both monitoring the degree of attenuation and safety testing.

With respect to actual production of biological products, inactivated polio vaccine was prepared in rhesus monkey kidney cell cultures. Later, live oral polio vaccine was prepared in similar cell cultures, and African green monkey kidney cell culture was also included as a suitable substrate for preparation of polio vaccines.

One possibility which is being explored currently is the use of the chimpanzee as a source of hepatitis B antigen (HB Ag) and antibody. Advances in this area of biologics manufacture are occurring rapidly.

It is obvious that tissues used in any stage of vaccine development and manufacture should be free from *all* extraneous agents. This has been more easily accomplished with smaller laboratory animals, such as: chickens, whose embryos are employed in the manufacture of live vaccines against yellow fever, measles, and smallpox; ducks, whose embryos are used in the manufacture of live rubella vaccine; dogs, whose kidneys are employed in live measles and rubella vaccines; and rabbits, whose kidneys are employed in the manufacture of rubella vaccine. For example, the flocks of chickens to be employed for vaccine manufacture must be free from *Salmonella pullorum,* avian tuberculosis, fowlpox, Rous sarcoma, avian leukosis, and other agents pathogenic for chickens. An equivalent degree of quarantine and maintenance of an isolated specific pathogen-free colony of nonhuman primates would be extremely difficult. The cost of such a venture would be probably prohibitively expensive. In addition, nonhuman primates are susceptible to human viruses, and an exchange of pathogens between the monkey and man would be difficult to control without the use of specially-constructed isolators.

Employing wild caught monkeys involves a constant, potential hazard. We must work with animals which may harbor such viruses as *Herpesvirus simiae* (B virus) and Marburg which are fatal for man. We must also be alert to recognize the yet unknown human pathogens. Many herpesviruses are known to inhabit some simian species as latent agents and produce overt disease in other monkeys [10]. Considering the pathogenicity of B virus for man, we must constantly be aware that these other simian herpesviruses are potential human pathogens. The potential hazard of employing wild-caught monkeys as a source of tissue for vaccine production is considerably reduced but not eliminated by the requirement that monkeys be held in quarantine for at least six weeks prior to their use [6]. Cross-infection among these animals is known to occur during this period and this would tend to perpetuate a potentially hazardous infectious agent in the colony.

Because of these and other problems, the development and employment of nonhuman primate diploid cell strains for vaccine manufacture appears to be a reasonable alternative. Once the diploid cell strain and the vaccine seed virus have been exhaustively tested and its safety insured, it would be relatively simple to perform the necessary control tests on the final vaccine. In fact, as a follow-up of recommendations made during the 1967 conference on cell cultures for virus vaccine production, held at the US Public Health Service, National Institutes of Health [11], the Division of Biologics Standards supported a program for development of new diploid cell lines from both rhesus and African green monkeys. PETRICCIANI *et al.* [14] described the results of this program and conclude that it was 'possible to develop populations of cells from subhuman primates which meet basic requirements for use in the production of human biologics'.

Extreme care goes into the selection of viruses to be used in the production of live virus vaccines to ensure safety and immunogenicity. In the past, less care went into the selection of cell substrates used for vaccine production. The extensive safety tests performed on each batch of vaccine were relied upon to detect extraneous agents and other potentially harmful materials which may have been introduced by the cell substrate or during virus propagation. This system has worked for over 25 years. However, now with the improved technology of growing, characterizing, and evaluating cells in continuous culture, it would appear reasonable to place the same degree of care to the development and selection of standardized cell substrates as put into the selection of the virus strains used for vaccine production [13]. In this regard, standardized nonhuman primate diploid cells would be a considerable improvement over primary cell cultures of tissues from wild-caught monkeys.

Vaccine Control Work

The tissues of nonhuman primates to be used for vaccine control work (such as determining potency of live virus vaccines and detecting extraneous agents) would necessarily have to be derived from healthy quarantined monkeys. The comments just made concerning the use of such tissues for vaccine manufacture would also apply here. And, again, nonhuman primate diploid cell strains could eventually be employed for this aspect of vaccine control work.

Nonhuman primates are essential to safety (neurovirulence) testing of live virus vaccine strains. At the present time, neurovirulence tests are performed on all live virus vaccines except smallpox. Although changes in such requirements might occur in the future, neurovirulence testing of live virus vaccine strains where the property of neurovirulence is intrinsic to the virus (e.g. polio and yellow fever viruses) would be a necessary part of safety testing. With the yellow fever 17D vaccine, rhesus monkeys are used also to monitor the degree of viscerotropism by measuring viremia and to determine potency by testing the neutralizing antibody response.

It is difficult to conceive an alternative to using nonhuman primates for many aspects of vaccine control work, especially for neurovirulence testing. Consequently, until such time when breeding and maintaining sufficient numbers of specific-pathogen-free monkeys becomes feasible, we will have to continue to use wild-caught monkeys. This will necessarily require a constant careful monitoring of procedures employed in trapping, maintaining at local 'staging' compounds, and shipping to final destination. Ultimately, nonhuman primates must be satisfactorily quarantined to make them both suitable for vaccine control work and safe for those who must handle them.

The Importance of Adequate Quarantine

Several reviews have emphasized the occurrence of recent epizootics of infectious diseases, latent infections as well as the comparative virology of nonhuman primates as related to man [7, 16]. Considering the source of infection, a microbial disease in a nonhuman primate may be an infection natural to the monkey with man being an accidental host, or the disease may be natural to man, acquired by the monkey and transmitted back to man. Examples of natural simian diseases have included simian herpes, monkeypox, and probably tuberculosis in some instances. The acquired infections might include viral hepatitis, measles, shigellosis, and tuberculosis. From the viewpoint of human medicine, both natural and acquired simian infections are important. A listing of some nonhuman primate infectious diseases associated with more memorable events include: Marburg virus disease [5]; B virus

(Herpesvirus simiae) [8], poxvirus infections, such as those caused by monkeypox [9], Yaba [1] and Yaba-like [4] viruses; infectious hepatitis [3]; simian hemorrhagic fever [17]; tuberculosis [15]; and shigellosis [2].

The threat of human infection from contact with nonhuman primates can be considerably reduced by an adequate quarantine. The US Public Health Service requires that monkeys used as a source of tissue in vaccine manufacture 'shall be maintained in quarantine for at least six weeks prior to use ...', and 'only monkeys that have reacted negatively to tuberculin at the start of the quarantine period and again within two weeks prior to use shall be used in the manufacture of vaccines' [18]. The practice at the National Institutes of Health Primate Quarantine Unit is to tuberculin test all animals every two weeks and keep them in quarantine for at least six weeks or until the tuberculin test is negative for all animals on at least two successive tests. All positive reactors are destroyed. This procedure of quarantine has proved satisfactory for both research and vaccine control work.

The health of the colony should be constantly supervised also beyond the quarantine period. Sick monkeys should be diagnosed and treatment instituted when feasible, and all dead animals necropsied to determine the cause of death.

References

1 BEARCROFT, W.G.C. and JAMIESON, M.F.: An outbreak of subcutaneous tumors in rhesus monkeys. Nature, Lond. *182:* 195–196 (1958).

2 CARPENTER, K.P.: Human and simian shigellosis; in GRAHAM-JONES Some diseases of animals communicable to man in Britain, pp.35–46 (Pergamon Press, London 1968).

3 DEINHARDT, F.: Hepatitis in subhuman primates and the hazards to man; in BALNER and BEVERIDGE Infections and immunosuppression in subhuman primates, pp.55–63 (Munksgaard, Copenhagen 1970).

4 ESPAÑA, C.: A pox disease of monkeys transmissible to man; in GOLDSMITH and MOOR-JANKOWSKI Medical primatology 1970, pp.694–708 (Karger, Basel 1971).

5 HENNESSEN, W.: Epidemiology of Marburg virus disease; in BALNER and BEVERIDGE Infections and immunosuppression in subhuman primates, pp.35–38 (Munksgaard, Copenhagen 1970).

6 KALTER, S.S. and HEBERLING, R.L.: Viral flora of tissue sources – simian and human. Nat. Cancer Inst. Monogr. No. 29, pp. 149–160 (US Department of Health, Education, and Welfare, Public Health Service, Bethesda, Md. 1968).

7 KALTER, S.S. and HEBERLING, R.L.: Comparative virology of primates. Bact. Res. *35:* 310–364 (1971).

8 KEEBLE, S.A.: B virus infection in man and monkey; in GRAHAM-JONES Some diseases

of animals communicable to man in Britain, pp. 183–188 (Pergamon Press, London 1968).

9 McConnell, S.: Simian pox viruses; in Balner and Beveridge Infections and immunosuppression in subhuman primates, pp. 83–86 (Munksgaard, Copenhagen 1970).

10 Melendez, L.V.; Hunt, R.D.; Daniel, M.D., and Trum, B.F.: New World monkeys, herpes viruses, and cancer; in Balner and Beveridge Infections and immunosuppression in subhuman primates, pp. 111–117 (Munksgaard, Copenhagen 1970).

11 Merchant, D.J.: Cell cultures for virus vaccine production. Nat. Cancer Inst. Monogr. No. 29, (US Department of Health, Education, and Welfare, Public Health Service, Bethesda, Md., 1968).

12 Parkman, P.D.; Meyer, H.M., jr.; Kirschstein, R.L., and Hopps, H.E.: Attenuated rubella virus. I. Development and laboratory characterization. New Engl. J. Med. *275:* 569–574 (1966).

13 Perkins, F.T.: The need for a standardized cell substrate for virus vaccine production. Jap. J. med. Sci. Biol. *24:* 329–344 (1971).

14 Petricciani, J.C.; Hopps, H.E., and Lorenz, D.E.: Subhuman primate diploid cells. Possible substrates for production of virus vaccines. Science *174:* 1025–1027 (1971).

15 Schmidt, L.H.: Control of tuberculosis in nonhuman primates; in Balner and Beveridge Infections and immunosuppression in subhuman primates, pp. 9–19 (Munksgaard, Copenhagen 1970).

16 Tauraso, N.M.: Review of recent epizootics in primate colonies and their relation to man. Lab. anim. Sci. (in press).

17 Tauraso, N.M.; Myers, M.G.; McCarthy, K., and Tribe, G.W.: Simian hemorrhagic fever; in Balner and Beveridge Infections and immunosuppression in subhuman primates, pp. 101–109 (Munksgaard, Copenhagen 1970).

18 US Public Health Service Regulations for Biological Products. Title 42, part 73, publ. 437 (Department of Health, Education, and Welfare, Washington, D.C., revised September 1970).

Author's address: Dr. Nicola M. Tauraso, Department of Health, Education, and Welfare, Public Health Service, National Institutes of Health, Division of Biologics Standards, Laboratory of Virology and Rickettsiology, *Bethesda, MD 20014* (USA)

Viral Oncology

Medical Primatology 1972. Proc. 3rd Conf. exp. Med. Surg. Primates, Lyon 1972, part III, pp. 132–133 (Karger, Basel 1972)

Viral Oncology

Review and Critique

F. DEINHARDT

Departments of Microbiology, Rush-Presbyterian-St. Luke's and University of Illinois Medical Centers, Chicago, Ill.

This chapter will review current knowledge and report recent results of experimental studies with oncogenic viruses in nonhuman primates. Four categories of viruses will be considered:

(1) Viruses isolated from nonhuman primates which are not known to cause malignant disease in primates but which transform cells in culture and induce tumours in some nonprimate animals, e.g. SV-40 or some of the primate adenoviruses.

(2) Oncogenic viruses of other animal species which can also induce tumours in nonhuman primates, e.g. Rous sarcoma virus and feline sarcoma viruses.

(3) Nonhuman primate viruses causing nonmalignant tumours or pox-like diseases, e.g. Yaba virus and Tana poxvirus.

(4) DNA or RNA containing nonhuman primate viruses, both naturally occurring and oncogenic in primates.

Two recent findings are of particular interest. The first primate C-type RNA virus isolated, simian sarcoma virus type 1 (*Lagothrix* sp.) (SSV-1), has now been almost completely characterized and its biological cycle, i.e. isolation from a tumour, growth in cell culture, tumour induction in primates with cell-free virus and subsequent reisolation of the virus, has been completed experimentally. SSV-1 has its own nontransforming, associated virus and it is similar in every respect to other known C-type RNA viruses of mammalian and avian origin. Other 'C-type' or 'B-type' RNA viruses have already been isolated from other primate tumours but their relationship to the tumour from which they were isolated must still be regarded as uncertain until definite proof of their oncogenicity has been obtained. Despite the results reported, this proof is still lacking. The second interesting finding is that herpesviruses without (or more probably, with very low) pathogenicity for the natural nonhuman primate host species may induce malignant lymphomas or leukemias in other nonhuman primates. *Herpesvirus saimiri* (HVS), the only virus of this group adequately studied until now, has many similarities with Epstein-Barr virus of man, in its epidemiology, natural transmission and host-cell virus interrelationships. It provides, therefore, an excellent model for the evaluation of the relationships of primate herpesviruses and neoplasia. The question has been raised whether herpesviruses themselves are oncogenic or whether they activate an underlying 'RNA oncogene'. If the second alternative is correct, then HVS is the most efficient 'oncogene-activator' ever observed, for every white-lipped marmoset, irrespective of age, develops neoplastic disease within days of inoculation. Space to discuss the arguments for and against the proposal that all tumours are caused by activation of an RNA oncogene is lacking, but I would like to re-emphasize that caution must be used in the interpretation of isolated pieces of data. Careful and extensive hybridization studies between the DNA products of RNA virus reverse transcriptases and the RNA or DNA of various tumours are necessary before further conclusions about the possible interrelationships of herpesviruses, C-type viruses and tumours can be drawn. The demonstration of enzyme activity alone, for example, in a tumour cell line derived from an HVS-induced tumour, does not prove that this activity is due to an RNA-directed oncornavirus enzyme, unless one at least demonstrates that the activity is directed by a 70S RNA. In this respect the studies presented in this chapter are potentially of great importance. However, so far the data allow us to speculate only and not to draw conclusions because insufficient proof has been offered for the nature of the enzyme in the HVS-induced tumour cell line.

The increase in activity and the progress in the study of oncogenic viruses in nonhuman primates is most encouraging but it is necessary to guard against too rapid conclusions. It is already clear that as the dust of the present hyperactivity in some areas of cancer research settles, a few candidate viruses, enzymes and virus-like particles will be lost, and I hope that none of the agents, enzymes and particles discussed here will belong to this group.

Author's address: Dr. FRIEDRICH DEINHARDT, Departments of Microbiology, Rush-Presbyterian-St. Luke's Medical Center, 1753 West Congress-Parkway, *Chicago, IL 60612* (USA)

Medical Primatology 1972. Proc. 3rd Conf. exp. Med. Surg. Primates, Lyon 1972, part III, pp. 134–142 (Karger, Basel 1972)

Oncogenicity of *Herpesvirus saimiri* Induced Lymphoma and the DNA Polymerases of the Lymphoma Derived Cell Line and *Herpesvirus saimiri*[1]

D. V. Ablashi, W. F. Loeb, G. R. Armstrong, Stringner S. Yang, Marion G. Valerio and R. H. Adamson

National Cancer Institute and Litton Bionetics, Inc., Bethesda, Md.

Introduction

The oncogenic property of *Herpesvirus saimiri* (HVS) to induce malignant lymphoma with lymphocytic leukemia in owl monkeys [2, 6] and marmoset monkeys [10] has been well documented. The *in vitro* rescue of the HVS genome has also been reported [2, 10]. In addition, Wolfe *et al.* [10] described development of lymphoma with leukemia in marmosets and transfer of the HVS genome from donor to recipient upon inoculation of minced lymphoid tissue. Recently, long-term cell cultures from lymphoid tissues of HVS-infected marmosets have been established [3, 9]. In this brief communication the following studies in owl monkeys are reported:

(1) *In vivo* induction of lymphoma without frank leukemia and detection of the HVS genome upon inoculation of lymphoid cells from an HVS-infected monkey.

(2) Establishment and characterization of cell culture from HVS-induced lymphoma cells.

(3) Activity of endogenous RNase sensitive DNA polymerase (RSDP) from the above cell culture.

1 Conducted under USPHS contract NIH-NCI 71–2025.

I. In vivo *Studies with Lymphoma Cells*

A male owl monkey (174 H) developed malignant lymphoma with a lymphocytic leukemia upon inoculation of HVS [2]. By use of a tissue grinder, a cell suspension was prepared from the mediastinal mass and the retroperitoneal mass which consisted of fused sublumbar and pelvic lymph nodes. The suspension in Hanks' BME containing 2% inactivated fetal calf serum with penicillin and streptomycin was inoculated i.m. and i.p. into another owl monkey (223 H). Monkey 223 H had no clinical signs of illness until seven months postinoculation. At this time an abdominal mass was palpated which was clinically identified as a lymphomatous mesenteric lymph node. From the time of inoculation until death (285 days) there were no clinical or hematological signs of frank leukemia.

No HVS could be isolated from the peripheral blood upon cultivation with owl monkey kidney (OMK) cells before 199 days postinoculation. Virus isolated at that time was identified by neutralization as HVS. HVS was also isolated from the cell cultures of mesenteric lymph nodes and kidney harvested at necropsy and by cocultivation of these cells with OMK cells.

The serology indicated development of a neutralizing HVS antibody ($\geq 1{:}16$) detected at 235 and 284 days postinoculation.

Grossly, a tumor mass consisting of fused mesenteric lymph nodes was observed, but peripheral lymph nodes were only slightly enlarged. No tumors were observed at sites of i.m. inoculation. Histopathologic examination of small intestines and mesenteric lymph nodes confirmed the diagnosis of lymphoma (fig. 1). The detailed hematologic, pathologic, serologic, and virologic studies will be reported elsewhere [4].

Inoculation of lymphoid cells from HVS-infected marmosets reported by WOLFE *et al.* [10] produced lymphocytic leukemia as well as lymphoma, but inoculation of lymphoid cells in this animal produced only lymphoma. The incubation periods of HVS-induced neoplasia in owl monkeys as well as in marmosets thus far observed were much shorter than those in this study [2, 6, 10]. The presence of HVS genome in the peripheral blood of virus inoculated animals in our studies [2] and those reported by others [10] has been detectable as early as 14 days. No tumors were observed at site of i.m. inoculation in this monkey. As both of the monkeys (donor and recipient) were male, no cytogenetic studies were possible to detect the origin of tumor cells. This study suggests that a process analogous to *in vitro* rescue of HVS may have occurred *in vivo*. Development of neoplasia, virus isolation and seroconversion may be dependent upon concentration of HVS and species of host animal.

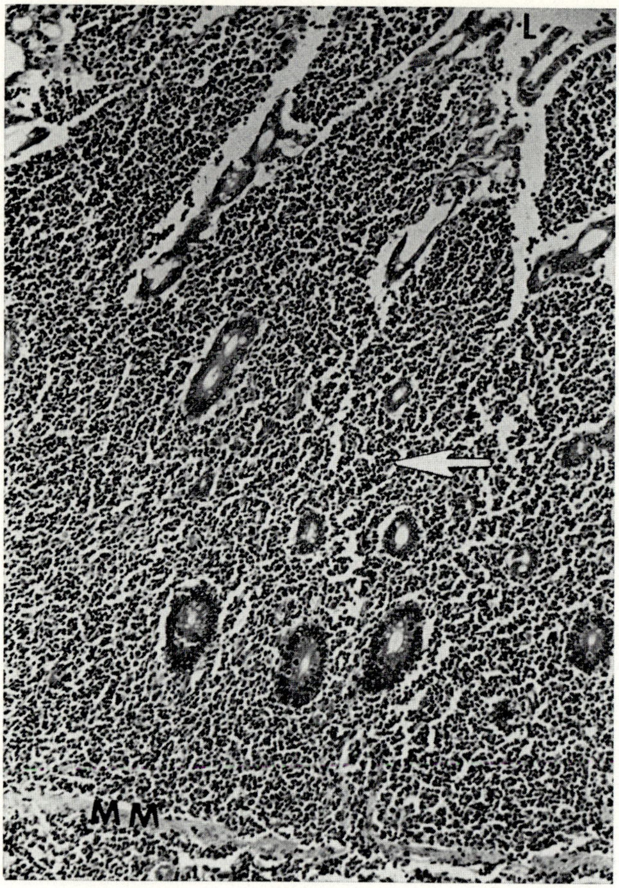

Fig. 1. Small intestine of monkey 223 H showing extensive infiltration of the lamina propria (arrow) and muscularis mucosae (MM) by neoplastic lymphocytes. Intestinal lumen is designated by 'L'. HE; × 100.

II. Establishment and Characterization of Cell Culture from Lymphoma Cells

A cell culture was started from thoroughly washed and trypsinized cells of the lymphoid mass of monkey 174 H, according to the method of Ablashi *et al.* [2]. The cells grew in suspension in the beginning, aggregating in clumps and morphologically appeared to be lymphoid. Later on, most of the floating cells formed a monolayer and the rest of them remained in suspension. The attached cells consisted of epitheloid and varying sizes of rounded cells (fig. 2). The viability count of each passage remained 1.1 × 10^7 cells/ml (table I). Both multinucleated and giant cells were observed in the cell culture (fig. 2). No trypsinization was required for subculture. When the floating cells were harvested and seeded by themselves, they also formed a monolayer consisting of epitheloid and rounded cells. The culture was designated as AA (Ablashi and Armstrong).

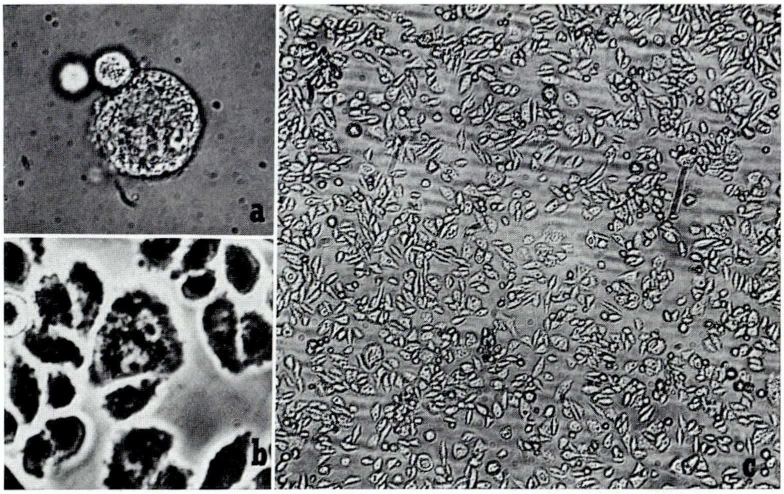

Fig. 2a–c. a A giant and a small size lymphoid cell observed in suspension cell cultures from P2. × 125. *b* A multinucleated giant cell observed in a monolayer from P7 (phase contrast; × 325). The other cells surrounding the giant cells are irregular in shape, varying from round to elliptical. *c* A monolayer from P7 of AA cells showing epithelioid and rounded cells of varying sizes. × 125.

The cytogenetics studies revealed that passages (P) 1–4 contained 54 chromosomes which is the normal diploid number for owl monkeys. This number shifted to 62 in P7 (fig. 2d). No significant morphologic changes of chromosomes were seen in AA cells from P3 to P4. However, in P7 (attached cells) and P15 (floating cells) 19 and 34%, respectively, of the metaphase spreads had structural aberrations consisting of infrequent breaks, chromosome pulverization and dicentric chromosomes (table II).

Even though the origin of the AA cells was from tumor tissue, the chromosomal changes suggest possible further cell transformation after P4. The other findings in support of transformation were: significant increase in cell density, production of more CO_2, growth in soft agar, and greater increase in multinucleated giant cells in later passages.

Table I. Isolation of HVS from AA cells grown *in vitro*

Passage	Passage	HVS detection		
level	days	IF	EM	cocultivation
Primary[1]	0	+	–	+
P4[2]	105	+	–	+
P5[2]	112	–	–	–
P7[2]	135	–	–	–
P15[2]	204	–	ND	–
P18[2]	230	–	ND	–
P34[2]	336	–	–	–

– = No virus or no viral antigen was detected; + = HVS was isolated or HVS antigen was detected.

1 3.5×10^6 viable cells/ml.

2 Average number of viable cells in P1–P34 was 1.1×10^7/ml.

d

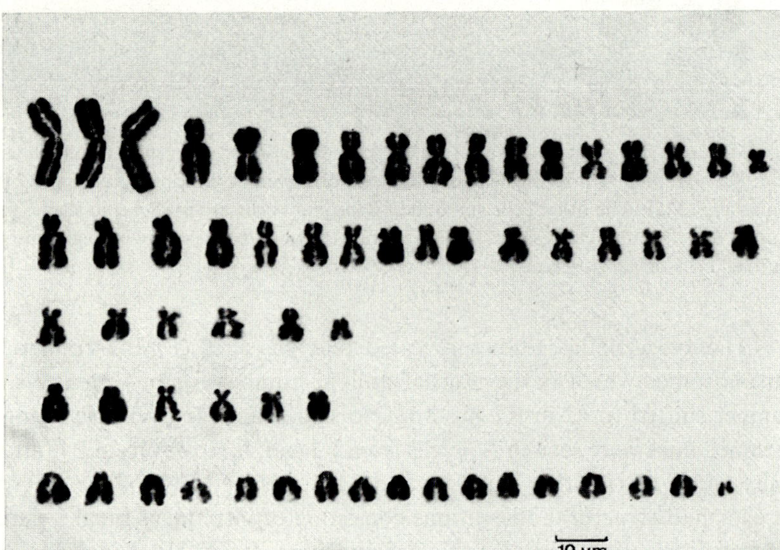

Fig. 2d. Karyotype obtained from P7 of AA cells showing the absence of secondary constriction on the subtelocentric marker chromosome normally present in owl monkey metaphase spread.

Table II. Cytogenetic analysis of AA cells from various passages

Passage	Analysis	Model No.	Number of cells with chromosome aberration							
			break	fragment	rearrangement	dicentric	ring	pulverization	> 10[1]	% aberration[2]
3	100	54	0	0	0	0	0	0	0	0
4	100	54	0	0	0	0	0	0	0	0
7	100	62	1	10	4	8	0	1	0	19
15+	50	62	3	15	6	8	1	2	11	34

+ = Composed of floating cells from previous passage that attached and formed a monolayer.
1 10 = Cells having greater than ten aberrations.
2 % aberration excluding gaps.

Virologic studies presented in table I show detection of HVS genome by immunofluorescence (IF) and cocultivation [2] only up to P4. Ultrastructural (EM) studies failed to demonstrate HVS in any of the passages. It is possible that the cells producing HVS may have degenerated after P4. It is also possible that the viral genome cannot be rescued by present methods employed. The detailed studies of this cell line will be reported elsewhere. This cell culture is different from most of those reported from marmosets, as it did not produce HVS after P4 [3, 9]. However, one lymphoid cell line derived recently has been shown to be negative for both membrane and internal HVS antigens as well as infectious HVS although virus can be rescued by cocultivation with vero cells [8].

III. RSDP Activity from AA Cultures

RSDP activity in culture media at P11 of AA cells with and without iododeoxyruidine treatment (20 μg/ml) was investigated. Samples of 50-ml culture media were harvested at specified times (fig. 3) and centrifuged at 15,000 *g* to remove cellular debris, then filtered (0.45 nm) prior to further centrifugation at 105,000 *g* for two hours. The pellets were washed with phosphate buffered saline (PBS) once prior to disruption by 0.015% triton X100 and assayed for RSDP activity. Assays for DNA polymerase have been described earlier [11]. In the final volume of 50 μl, the assay contained tris-HCl buffer (pH 8.0 and 2.5 μM) Mg acetate 0.3 μmole, dithiothreitol 0.4 μmole,

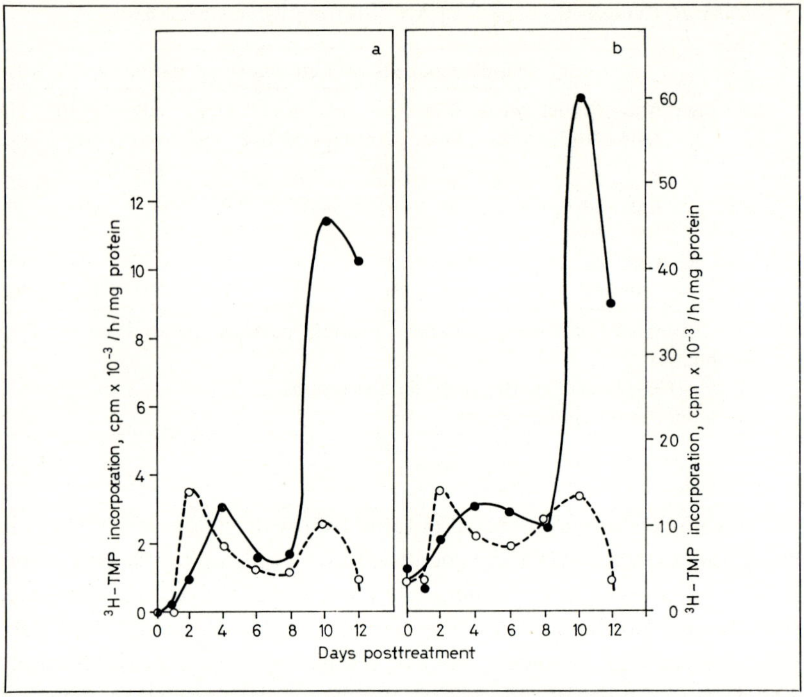

Fig. 3. Release of RSDP activities from AA-11 cells with or without IUDR treatment. All experimental conditions were described in the text. (a) Depicts endogenous RSDP activities. (b) Depicts dT^{12}.rA stimulated RSDP activities. ● = Untreated RSDP activities; ○ = IUDR-treated activities.

NaCl 3 μmole, 5 μCi of tritiated thymidine triphosphate (3HTTP, 17.0 mCi/μM from New England Nuclear) and approximately 100–150 μg of protein from lysed 105,000 *g* pellet. Both an endogenous and an oligo-dT^{12}. poly rA (25 μg/ml from Collaborative Research) stimulated reaction were followed.

The pellets (105,000 *g*) prepared from AA cells of P4 and P7 had no RSDP activity. RSDP activities, whether endogenous or stimulated by dT^{12}.rA, in P11 appeared in a biphasic pattern (fig. 3). An initial peak on day 4 was detected and followed by a second peak on day 10. The pellets from P11 containing IUDR showed no augmentation of the initial peak of RSDP activity, the second peak of RSDP activity (day 10) was apparently suppressed. In contrast induction of virus production by IUDR at the above dose level has been reported in nonproducing murine cells containing murine leukemia virus genome [1, 5]. Comparison of RSDP from AA cells with HVS DNA

Table III. A comparison of some biochemical properties of RSDP from AA-11 culture medium with HVS DNA polymerase[1]

Conditions	^{3}H-TMP incorporation cpm/15 min reaction/50 μl	
	RSDP	HVS DNA polymerase
Complete	857	2,203
Minus triton X100	78	105
Minus $MgCl_2$	67	90
Minus dithiothreitol	53	72
Minus dATP, dGTP, dCTP	136	310
Preincubation with 1.0 μg RNase (30 min)	218	2,374
Complete plus dT^{12}.rA 25 μg/ml	5,683	4,006
Complete plus dT^{12}.dA 25 μg/ml	1,862	4,461

1 All assay conditions were described in the text. RNase digestion was carried out at 37 °C in 50 mM tris-HCl, pH 7.2, 50 mM NaCl.

polymerase was carried out (table III). The 105,000 *g* pellet from P11 cells and partially-purified HVS both required triton X100 treatment for the polymerase assay. Both polymerase activities were dependent on Mg^{++}, dithiothreitol and presence of 4-deoxynucleoside triphosphates. Activities of RSDP but not of HVS DNA polymerase were sensitive to an earlier RNase digestion. Also, RSDP exhibited much greater preference for dT^{12}.rA rather than dT^{12}.dA. HVS DNA polymerase, on the other hand, showed equivalent preference for both synthetic templates, indicating that it is primarily a DNA dependent DNA polymerase and supporting the evidence that our HVS pool did not contain a possible type C virus.

Our further data indicate that this RSDP activity banded at a density of 1.16 g/ml as compared to the density of 1.27–1.28 g/ml of HVS [7].

Detailed descriptions of the above studies will be reported elsewhere.

The above data suggest that HVS might have stimulated induction of oncogenicity of AA cells and the release of an RSDP activity in the later passages.

All of these studies indicate significant discrepancies between the formation of complete virus particles and the pathologic, cytologic and biochemical manifestations attributed to HVS. If indeed all of these manifestations are exclusively induced by HVS, this to a great degree explains the failure to isolate virus from certain primate neoplasms. This and alternative hypotheses are currently under investigation.

References

1 AARONSON, S.A.; TODARO, G.J., and SCOLNICK, E.M.: Induction of murine 'C' virus from clonal line of virus free Balb 3T3 cells. Science *174:* 157 (1971).

2 ABLASHI, D.V.; LOEB, W.F.; VALERIO, M.G.; ADAMSON, R.H.; ARMSTRONG, G.R.; BENNETT, D.G., and HEINE, U.: Malignant lymphoma with lymphocytic leukemia induced in owl monkeys by *Herpesvirus saimiri.* J.nat.Cancer Inst. *47:* 837–855 (1971).

3 FALK, L.A.; WOLFE, L.G.; HOEKSTRA, J., and DEINHARDT, F.: Demonstration of *Herpesvirus saimiri* associated antigens in peripheral lymphocytes from infected marmosets during *in vitro* cultivation. J.nat.Cancer Inst. *48:* 523–530 (1971).

4 LOEB, W.F.; VALERIO, M.G.; ABLASHI, D.V., and ARMSTRONG, G.R.: Lymphoma induction and virus isolation from an owl monkey inoculated with lymphoma cells induced by *Herpesvirus saimiri* (in preparation).

5 LOWY, D.R.; ROWE, W.P.; TEICH, N., and HARTLEY, J.W.: Murine leukemia virus. High-frequency activity *in vitro* by 5-iodoleoxyuridine and 5-bromodeoxyuridine. Science *174:* 155–156 (1971).

6 MELENDEZ, L.V.; HUNT, R.D.; DANIEL, M.D.; BLAKE, B.J., and GARCIA, F.G.: Acute lymphocytic leukemia in owl monkeys inoculated with *Herpesvirus saimiri.* Science *171:* 1161–1163 (1971).

7 RABIN, H. and PARSONS, J.A.: Personal commun.

8 RABIN, H. and PEARSON, G.: Personal commun.

9 RABSON, A.S.; O'CONNOR, G.R.; LORENZ, D.E.; KIRSCHSTEIN, R.L.; LEGALLIS, F.Y., and TOMMIE, T.S.: Lymphoid cell culture line derived from lymph node of marmoset infected *Herpesvirus saimiri.* Preliminary report. J.nat.Cancer Inst. *46:* 1099–1109 (1971).

10 WOLFE, L.G.; FALK, L.A., and DEINHARDT, F.: Oncogenicity of *Herpesvirus saimiri* in marmoset monkeys. J.nat.Cancer Inst. *47:* 1145–1162 (1971).

11 YANG, S.S.; HERREA, F.; SMITH, R.G.; REITZ, M.; LANCINI, G.; TING, R., and GALLO, R.: Rifamycin antibiotics. Inhibition of Rauscher (murine) leukemia virus reverse transcriptase and of purified DNA polymerase from human normal and leukemic lymphoblasts. J.nat.Cancer Inst. *49:* 7–25 (1972).

Authors' addresses: D.V. ABLASHI, G.R. ARMSTRONG and R.H. ADAMSON, National Cancer Institute, *Bethesda, MD 20014;* W.F. LOEB and MARION G. VALERIO, Department of Pathology, Litton Bionetics, Inc., 5510 Nicholson Lane, *Kensington, MD 20795;* STRINGNER S. YANG, Department of Experimental Oncology, Litton Bionetics, Inc., 7300 Pearl Street, *Bethesda, MD 20014* (USA)

Medical Primatology 1972. Proc. 3rd Conf. exp. Med. Surg. Primates, Lyon 1972, part III, pp. 143–150 (Karger, Basel 1972)

Studies on Oncogenic Properties of a Virus Isolated from the Monkey Breast Tumor

H. Chopra, D. Fine, R. Pienta and N. Woodside

National Cancer Institute (NIH) and Litton Bionetics Inc., Bethesda, Md.

Introduction

A new virus morphologically resembling the known oncogenic viruses of other animal species was detected by electron microscopy in a spontaneous breast tumor of a rhesus monkey [1]. The virus was isolated [2], and propagated [3] by cocultivation with monkey embryo cells and was subsequently demonstrated to infect monkey, chimpanzee and human cell lines [4]. The virus was shown to be different morphologically and serologically from the known oncogenic RNA viruses and simian foamy viruses [5]. The present report will summarize morphological, biochemical, and *in vitro* transforming characteristics of this virus which may suggest its oncogenic potential.

Material and Methods

A breast tumor developed spontaneously in a rhesus monkey *(Macaca mulatta)* at Mason Research Institute, Worcester, Mass. (USA). The clinical history, histopathology and endocrinologic milieu of the monkey bearing the tumor were recently reported [14]. Similarly, the techniques employed to process tumor tissue for electron microscopy and tissue culture studies were described previously in detail [2–4].

Cell-free virus (1×10^6 TCID) was inoculated into several simian cell lines including rhesus foreskin cells (rhfs) in which a specific cytopathic effect (CPE) developed one to 30 days following infection.

The transformation of the virus-infected monkey foreskin cells was investigated by means of the soft agar technique of MacPherson [13]. The virus-infected rhfs cells were trypsinized, and suspensions of single cells (1×10^3 to 1×10^5 cells/60 mm plate) were seeded into semisolid agar medium which consisted of modified McCoy's 5a medium containing a final concentration of 0.33 % agar, 10 % fetal calf serum, 10 % tryptose phosphate broth and antibiotics. This cell suspension was overlayed onto a base layer of medium containing 0.5% agar. The uninfected rhfs control cells were processed in a similar manner.

The plates were incubated at 37 °C in a 5-percent CO_2 humid incubator and refed with semisolid agar medium at seven- to ten-day intervals. By three to four weeks, numerous colonies developed and grew in the plates seeded with the infected cells. To confirm the presence of transformed cells, sublines of cells isolated from colonies in semisolid agar medium were grown in 'factor-free' medium which consisted of Dulbecco's modified medium supplemented with 10% agamma calf serum previously heated at 70 °C for 30–45 min. This treatment destroys growth factors required for the growth of normal nonmalignant cells.

Results

Electron microscopy of thin sections of the monkey breast tumor biopsy revealed small groups of epithelial cells. A large number of virus particles were observed as dark granules on the cell surfaces and in the intercellular spaces (fig. 1). At higher magnification, these extracellular virus particles were seen budding from the cell surface (fig. 2). They were spherical or oval particles, measuring 100–120 nm in diameter. In the cytoplasm another category of particles measuring 60–95 nm in diameter was observed, which appeared to be incorporated into the budding extracellular virus. The mature extracellular virus consisted of an outer unit membrane and an inner central nucleoid.

The cell-free virus, isolated by cocultivation of tumor tissue with the monkey embryo cells, infected monkey lung and chimpanzee lung cells as well as human embryo and human lymphoblastic (NC-37) culture. Long-term propagation of this virus in human embryo and in human lymphoblasts has shown that while the virus continues to develop intracytoplasmically as type A particles, the extracellular virus shows morphological variation in consisting of an eccentric nucleoid, thus resembling type B particles of mouse mammary tumor virus (fig. 3).

The infectivity of cell lines such as monkey embryo, monkey lung, chimpanzee lung, human embryo and human lymphoblast (NC-37) cells was

---

Fig. 1. Low power electron micrograph of monkey breast tumor epithelial cells. Note virus particles (arrows) in the intercellular spaces. × 58,000.

Fig. 2. Electron micrograph showing an intracytoplasmic (arrow) and budding forms of virus particles. × 81,500.

Fig. 3. Extracellular virus with eccentric nucleoids, resembling type B mouse mammary tumor virus. × 92,000.

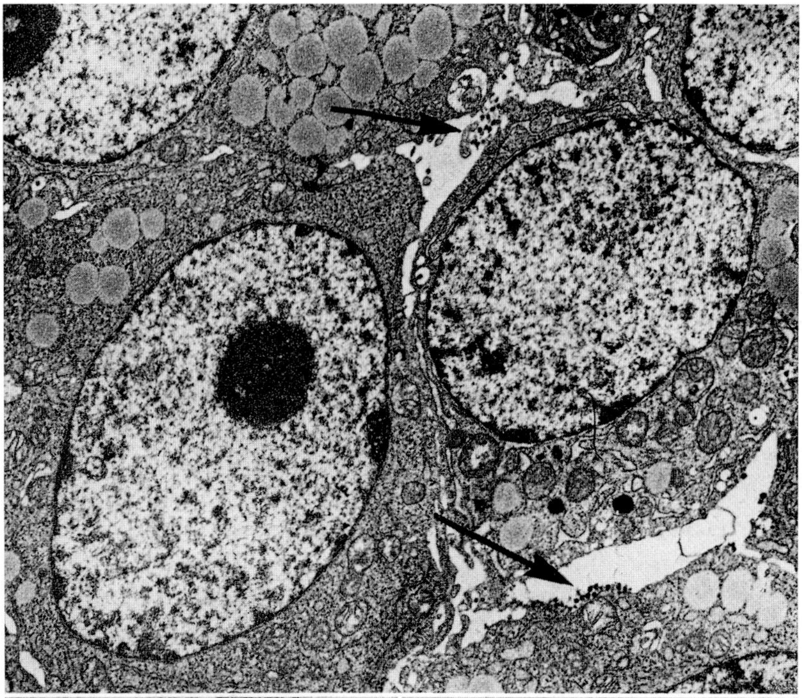

1

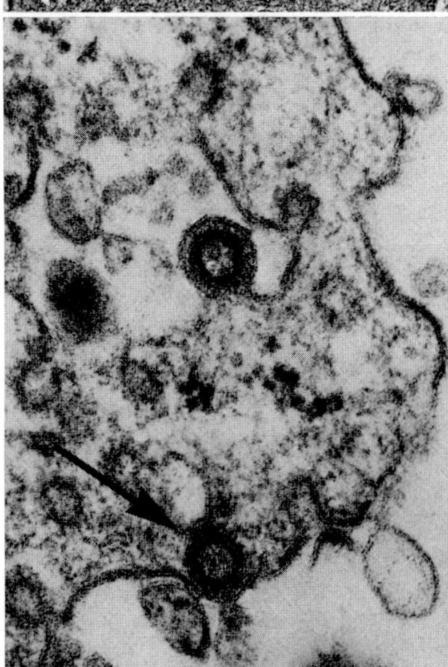

2

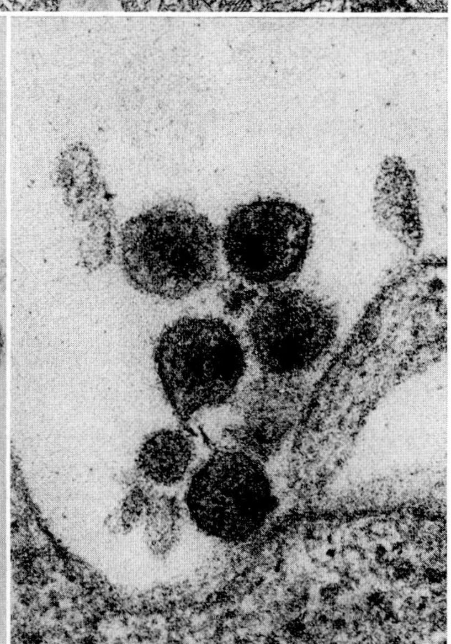

3

demonstrated by electron microscopy without any apparent CPE. However, the infected cell cultures of rhfs have demonstrated specific CPE within a few hours. The CPE was characterized by multiple nuclei clustered within the affected cells and surrounded by a large cytoplasmic area (fig. 4 and 5). The CPE was consistently observed in the infected rhfs cells and thus provides an assay system for virus detection and quantitation.

The rhfs cells infected with the virus and subsequently isolated from semisolid agar differed in morphology from the original foreskin cells. They appeared to be transformed, having lost contact inhibition, and grew in clumps. Furthermore, they satisfy several other criteria for *in vitro* transformation in that they grow in semisolid agar and in 'factor-free' medium. In semisolid agar numerous colonies developed and grew in the plates seeded with infected cells (fig. 6). The uninfected cells failed to grow in semisolid agar layer.

Cells from individual colonies were suspended in the culture medium and replated into a plastic flask. Seven sublines of transformed cells were established from these soft agar isolates.

Electron microscopy has revealed these cells to be more epitheloid with well-developed endoplasmic reticulum and Golgi apparatus. Each of these subline cultures has been found to release infectious virus (fig. 7 A and B). Cytogenetic analysis of the transformed sublines showed extensive polyploidy as compared to the control cultures.

Several clones of transformed cells were inoculated into newborn rhesus monkeys to study their tumorigenic potential. When approximately 2×10^6 cells from each of the sublines were inoculated s.c., palpable masses were observed as early as six days postinoculation. The masses increased in size but in all cases regressed over a period of two weeks. The biopsied material from these masses and enlarged lymph nodes revealed the presence of infectious virus by electron microscopy.

Other rhesus monkeys inoculated with cell-free virus have to date failed to develop any tumors. Using *in vitro* tissue culture assays and electron microscopy, we have found proliferation of infectious virus in hyperplastic lymph

---

Fig. 4. Light micrograph of uninfected control rhesus monkey foreskin cells. × 64.

Fig. 5. Rhesus monkey foreskin cell culture showing cytopathic effects. × 130.

Fig. 6. Light micrograph showing colonies of transformed cells growing in semisolid agar. × 70.

Fig. 7 a Electron micrograph of the transformed multinucleated rhesus foreskin cell. × 2,240. *b* Extracellular virus observed on the surface of a transformed cell. × 42,000.

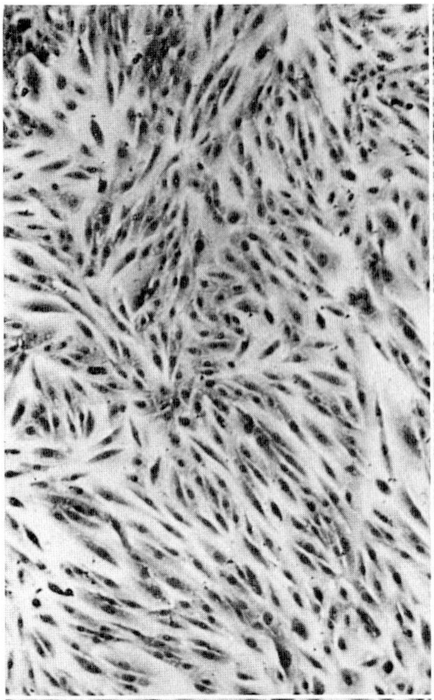

4

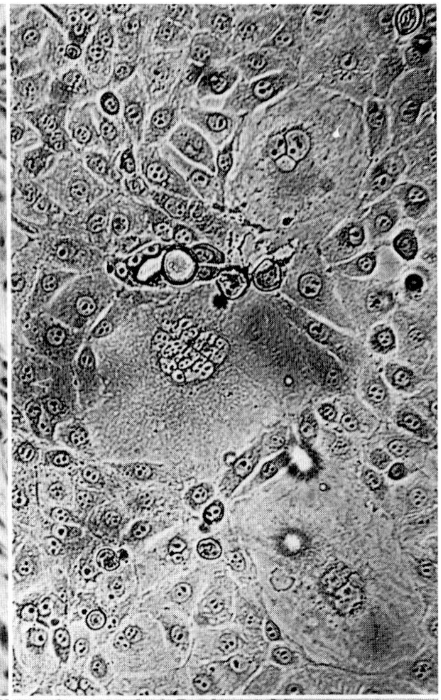

5

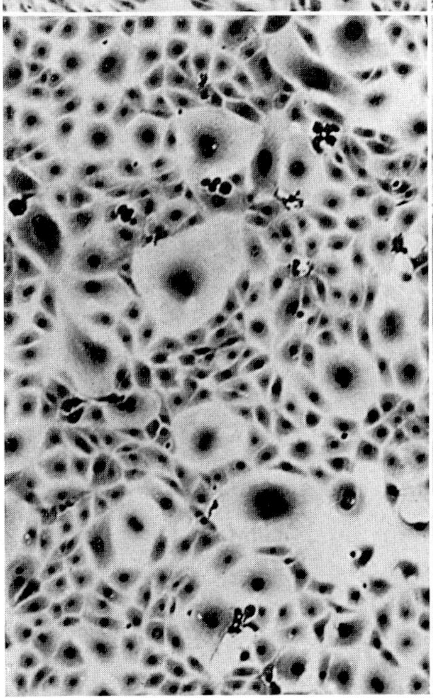

6

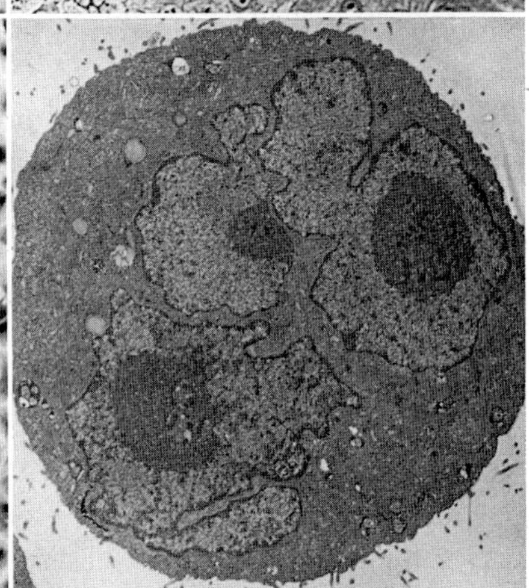

7a

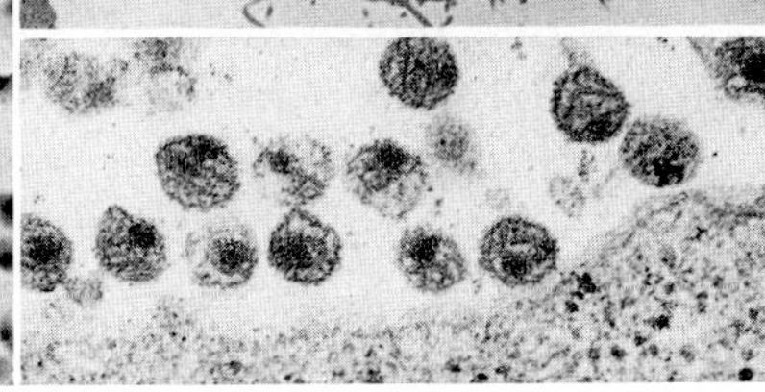

7b

nodes of the inoculated infant rhesus monkeys. Although prolonged lymphadenopathy has been observed in the monkeys inoculated with the virus, there is no indication of breast infection, as their milk secretions have failed to show any infectious virus by electron microscopy or by *in vitro* assay system.

Discussion

The discovery and successful propagation of a virus from the spontaneous breast tumor of a rhesus monkey has resulted in the first isolation of virus from a solid tumor in a primate [1, 2]. The virus in the monkey tumor cells develops in a pattern similar to the mouse mammary tumor virus (MTV) which is known to be the causative agent, in that they are first observed in the cytoplasm as doughnut-shaped intracytoplasmic A particles which bud off extracellularly from the cell surface. During propagation of this virus in monkey embryo and human lymphoblast cells (NC-37), this virus has come to resemble morphogenically type B virus particles of mouse MTV in consisting of an outer unit membrane and eccentric nucleoid [7, 12]. Thus, morphologically this virus shows characteristics of the known oncogenic RNA viruses [11]. Nevertheless, it is demonstrated that this agent is distinct from the simian foamy viruses [5].

The characterization of the product synthesization suggests that this virus may possess many of the biochemical and biophysical features common to the known oncogenic RNA viruses of other species [19]. It has a buoyant density of 1.16 g/ml, and contains 60–70S RNA [15, 17]. The presence of three DNA polymerase activities, including the RNA instructed DNA polymerase, has been demonstrated in the monkey tumor virus [17, 19]. This finding is considered most significant in view of the fact that the presence of RNA-instructed DNA polymerase has been observed in all 27 isolates of oncogenic RNA viruses. Whereas the presence of RNA instructed DNA polymerase in the virion is not proof of its oncogenic potential, one cannot ignore the observation that all the oncogenic RNA viruses from numerous species possess this enzyme activity. Further, the DNA product synthesized from the viral RNA *in vitro* has been used in molecular hybridization studies to probe for complementary or homologous RNA structures of viral origin unique to human neoplasm with particular emphasis on human breast tumors [18].

Infectivity of cell cultures of primate species [4] and demonstration of CPE in several monkey and human cell lines [8] appear to be the first demonstration of biological activity of this virus. However, in absence of any tumor induction by cell-free virus as yet, *in vitro* transformation of rhfs cells is the most significant biological activity of the virus demonstrated so far [16]. In our preliminary studies, transformed cells inoculated into newborn rhesus monkeys demonstrated tumorogenic potentials by developing palpable masses at the site of inoculation [9].

The monkey tumor virus has demonstrated morphological, biophysical and biochemical properties common to the viruses having known oncogenic potential [6]. Furthermore, the *in vitro* transformation of rhfs by this virus and the subsequent demonstration of the potential tumorogenic activity by the virus transformed cells indicates its probable oncogenic nature. However, studies are in progress to demonstrate a direct etiological relationship of the virus to the monkey breast cancer.

References

1 Chopra, H.C.: Electron microscopic detection of an oncogenic-type virus in a monkey breast tumor. Proc.amer.Ass.Cancer Res. *11:* 16 (1970).

2 Chopra, H.C. and Mason, M.M.: A new virus in a spontaneous mammary tumor of a rhesus monkey. Cancer Res. *30:* 2081–2086 (1970).

3 Chopra, H.C.; Zelljadt, I.; Jensen, E.M.; Mason, M.M., and Woodside, N.J.: Infectivity of cell cultures by a virus isolated from a monkey mammary carcinoma of a rhesus monkey. J.nat.Cancer Inst. *46:* 127–137 (1971).

4 Chopra, H.C., Zelljadt, I.; Woodside, N.J., and Walling, M.J.: Studies on virus particles resembling oncogenic RNA viruses in monkey breast carcinoma. Cancer *28:* 1406–1414 (1971).

5 Chopra, H.C.; Hooks, J.J.; Walling, M.J., and Gibbs, C.J.: Morphology of simian foamy viruses, with particular reference to virus isolated from spontaneous tumor of a rhesus monkey. J.nat.Cancer Inst. *48:* 451–463 (1972).

6 Chopra, H.C. and Oie, H.K.: Possible etiological role of virus particles detected in rat and monkey mammary tumors. J.nat.Cancer Inst. *48:* 1059–1065 (1972).

7 Chopra, H.C.: Oncorna type virus particles in a tumor of a rhesus monkey; in Chieco-Bianchi and Dutcher Proc. 5th Int.Symp. on comparative Leukemia Research, Padova 1971. Bibl.haemat., vol.39, pp.228–235 (Karger, Basel 1972).

8 Fine, D.L.; Landon, J.C., and Kubicek, M.T.: Simian tumor virus isolate: Demonstration of cytopathic effects *in vitro*. Science *174:* 420–421 (1971).

9 Fine, D.L.; Pienta, R.J.; Kubicek, M.T.; Landon, J.C.; Chopra, H.C., and Valerio, M.G.: Recovery of infectious virus from tissues of *Macaca mulatta* inoculated with Mason-Pfizer monkey virus transformed cells. Proc.Amer.Soc.Microbiol. (abstract) 211 (1972).

10 Jensen, E.M.; Zelljadt, I.; Chopra, H.C., and Mason, M.M.: Isolation and propagation of a new virus from a spontaneous mammary carcinoma of a rhesus monkey. Cancer Res. *30:* 2388–2393 (1970).

11 KRAMARSKY, B.; SARKAR, N.H., and MOORE, D.H.: Ultrastructural comparison of a virus from a rhesus monkey mammary carcinoma with four oncogenic RNA viruses. Proc. nat. Acad. Sci., Wash. *68:* 1603–1607 (1971).

12 MANNING, J.S. and HACKETT, A.J.: Morphological and biophysical properties of the Mason-Pfizer monkey virus. J. nat. Cancer Inst. *48:* 417–422 (1972).

13 MACPHERSON, I.: Agar suspension culture for quantitation of transformed cells; in ABEL and SALZMAN, Fundamental techniques in virology, pp. 214–222 (Academic Press, New York 1969).

14 MASON, M.M.; BOGDEN, A.E.; ILIEVSKI, V.; ESBER, H.J.; BAKER, J.R., and CHOPRA, H.C.: History of a rhesus monkey adenocarcinoma containing virus particles resembling oncogenic RNA viruses. J. nat. Cancer Inst. *48:* 1323–1331 (1972).

15 NOWINSKI, R.C.; EDYNAK, E., and SARKAR, N.H.: Serological and structural properties of Mason-Pfizer monkey virus isolated from the mammary tumor of a rhesus monkey. Proc. nat. Acad. Sci., Wash. *68:* 1608–1612 (1971).

16 PIENTA, R.J., FINE, D.L.; HURT, T.; SMITH, C.K.; LANDON, J.C., and CHOPRA, H.C.: Transformation of rhesus foreskin cells by Mason-Pfizer monkey virus. J. nat. Cancer Inst. *48:* 1913–1917 (1972).

17 SCHLOM, J. and SPIEGELMAN, S.: DNA polymerase activities and nucleic acid components of virions isolated from a spontaneous mammary carcinoma of a rhesus monkey. Proc. nat. Acad. Sci., Wash. *68:* 1613–1617 (1971).

18 SCHLOM, J. and SPIEGELMAN, S.: Detection of high molecular weight RNA in particles from human milk. Science *175:* 542–544 (1971).

19 SPIEGELMAN, S.; BURNY, A.; DAS, M.R.; KEYDAR, J.; SCHLOM, J.; TRAVNICEK, M., and WATSON, K.: Characterization of the products of RNA directed DNA polymerases in oncogenic RNA viruses. Nature, Lond. *227:* 563–567 (1970).

Authors' address: Dr. H. CHOPRA, Dr. D. FINE, Dr. R. PIENTA and N. WOODSIDE, National Cancer Institute (NIH) and Litton Bionetics Inc., *Bethesda, MD 20014* (USA)

Medical Primatology 1972. Proc. 3rd Conf. exp. Med. Surg. Primates, Lyon 1972, part III, pp. 151–158 (Karger, Basel 1972)

Epidemiology of *Herpesvirus saimiri* Infection in Squirrel Monkeys[1]

L. Falk, L. Wolfe and F. Deinhardt

Departments of Microbiology, Rush-Presbyterian-St. Luke's and University of Illinois Medical Centers, Chicago, Ill.

Introduction

Herpesvirus saimiri (HVS), isolated originally from kidney cell cultures of squirrel monkeys *(Saimiri sciureus)* [13] has been shown to be oncogenic for five genera of nonhuman primates (table I). The experimentally-induced lymphoproliferative disease in susceptible primate species ranges from lymphoma to lymphocytic leukemia. We studied the disease experimentally-induced by HVS in cotton-topped *(Saguinus oedipus)* and white-lipped *(S. nigricollis, S. fuscicollis)* marmosets [23], and during the course of these studies found that HVS was carried *in vivo* in a repressed state in lymphocytic

Table I. Susceptibility of nonhuman primate genera to *Herpesvirus saimiri*

Species	Susceptibility[1]	Reference
Saguinus (marmoset)		
oedipus	27/27, 24/24	11, 23
fuscicollis	4/4	23
nigricollis	4/4	23
Aotus trivirgatus (owl)	9/14, 5/5	16,1
Ateles geoffroyi (red spider)	2/6	12
Cebus albifrons (cinnamon ringtail)	4/4	14
Cercopithecus aethiops (African green)	2/6	15

1 Number developing disease/number inoculated.

1 Supported by research contract No. NIH 71-2032, within the Special Virus Cancer Program, NCI, training grant No. TOI-AI-2053, NIAID, and grant No. RR-05477, General Research Support Branch, RFR, NIH, USPHS.

cells. Examination of fresh neoplastic tissues or peripheral lymphocytes immediately after removal from the animals showed no inclusion bodies, viral antigens or viral particles [23], but when the neoplastic cells were grown as explant cultures, or cocultivated with susceptible indicator cells, HVS-associated antigens [3], viral particles and inclusion bodies were demonstrated. The finding that HVS was apparently carried only in lymphocytic cells in marmosets led us to investigate whether there might be a similar association of HVS with lymphocytes in the natural host, squirrel monkeys.

Isolation of HVS from Squirrel Monkeys

In a preliminary study [4] a group of ten squirrel monkeys exhibited at a local zoo was studied. These animals were pets, given to the zoo by individuals of the community; all monkeys were active and showed no overt disease. Heparinized blood was collected for hematologic, virologic and serologic studies. No hematologic abnormalities were observed: total leukocyte counts ranged from 8,300 to 17,000 mm^3 with absolute lymphocyte counts of 200 to 6,540 mm^3. By cocultivation with Vero cell cultures, virus was recovered from six of ten whole blood samples and from five of six lymphocyte samples separated from whole blood on Ficoll-Hypaque (FH) gradients [3, 22]. Virus was not isolated from FH cell-pellets containing erythrocytes and polymorphonuclear leukocytes, or from cell-free extracts of whole blood, lymphocytes or FH cell-pellets. The isolates were shown to be antigenically similar or identical to HVS by virus neutralization and indirect fluorescent antibody (FA) tests. Marmoset and guinea pig anti-HVS sera reacted positively with each of the isolates, but no virus neutralization or FA staining was obtained using antiserum to herpes simplex virus or *Herpesvirus platyrrhinae* [9]. Serum HVS antibodies were detected in four of six animals by FA and neutralization tests.

Similar results were obtained with a group of eight animals recently imported from South America by a pet shop. HVS was isolated from peripheral lymphocytes of six and antibodies were demonstrable in six of the eight monkeys.

We also studied a large number of colony-born and recently-imported squirrel monkeys, as well as imported squirrel monkeys that had been housed in the colony for several years. Blood samples for virus isolation and serological studies were collected from 129 monkeys. Results of virus isolation are summarized in table II. Virus was not isolated from five monkeys ≤ 2

Table II. Isolation of *Herpesvirus saimiri* from a colony of squirrel monkeys

Age	Virus isolation		
	total isolates	lymphocytes	whole blood
≤ 2 months	0/5	ND	0/5
≤ 1 year	7/16 (44)[1]	6/15 (40)	3/16 (19)
≥ 2 years	8/19 (42)	4/5 (80)	7/19 (37)
≥ 3 years	33/67 (49)	10/11 (91)	24/67 (36)
? (imported)	*7/22* (32)	*3/4* (75)	5/22 (30)
	55/129 (43)	23/35 (66)	33/129 (30)

1 % of monkeys from which virus was isolated.

months old; but virus was isolated from 48 monkeys ranging in age from ≤ 1 year to ≥ 3 years of age and from seven recently-imported monkeys of unknown age. The more frequent isolation of virus from separated lymphocytes (23/35) compared to virus isolation from whole blood (33/129) confirmed previous studies [4]. The frequency of virus isolation from lymphocytes indicated that a greater percentage of monkeys ≥ 2 years of age were latently infected with HVS than monkeys ≤ 1 year old.

Serum samples from the squirrel monkeys were evaluated for HVS antibodies by indirect FA tests (table III). Serum from two monkeys ≤ 2 months and ten of 16 monkeys ≤ 1 year old had no measurable levels of antibodies, but all monkeys ≥ 2 years old were seropositive.

One isolate, SM No. 11, was evaluated for oncogenicity in two cotton-topped and two white-lipped marmosets. The four experimentally-infected

Table III. Serum antibody titers to *Herpesvirus saimiri* in a colony of squirrel monkeys

Age	Number of monkeys	Number with HVS antibody titers[1]			
		< 4	4–16	32–64	128
≤ 2 months	2	2			
≤ 1 year	16	10	4	2	
≥ 2 years	19		12	5	2
≥ 3 years	67		13	48	6
? imported	22	6	7	9	

1 Reciprocal of serum dilution giving positive staining in indirect fluorescent antibody tests.

marmosets developed a fatal lymphoproliferative disease and died 18–26 days postinoculation (p.i.). HVS was isolated from each of the marmosets, and lymphoblastoid cell lines were established from lymphoid tissues of two of the marmosets [5]. Gross and microscopic features of the disease were identical with those described previously [23].

Experimental Infection of Squirrel Monkeys with HVS

The high incidence of latent HVS infection in older monkeys, whether imported or colony-born, makes it almost impossible to study the expression of primary experimental infection in this species. Therefore, seven virus and antibody negative colony-born squirrel monkeys, approximately four to six months old, were generously supplied by Dr. T. CLARKSON, Bowman Gray School of Medicine, Winston-Salem, N.C. Blood samples were collected at weekly intervals for three weeks for hematologic, virologic and serologic studies. None of the animals showed abnormal hematologic values, HVS was not isolated from their peripheral lymphocytes and all were seronegative. The animals were divided into three groups: Group 1 animals were inoculated with $10^{4.7}$ $TCID_{50}$ of the prototype strain of HVS (originally obtained from Dr. MELENDEZ); group 2 animals were uninoculated, and caged with group 1 monkeys; and group 3 animals were uninoculated and were isolated from animals of group 1 and 2. Blood samples were collected at three- to 18-day intervals p.i. for hematologic, virologic and serologic studies. Throat and rectal swabs were also collected for virus isolation.

HVS was not isolated up to seven days p.i. from lymphocytes of any monkey. Virus was first isolated from group 1 monkeys at 17–24 days p.i. and at subsequent intervals thereafter (table IV). Both cagemate controls

Table IV. Isolation of *Herpesvirus saimiri* from experimentally-infected squirrel monkeys

Group No.	Number of monkeys	Days postinoculation							
		7	17	24	31	42	52	60	78
1	3	0[1]	2	3	3	3	3	2	2
2	2	0	0	0	0	0	0	1	2
3	2	0	0	0	0	0	0	0	0

1 Number of virus-positive monkeys.

(group 2) remained virus negative until virus was isolated from one cagemate at 60 days p.i. and at 78 days from both cagemates. The two group 3 controls, isolated from group 1 and 2, remained virus negative up to the last observation period. Attempts to isolate virus from throat and rectal swabs from animals of all three groups were unsuccessful.

Seroconversion (table V) in group 1 monkeys occurred at approximately the same p.i. intervals (24 days) that HVS was first isolated from their peripheral lymphocytes. Up to 52 days p.i. seroconversion was not evident in any monkeys of group 2 and 3.

Table V. Seroconversion in *Herpesvirus saimiri* experimentally-infected squirrel monkeys

Group No.	Number of monkeys	Days postinoculation						
		0	7	14	24	31	42	52
1	3	0[1]	0	0	3	3	3	3
2	2	0	0	0	0	0	0	0
3	2	0	0	0	0	0	0	0

1 Number of seropositive monkeys.

Throughout the entire observation period, no hematologic abnormalities were detected; total leukocyte and differential counts were similar in monkeys of each group and were comparable to the preinoculation baseline determinations, and the animals did not develop any clinical disease.

Discussion

Previous studies showed that 88% of adult, wild-caught squirrel monkeys are seropositive for HVS antibodies [2]. The findings reported here show that, in addition to the high percentage of seropositive squirrel monkeys, an approximately equal number of imported and colony-born squirrel monkeys are latently infected with HVS. Results of the colony study suggest that latent infections are a direct result of horizontal transmission of HVS sometime during the first year of life. Virus could not be isolated from 12 monkeys less than six months old and nine of nine tested were seronegative. Virus was isolated from seven of 16 monkeys approximately one year old, but only 38% were seropositive. All colony monkeys two years old, or older, were seropositive. Once infected, monkeys probably remain latently infected for the rest of their lives.

More direct evidence for horizontal transmission was obtained from the cagemates of the experimentally-infected squirrel monkeys. The two cagemate controls were virus positive at 36 and 54 days after HVS was first isolated from the infected monkeys. The possibility that the monkeys were already latently infected, even though the assay procedure did not detect the infection, cannot be excluded; but the fact that monkeys isolated from the infected monkeys remained virus negative argues against this possibility.

One question unresolved by our studies is the manner by which HVS is transmitted, i.e. whether transmission is cell-free or cell-associated. Attempts to isolate virus from throat and rectal swabs were unsuccessful, but again the sensitivity of available assay methods for detecting small amounts of virus is questionable. HVS is not transmitted horizontally from experimentally-infected marmosets to their cagemate controls: uninfected marmosets have been housed with infected animals for periods up to ten months, but virus was not isolated from their lymphocytes, nor was seroconversion demonstrated [23].

HVS, like a number of other herpesviruses of nonhuman primates, *Herpesvirus simiae* [20], *Herpesvirus platyrrhinae* [9] and *Herpesvirus ateles* [10] apparently cause no or only a subclinical disease in their natural host, but severe disease in closely-related species. Study of HVS is important because of the association of a number of herpesviruses with malignant disease. The oncogenic Marek's disease virus of chickens [18] and rabbit lymphoma herpesvirus [8] are carried, similar to HVS, latently in the lymphocytes of their natural hosts in which under certain conditions they also cause malignant disease. In addition, Epstein-Barr virus of man, the etiological agent of infectious mononucleosis [6], has been implicated as the cause of Burkitt's lymphoma [7] and nasopharyngeal carcinoma [21], and recently an association of herpes simplex virus type II with cervical carcinoma has been considered [17, 19].

Studies of the mechanisms which determine the outcome of host cell-HVS interactions in the persistent latent infections *versus* the malignant lymphoproliferative disease, and also the repression of viral genome functions *in vivo* but almost immediate derepression when infected cells are grown *in vitro,* are, therefore, important as they may help in understanding the association of herpesviruses and the development of neoplasms.

Acknowledgements

We thank the Board of Health, City of Chicago, for providing space for housing many of our experimental animals and all members of our department for their contribution to this study.

References

1 ABLASHI, D.V.; LOEB, W.F.; VALERIO, M.G.; ADAMSON, R.H.; ARMSTRONG, G.R.; BENNETT, D.G., and HEINE, V.: Malignant lymphoma with lymphocytic leukemia in owl monkeys induced by *Herpesvirus saimiri*. J.nat.Cancer Inst. *47:* 837–856 (1971).

2 DEINHARDT, F.; FALK, L.; MARCZYNSKA, B.; SHRAMEK, G., and WOLFE, L.: *Herpesvirus saimiri*. A simian counterpart of Epstein-Barr virus of man? In CHIECO-BIANCHI and DUTCHER Proc. 5th Int. Symp. on Comparative Leukemia Research, Padova 1971. Bibl. haemat., vol 39 (Karger, Basel, in press).

3 FALK, L.A.; WOLFE, L.G.; HOEKSTRA, J., and DEINHARDT, F.: Demonstration of *Herpesvirus saimiri*-associated antigens in peripheral lymphocytes from infected marmosets during *in vitro* cultivation. J.nat.Cancer Inst. *48:* 523–530 (1972).

4 FALK, L.A.; WOLFE, L.G., and DEINHARDT, F.: Isolation of *Herpesvirus saimiri* from blood of squirrel monkeys *(Saimiri sciureus)*. J.nat.Cancer Inst. *48:* 1499–1505 (1972).

5 FALK, L.A.; MARCZYNSKA, B.; WOLFE, L., and DEINHARDT, F.: Characterization of lymphoid cell lines established from *Herpesvirus saimiri* (HVS)-infected marmosets. Abstracts of the Annual Meeting of the American Society for Microbiology, p. 191 (1972).

6 HENLE, G.; HENLE, W., and DIEHL, V.: Relation of Burkitt's tumor-associated herpes-type virus to infectious mononucleosis. Proc.nat.Acad.Sci. *59:* 94–101 (1968).

7 HENLE, G.; HENLE, W.; CLIFFORD, P.; DIEHL, V.; KAFUKO, G.W.; KIRYA, B.G.; KLEIN, G.; MORROW, R.H.; MUNUBE, G.M.R.; PIKE, P.; TUKEI, P.M., and ZIEGLER, J.: Antibodies to EB in Burkitt's lymphoma and control groups. J.nat.Cancer Inst. *43:* 1147–1157 (1969).

8 HINZE, H.C.: New member of the Herpesvirus group isolated from wild cottontail rabbits. Infect.Immun. *3:* 350–354 (1971).

9 HOLMES, A.W.; CALDWELL, R.G.; DEDMON, R.E., and DEINHARDT, F.: Isolation and characterization of a new Herpes virus. J.Immunol. *92:* 602–610 (1964).

10 HULL, R.N.; DWYER, A.C.; HOLMES, A.W.; NOWAKOWSKI, E.; DEINHARDT, F.; LENNETTE, E.H., and EMMONS, R.W.: World Health Organization Scientific Publication No. 235, pp. 137–144 (1972).

11 HUNT, R.D.; MELENDEZ, L.V.; KING, N.W.; GILMORE, C.E.; DANIEL, M.D.; WILLIAMSON, M.E., and JONES, T.C.: Morphology of a disease with features of malignant lymphoma in marmosets and owl monkeys inoculated with *Herpesvirus saimiri*. J.nat.Cancer Inst. *44:* 447–465 (1970).

12 HUNT, R.D.; MELENDEZ, L.V.; KING, N.W., and GARCIA, F.G.: *Herpesvirus saimiri* malignant lymphoma in spider monkeys. J.med.Prim. *1:* 114–128 (1972).

13 MELENDEZ, L.V.; DANIEL, M.D.; HUNT, R.D., and GARCIA, F.G.: An apparently new herpesvirus from primary kidney cultures of the squirrel monkey *(Saimiri sciureus)*. Lab.anim.Care *18:* 374–381 (1968).

14 MELENDEZ, L.V.; HUNT, R.D.; DANIEL, M.D.; FRASER, C.E.O.; GARCIA, F.G., and WILLIAMSON, F.D.: Lethal reticuloproliferative disease induced in *Cebus albifrons* monkeys by *Herpesvirus saimiri.* Int.J.Cancer *6:* 431–435 (1970).

15 MELENDEZ, L.V.; HUNT, R.D.; DANIEL, M.D., and TRUM, B.F.: New world monkeys, herpes viruses and cancer; in BALNER and BEVERIDGE Infections and immunosuppression in sub-human primates, pp.111–117 (Munksgaard, Copenhagen 1970).

16 MELENDEZ, L.V.; HUNT, R.D.; DANIEL, M.D.; BLAKE, B.J., and GARCIA, F.G.: Acute lymphocytic leukemia in owl monkeys *(Aotus trivirgatus)* inoculated with *Herpesvirus saimiri.* Science *171:* 1161–1163 (1971).

17 NAHMIAS, A.J.; NAIB, Z.M., and JOSEY, W.E.: Association of genital herpesvirus with cervical cancer. Int.Virol. *1:* 187–188 (1969).

18 NAZERIAN, K.; SOLOMON, J.J.; WITTER, R.L., and BURMESTER, B.R.: Studies on the etiology of Marek's disease. II. Finding of a herpesvirus in cell culture. Pro.Soc.exp. Biol.Med. *127:* 177–182 (1968).

19 RAWLS, W.E.; TOMPKINS, W.A.F., and MELNICK, J.L.: The association of herpesvirus type 2 and carcinoma of the uterine cervix. Amer.J.Epidem. *89:* 547–554 (1969).

20 SABIN, A.B.: Studies on the 'B' virus. I. The immunological identity of a virus isolated from a human case of ascending myelitis associated with visceral necrosis. Brit.J.exp. Path. *15:* 248–279 (1934).

21 DESCHRYVER, A.; FRIBERG, S.; KLEIN, G.; HENLE, W.; HENLE, G.; DE-THE, G.; CLIFFORD, P., and HO, H.C.: Epstein-Barr virus-associated antibody patterns in carcinoma of the post-nasal space. Clin.exp.Immunol. *5:* 443–459 (1969).

22 THORSBY, E. and BRATLIE, A.: A rapid method for preparation of pure lymphocyte suspensions; in Histocompatability testing, pp.655–656 (Williams & Wilkins, Baltimore 1970).

23 WOLFE, L.G.; FALK, L.A., and DEINHARDT, F.: Oncogenicity of *Herpesvirus saimiri* in marmoset monkeys. J.nat.Cancer Inst. *47:* 1145–1162 (1972).

Authors' address: Drs. LAWRENCE FALK, LAUREN WOLFE and FRIEDRICH DEINHARDT, Departments of Microbiology, Rush-Presbyterian-St. Luke's and University of Illinois Medical Centers, *Chicago, IL 60612* (USA)

Medical Primatology 1972. Proc. 3rd Conf. exp. Med. Surg. Primates, Lyon 1972, part III, pp. 159–162 (Karger, Basel 1972)

Herpesvirus ateles Lymphoma in Cotton-Topped Marmosets

The Virus, the Disease, and Evidence for Horizontal Transmission

R. D. Hunt, L. V. Meléndez and B. F. Trum

New England Regional Primate Research Center, Harvard Medical School, Southborough, Mass.

Three viruses of nonhuman primate origin have been shown to cause malignancies in other nonhuman primate species. The first of these, *Herpesvirus saimiri* was isolated in 1968 and shown to cause malignant lymphoma and leukemia in cotton-topped marmosets *(Saguinus oedipus)* and owl monkeys *(Aotus trivirgatus)* [2, 4, 5]. These findings were later corroborated by other investigators [1, 10]. The virus is now known to be carried by squirrel monkeys *(Saimiri sciureus)* which have not been shown to suffer ill effects from the infection. We have also demonstrated that *H. saimiri* causes malignant lymphoma in spider monkeys *(Ateles geoffroyi)* and rabbits *(Oryctolagus cuniculus)* and a reticuloproliferative disorder in cebus monkeys *(Cebus albifrons)* and African green monkeys *(Cercopithecus aethiops)*. These studies are of particular significance for several reasons. They represented the first demonstration of a virus of monkey origin which is oncogenic in other monkey species; they represented the first oncogenic herpesvirus in a mammalian species and the first DNA virus to be associated with leukemia in mammalian species.

The wooly monkey *(Lagothrix lagothricha)* C-type virus isolated in 1971 by Theilen *et al.* [8] from a spontaneous fibrosarcoma and shown to induce fibrosarcoma in white-lipped marmosets *(Saguinus nigricollis* and *Saguinus fuscicollis fuscicollis)* by Wolfe *et al.* [9] represents another primate origin virus oncogenic in another primate species. These studies uncovered the first oncogenic C-type virus in nonhuman primates.

Herpesvirus ateles is the most recently-reported virus of primate origin which is oncogenic in a primate species [6, 7], and is the subject of this report.

Following the occurrence of lymphosarcoma in two human beings caring for spider monkeys in Guatemala, we initiated a program to study the indigenous viruses of this species. We were particularly interested in the possibility that *H. saimiri* was carried by these animals as this virus is oncogenic in such a wide spectrum of hosts. Although we did not isolate *H. saimiri* from spider monkeys, two new herpesviruses were uncovered, Guatemala isolate AT-46 isolated from a spider monkey in the Guatemala colony, and *H. ateles* isolated from a spider monkey imported to our laboratories from Guatemala [7]. Guatemala isolate AT-46 has not been shown to be pathogenic.

As previously reported, *H. ateles* meets all necessary physical, chemical, and ultrastructural criteria to be included in the herpesvirus group [7]. That the virus is a distinct agent and not related to *H. saimiri* is clearly shown by the following data. *In vitro* serum neutralization studies have shown no cross-reaction between *H. ateles* and *H. saimiri, H. simplex, H. suis,* infectious bovine rhinotracheitis virus, spider monkey herpesvirus (Lennette and Hull), AT-46, *H. aotus* type 1 and 2, and *H. saguinus*. *H. ateles* induces CPE in the following tissue cultures which are not susceptible to *H. saimiri,* rabbit kidney line, hamster heart, and goat synovial bursa and does not produce CPE in Vero cell line which is susceptible to *H. saimiri*. Another distinguishing feature is that *H. saimiri* induces lymphoma in rabbits, whereas *H. ateles* does not.

Recently we have studied 12 cotton-topped marmosets injected with approximately 10,000 $TCID_{50}$ of *H. ateles* which was prepared in an owl monkey kidney cell line. Three uninoculated marmosets were housed singly with three inoculated animals as contact controls. The inoculated animals died between 26 and 32 days after injection; nine of the 12 developed a peripheral blood picture of leukemia. The total white blood count 26 days after injection ranged from 13,900 to 24,900 (preinoculation values of 7,500–15,800) with absolute lymphocyte counts of 5,000–18,000 (preinoculation values of 1,900–5,200) of which 22–52% were lymphoblasts. The outstanding gross findings were marked enlargement of the spleen, thymus, and all lymph nodes. Microscopically the neoplastic cells were uniformly lymphoblasts. Mitotic figures were numerous and the cells invaded and replaced the entire cytoarchitecture of lymph nodes, spleen, and thymus. Extensive infiltration was also present in liver, adrenal, kidney, myocardium, heart, lungs, salivary gland, pancreas, choroid plexus and bone marrow.

Three of the contact controls remained in good clinical health, did not develop an abnormal peripheral blood picture, and upon sacrifice 230 days after the onset of the study, no lesion was seen indicative of either a viral infection or neoplastic disease.

One of the contact controls, however, died 86 days after the start of the study. The blood picture of this marmoset remained within normal limits until three days before death when the total white blood count was 28,400 with an absolute lymphocyte count of 8,804, of which 23% were lymphoblasts. Gross and histopathologic findings were those of malignant lymphoma, lymphoblastic type, identical in appearance to the malignancy seen in the inoculated animals. The occurrence of malignant lymphoma in this contact control is evidence of horizontal transmission of the disease. This has not been observed in studies with *H.saimiri.*

In comparison with *H.saimiri* lymphoma in cotton-topped marmosets, each example of *H.ateles* lymphoma has been of the lymphoblastic type and the total white blood cell count is much lower. Aside from these differences, the two malignancies are remarkably similar. The natural history of the two agents is also similar. Both are carried as latent infections in one species of primates (*H.saimiri* in squirrel monkeys and *H.ateles* in spider monkeys) and both cause leukemia and lymphoma in cotton-topped marmosets. The host range in which *H.saimiri* causes lymphoma is very broad; *H.ateles* has yet to be tested to determine if it is oncogenic in additional primate species. The demonstration that two herpesviruses can be carried by one species and cause cancer in other species, poses the intriguing question as to whether these or other oncogenic herpesviruses may behave as zoonoses.

In conclusion, *H.ateles,* which is carried by spider monkeys and which is distinct from *H.saimiri,* causes malignant lymphoma and leukemia in cotton-topped marmosets. Also, data is presented which suggests horizontal transmission of the virus and the disease between inoculated marmosets and a contact control.

References

1 Ablashi, D.V.; Loeb, W.F.; Valerio, M.G.; Adamson, R.H.; Armstrong, G.R.; Bennett, D.G., and Heine, V.: Malignant lymphoma with lymphocytic leukemia induced in owl monkeys by *Herpesvirus saimiri.* J.nat.Cancer Inst. *47:* 837–855 (1971).

2 Hunt, R.D.; Meléndez, L.V.; King, N.W.; Gilmore, C.E.; Daniel, M.D.; Williamson, M.E., and Jones, T.C.: Morphology of a disease with features of malignant lymphoma in marmosets and owl monkeys inoculated with *Herpesvirus saimiri.* J.nat.Cancer Inst. *44:* 447–465 (1970).

3 Hunt, R.D. and Meléndez, L.V.: Clinical, epidemiological and pathological features of cytocidal and oncogenic herpesviruses in South American monkeys. J.nat.Cancer Inst. (in press).

4 MELÉNDEZ, L.V.; DANIEL, M.D.; HUNT, R.D., and GARCIA, F.G.: An apparently new herpesvirus from primate kidney cultures of the squirrel monkey *(Saimiri sciureus)*. Lab.anim.Care *18:* 374–381 (1968).

5 MELÉNDEZ, L.V.; HUNT, R.D.; DANIEL, M.D.; GARCIA, F.G., and FRASER, C.E.O.: *Herpesvirus saimiri* II. An experimentally induced malignant lymphoma in primates. Lab.anim.Care *19:* 378–386 (1969).

6 MELÉNDEZ, L.V.; HUNT, R.D.; KING, N.W.; BARAHONA, H.H.; DANIEL, M.D.; FRASER, C.E.O., and GARCIA, F.G.: A new lymphoma virus of monkeys. *Herpesvirus ateles.* Nature New Biol. *235:* 182–184 (1972).

7 MELÉNDEZ, L.V.; CASTELLANOS, H.; BARAHONA, H.H.; DANIEL, M.D.; HUNT, R.D.; FRASER, C.E.O.; GARCIA, F.G., and KING, N.W.: Two new herpesviruses from spider monkeys *(Ateles geofroyi)*. J.nat.Cancer Inst. (in press).

8 THEILEN, G.H.; GOULD, D.; FOWLER, M., and DUNGWORTH, D.L.: C-type virus in tumor tissue of a wooly monkey (*Lagothrix* spp.) with fibrosarcoma. J.nat.Cancer Inst. *47:* 881–889 (1971).

9 WOLFE, L.G.; DEINHARDT, F.; THEILEN, G.H.; RABIN, H.; KAWAKAMI, T., and BUSTAD, L.K.: Induction of tumors in marmoset monkeys by simian sarcoma virus type 1 *(Lagothrix)*. A preliminary report. J.nat.Cancer Inst. *47:* 1115–1120 (1971).

10 WOLFE, L.G.; FALK, L.A., and DEINHARDT, F.: Oncogenicity of *Herpesvirus saimiri* in marmoset monkeys. J.nat.Cancer Inst. *47:* 1145–1162 (1971).

Authors' address: Dr. R. HUNT, Dr. L.V. MELÉNDEZ and Dr. B. F. TRUM, New England Regional Primate Research Center, *Southborough, MA 01772* (USA)

Medical Primatology 1972. Proc. 3rd Conf. exp. Med. Surg. Primates, Lyon 1972, part III, pp. 163–168 (Karger, Basel 1972)

Characterization of a C-Type Virus Associated with Gibbon Lymphosarcoma

T. G. Kawakami, Patricia M. Buckley and Sally D. Huff

Comparative Oncology Laboratory, University of California, Davis, Cal.

Oncogenic RNA viruses have been established as the causal agents of leukemia and fibrosarcoma in feline and murine species and have been characterized [2, 5]. Viral agents with similar morphology were found associated with a spontaneous woolly monkey fibrosarcoma (SSV-1) [11] and a gibbon lymphosarcoma [4, 9]. SSV-1 when inoculated into newborn marmosets induced fibrosarcoma; thus demonstrating the oncogenicity of the agent [12]. *In vitro* studies on SSV-1 and gibbon lymphosarcoma viruses indicate that both agents infect cells in culture and possess morphologic characteristics similar to known C-type viruses [3, 4]. Reported here is further evidence that the gibbon lymphosarcoma virus has other characteristics in common with known oncogenic RNA viruses.

Material and Methods

Tissue cultures of gibbon and feline lymphoid cells initiated from spontaneous lymphosarcoma were propagated in Liebovitz medium supplemented with 15% v/v heat inactivated fetal calf serum as previously described [4, 10]. The cultures were propagated by dividing the culture 1:2 once a week and adding fresh medium. The viruses were concentrated from spent tissue culture fluid by rate-flow zonal ultracentrifugation (Beckmann L-4 with B-16 rotor). The concentrated viruses were either further purified or used directly for various studies.

Tissue culture cells for electron microscopic examination were fixed in 2% glutaraldehyde in Millonig's buffer for two hours followed by one hour postfixation in 1% osmium tetroxide. Ultrathin sections were doubly stained with uranyl acetate and lead citrate and were examined in a Phillips EM 200 electron microscope.

Isotopic labeling aided in determining the nucleic acid and buoyant density of the virus. Two to 10 μC/ml of ^{3}H-uridine was added to actively growing cultures for 20 h at which time the virus was concentrated from the supernatant by differential centrifugation. Buoyant density of the virus was determined by isopycnic centrifugation in sucrose gradient in the presence of standard density beads.

Immunodiffusion tests were conducted using immune sera prepared in steers against SSV-1 and feline fibrosarcoma viruses (FSV). Sera were obtained following hyperimmunization of the animals with virus-infected autochthonous cells. Serum samples were heat-inactivated at 56 °C for 30 min and used in immunodiffusion plates containing buffered 1 % purified agar. All viral antigens were treated with ether prior to use. Plates were incubated at room temperature and the results recorded after 24 and 48 h.

RNA-DNA polymerase immunoinhibition assays were conducted under conditions previously described [1]. A typical test used 4 μg of purified detergent-treated virions incubated together with 50–350 μg of serum protein and synthetic RNA-DNA hybrid template.

Results and Discussion

Electron microscopic examination of the gibbon lymphoid cells propagated *in vitro* showed the presence of large numbers of extracellular C-type particles associated with the cells. Figure 1 shows a typical cell with associated extracellular virions. The mature particles measured approximately 100 nm in diameter with an electron-dense nucleoid measuring approximately 85 nm. Budding forms were observed infrequently on the plasma membrane.

Tritiated-uridine incorporation studies indicated that the isotope was incorporated into particles which banded at 1.16 g/cm^3 upon isopycnic centrifugation. Figure 2 shows a representative curve from an experiment in which labelled particles corresponded in position to a bead with known density of 1.16 g/cm^3. A virus band of comparable density used for antigen was observed to give a positive precipitin line in the presence of immune serum.

Immunodiffusion tests were conducted on purified ether-treated gibbon and other known oncogenic C-type viruses in the presence of immune sera. Table I summarizes the results of these experiments. A contiguous precipitin line was observed with both gibbon and SSV-1 viruses but failed to appear with antigens from feline or murine C-type viruses tested in the presence of anti-SSV-1 virus serum. On the other hand, a precipitin line developed only with the feline leukemia virus antigen in the presence of anti-FSV serum.

The RNA-DNA polymerase immunoinhibition test conducted on purified gibbon, SSV-1 and feline C-type virus polymerases showed that inhibition of the polymerases of the feline or simian species by immune serum protein was highly selective. Table II shows the results of tests conducted on the gibbon, SSV-1 and feline C-type virus polymerases in the presence of either anti-SSV-1 or anti-FSV serum protein under identical conditions. The anti-

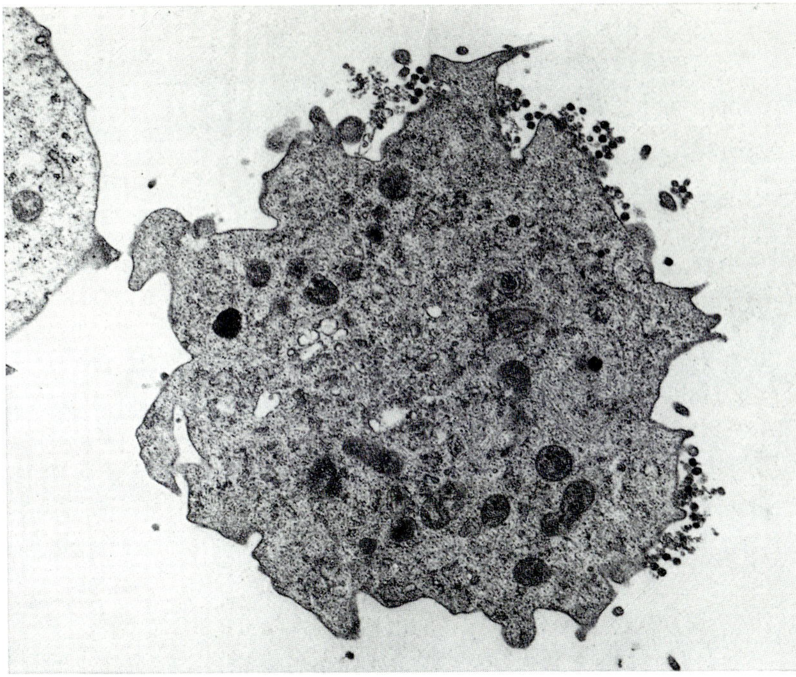

Fig. 1. Electron micrograph of a gibbon lymphoid cell propagated *in vitro* with associated mature viral particles.

Table I. Results of immunodiffusion tests

C-Type virus antigen	Precipitin line formation in the presence of immune serum	
	FSV	SSV
Gibbon	–	+
Woolly monkey	–	+
Feline	+	–
Murine	–	–

SSV-1 serum selectively inhibited the gibbon and SSV-1 virus polymerases 80–90% compared to the control when 75–300 μg of immune serum protein was present, while the feline leukemia virus polymerase was not inhibited. On the other hand, anti-FSV serum protein tested under similar conditions markedly inhibited the feline leukemia virus polymerase but failed to show any effect upon the gibbon and SSV-1 C-type viruses.

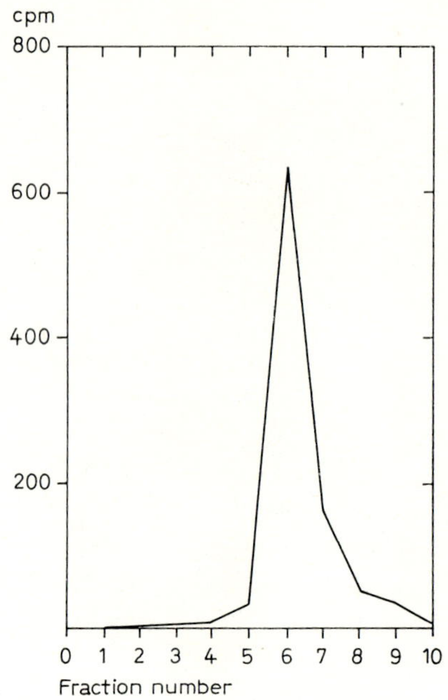

Fig. 2. Graph showing distribution of ^{3}H-uridine labelled particles isolated from a gibbon lymphoid culture in sucrose gradient with a peak at a density of 1.16 g/cm^{3}.

Results of the present study based on morphologic, physical, immunologic, and RNA-DNA polymerase inhibition tests indicate the newly-isolated gibbon C-type virus possesses characteristics of known RNA oncogenic viruses.

The morphology of known oncogenic C-type viruses has been described for the murine and feline species. These viruses typically replicate by budding from the cell membrane with resultant formation of a spherical viral particle

Table II. Results of RNA-DNA polymerase immunoinhibition test

C-Type virus RNA-DNA polymerase	% inhibition of RNA-DNA polymerase reaction in presence of immune serum	
	FSV	SSV
Gibbon	0	80
Woolly monkey	0	90
Feline	90	0

which possesses an envelope and an electron-dense nucleoid. The morphologic characteristics of the present agent are identical to those described in other species. The presence of the identical morphologic particles in the original tumor would support that the gibbon C-type virus is associated with the spontaneous tumor [4, 9].

Buoyant density of C-type viruses has been reported to be 1.16 g/cm^3. The feline leukemia virus isolated from the plasma was found to be between 1.14 and 1.16 g/cm^3 [2]. Tissue culture-propagated feline particles also have been demonstrated to have comparable density. The gibbon virus propagated *in vitro* from the lymphoid cells has the characteristic buoyant density of 1.16 g/cm^3 as demonstrated by isopycnic centrifugation of ^{3}H-uridine incorporated particles. The incorporation of ^{3}H-uridine into particles would indicate that these particles possess ribonucleic acid and are identical to the murine and feline oncornaviruses.

The major internal soluble protein of C-type viruses has been characterized in several species. The soluble protein is ether-stable and possesses a molecular weight of approximately 30,000 daltons. The intraspecific antigen of the murine, feline and hamster viruses has not been shown to cross-react [6]. The evidence from the present study indicates that the major ether-stable soluble protein in the gibbon C-type virus cross-reacts with SSV-1. The molecular size of the present protein was found to be comparable to known oncornaviruses in polyacrylamide gel electrophoresis. While an interspecific antigen common with other oncogenic C-type viruses has been reported for the two simian viruses, evidence presented in this study would indicate that the shared antigen is an intraspecific antigen. This is unlike the rodent family where unrelated species do not share a common intraspecific antigenic determinant. It is unclear whether this common characteristic is coincidental or arises from infection with a common agent.

RNA-DNA polymerase or reverse transcriptase has been shown to be a characteristic enzyme for C-type viruses. This enzyme has been reported to be associated with a few nononcogenic agents, but an immune serum specifically directed against a C-type virus polymerase appears to inhibit only enzymes of closely-related oncornaviruses. Thus, enzymes of murine B-type, visna and foamy viruses are unaffected [8]. Results of our polymerase inhibition studies would indicate that the two simian C-type viruses are closely related since both virus polymerases were equally inhibited by the anti-SSV-1 serum protein.

Although oncogenicity has not been demonstrated for the gibbon C-type virus, results from this study indicate that the newly-isolated agent has many characteristics of proven oncogenic agents. *In vivo* studies are in progress in an attempt to demonstrate oncogenicity of the agent.

References

1 AARONSON, S.A.; PARKS, W.P.; SCOLNICK, E.M., and TODARO, G.J.: Antibody to the RNA-dependent DNA polymerase of mammalian C-type RNA tumor viruses. Proc. nat. Acad. Sci. *68:* 920–924 (1971).

2 KAWAKAMI, T.G.; THEILEN, G.H.; DUNGWORTH, D.L.; MUNN, R.J., and BEALL, S.G.: 'C'-type viral particles in plasma of cats with feline leukemia. Science *158:* 1049 (1967).

3 KAWAKAMI, T.G.; BUCKLEY, P.M.; HUFF, S.D.; MCKAIN, D., and FIELDING, H.: A comparative study *in vitro* of a simian virus isolated from spontaneous woolly monkey fibrosarcoma and of a known feline fibrosarcoma virus; in CHIECO-BIANCHI and DUTCHER Proc. 5th Int. Symp. on Comparative Leukemia Research, Padova 1971 (Karger, Basel, in press).

4 KAWAKAMI, T.G.; HUFF, S.D.; BUCKLEY, P.; DUNGWORTH, D.L., and SNYDER, S.P.: C-type virus associated with gibbon lymphosarcoma. Nature New Biol. *235:* 170–171 (1972).

5 MOLONEY, J.B.: Biological studies on a lymphoid leukemia virus extracted from sarcoma 37. I. Origin and introductory investigation. J. nat. Cancer Inst. *24:* 933–951 (1964).

6 OROSZLAN, S.; FOREMAN, C.; KELLOFF, G., and GILDEN, R.V.: The group-specific antigen and other structural proteins of hamster and mouse C-type viruses. Virology *43:* 665–674 (1971).

7 PARKS, W.; SCOLNICK, E.M.; ROSS, J.; TODARO, G.J., and AARONSON, S.A.: Immunological relationships of reverse transcriptases from ribonucleic acid tumor viruses. J. Virol. *9:* 110–115 (1972).

8 SCOLNICK, E.M.; PARKS, W.P.; TODARO, G.J., and AARONSON, S.A.: Immunological characterization of primate C-type virus reverse transcriptases. Nature New Biol. *235:* 35–40 (1972).

9 SNYDER, S.P.; DUNGWORTH, D.L.; KAWAKAMI, T.G.; CALLAWAY, E., and LAU, D. T-L.: Two cases of lymphosarcoma in gibbons *(Hylobates lar)* with associated C-type virus. Submitted to J. nat. Cancer Inst.

10 THEILEN, G.H.; KAWAKAMI, T.G.; RUSH, J.D., and MUNN, R.J.: Replication of cat leukemia virus in cell suspension cultures. Nature *222:* 589–590 (1968).

11 THEILEN, G.H.; GOULD, D.; FOWLER, M.E., and DUNGWORTH, D.L.: C-type virus in tumor tissue of a woolly monkey *(Lagothrix* spp.) with fibrosarcoma. J. nat. Cancer Inst. *47:* 881 (1971).

12 WOLFE, L.G.; DEINHARDT, F.; THEILEN, G.H.; RABIN, H.; KAWAKAMI, T.G., and BUSTAD, L.K.: Induction of tumors in marmoset monkeys by simian sarcoma virus, type 1 *(Lagothrix)*. A preliminary report. J. nat. Cancer Inst. *47:* 1115 (1971).

Author's address: Dr. THOMAS G. KAWAKAMI, Comparative Oncology Laboratory and Department of Pathology School of Veterinary Medicine, University of California, *Davis, CA* (USA)

Medical Primatology 1972. Proc. 3rd Conf. exp. Med. Surg. Primates, Lyon 1972, part III, pp. 169–175 (Karger, Basel 1972)

Rhesus Monkey Lymphosarcoma[1]

Study of One Case

H. Rabin, V. G. Nelson, G. H. Theilen, C. Espana and E. Smith

Litton Bionetics, Inc., Kensington, Md., National Center for Primate Biology and School of Veterinary Medicine, University of California, Davis, Calif.

For the past three years malignant lymphoma has been reoccurring at the National Center for Primate Biology (NCPB), University of California, Davis [9]. Approximately 30 cases have been observed to date, mostly in rhesus monkeys, *Macaca mulatta*. The histories of the different cases are very variable and, so far, no common etiological factor has been identified. This paper presents the results of studies performed on one of these lymphosarcoma cases. Included in the paper are descriptions of the case history, the pathology, tumor cell cultures, a virus isolation from cultured tumor cells, and attempts to transmit the disease to other nonhuman primates.

A young, adult, wild-caught, female rhesus monkey arrived at the NCPB on July 25, 1968. In the fall of 1970, she was placed in an endocrine research program and on October 29, 1970, a bilateral ovariectomy was performed. Two weeks later, she was started on a long course of intermittent estrogen treatment in which 10 μg/day of 17-β-estradiol was administered in three sessions of 21, 20 and 43 days, each interspersed with two sessions of ten and 12 days each with no treatment. A uterine biopsy was performed on February 4, 1971, at which time she was treated with progesterone (norethisteronacetate, 1 mg). A second uterine biopsy was performed on February 18, 1971, at which time enlargement of the inguinal lymph nodes was first noted. A third uterine biopsy was performed on February 27, 1971, and enlargement both of the inguinal and the retroperitoneal lymph nodes was observed. At

1 Supported in part by USPH, NIH, NCI contracts NIH 71-2025 and NIH 70-2048 from the Special Virus Cancer Program.

this time the monkey was removed from the endocrine research program and held for further observation as a suspected lymphosarcoma case. Enlargement of the orbit of the eye was first noticed about June 1, 1971. Later, two other masses were detected, one on the midline of the abdomen and one on the mid-ventral section of the pelvis. One day prior to death, July 13, 1971, these masses measured in diameter approximately 2.3 cm for the orbital mass, 1.4 cm for the abdominal mass, and 3.0 cm for the pelvic mass. Figure 1 shows the appearance of the monkey with the three large masses clearly visible.

One day following surgery to remove portions of two of the masses, the monkey was in terminal condition, and was killed and necropsied. No large tumor-like masses other than those described were seen upon gross exami-

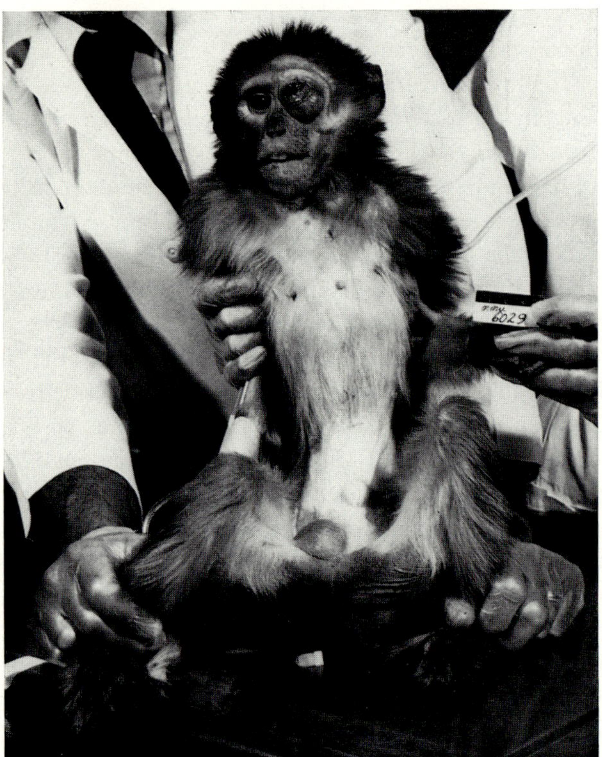

Fig. 1. Photograph of rhesus monkey one day prior to death showing tumors in the orbital, abdominal, and pelvic areas.

nation. Histopathologic examination confirmed that the three masses were lymphosarcomas and also revealed lymphosarcoma involving the heart, colon, small intestine and inguinal lymph nodes. Figure 2 illustrates the microscopic appearance of the tumor cells. Cells from the tumor masses were cultured *in vitro* at 37 °C in either McCoy's 5 A medium plus 10% fetal calf serum or Leibovitz L-15 medium plus 10% fetal calf serum. In culture, the cells grew very well over the first several days after initial seeding in each type of medium. Growth was virtually all in suspension where the cells formed large clumps. Dividing cells were relatively common. The appearance of the cells after seven days in culture is shown in figure 3. Chromosome counts performed on cells after ten days in culture revealed a modal number of 42, the normal diploid chromosome number of rhesus monkeys [3]. Electron

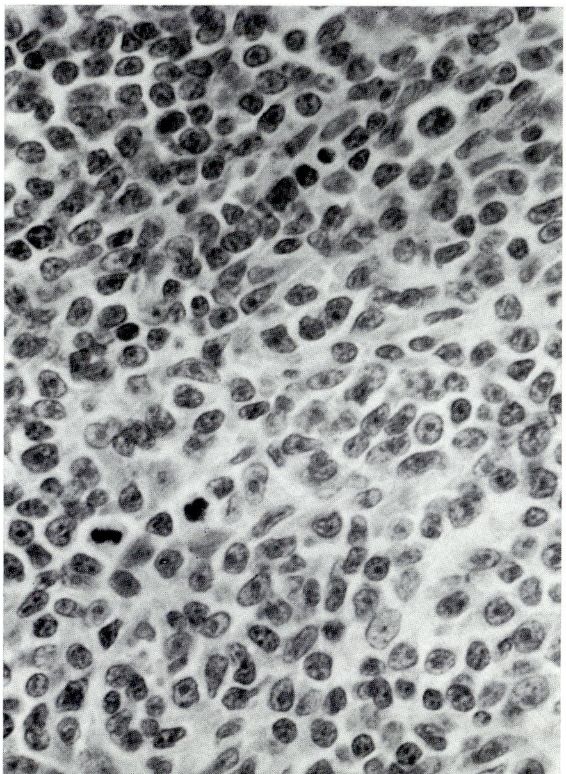

Fig. 2. Photomicrograph of a section of neoplasm showing typical tumor cells. HE. × 400.

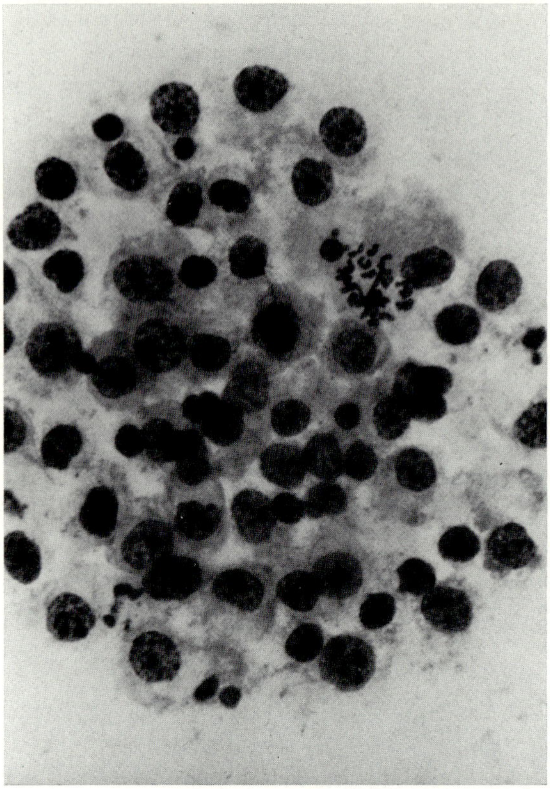

Fig. 3. Photomicrograph of cultured tumor cells after seven days *in vitro*. Giemsa. × 400.

microscopic examination of original tumor cells and of tumor cells after seven to 13 days in culture confirmed the general characteristics observed by light microscopy but did not reveal the presence of virus particles.

In an attempt to obtain a virus isolate, a cell extract was prepared by subjecting cultured cells 16 days after initial seeding to four cycles of alternate freezing and thawing. The extract was clarified by centrifugation and inoculated onto third passage African green monkey kidney (AGMK) cells. After four days of incubation at 37 °C, cytopathology, characterized by multinucleation typical of that described for foamyviruses [4], developed. Electron microscopic examination of infected AGMK cells revealed the presence of characteristic foamyvirus particles [1]. No such virus particles were seen in uninfected AGMK cells. Cytopathology, characterized by multinucleation, developed spontaneously in cultures of the tumor cells themselves at about three weeks after initial seeding and resulted in the eventual loss of all the cultures. The multinucleation-inducing agent has been found to produce typical cytopathology to low titer in cultures of rhesus monkey foreskin cells and human foreskin cells in addition to those of AGMK cells. Preliminary serological data obtained in collaboration with Drs. S. S. KALTER and R. L. HEBERLING of the Simian Virus Reference Laboratory, Southwest Foundation for Research and Education, indicate that this agent is related to simian foamyvirus, type 1.

Finally, efforts were made to transmit lymphosarcoma to other nonhuman primates. An earlier report indicated that one successful transmission of lymphosarcoma had been accomplished with fresh tumor cells from another lymphosarcoma case which had occurred at the NCPB [9]. Table I shows the various transmission experiments performed with fresh, cultured, or previously frozen (liquid nitrogen) tumor cells and a differentially centrifuged tumor extract prepared according to the general procedure of MOLONEY [8]. In these limited experiments primates of four different species, *M. mulatta, M. speciosa, Cercopithecus aethiops* and *Saimiri sciureus,* were inoculated. In addition, two types of immunosuppression were employed. Imuran, at approximately 3 mg/kg body weight given orally, was used with three animals. One juvenile, rhesus monkey was subjected to lethal whole body x-irradiation (950 rads) and antilymphocyte serum followed by bone marrow replacement with autologous, nonirradiated cells to which previously frozen lymphosarcoma cells were added. Although a large number of lymphosarcoma cells were administered in this latter test, the number of live tumor cells was relatively small due to the low viability of these cells when recovered from liquid nitrogen. No tumors have developed in any of these inoculated monkeys, to date. The surviving animals are being maintained under observation.

Further study of this and other cases of lymphosarcoma occurring in rhesus monkeys is deemed highly significant. The disease, in many of its pathologic features, resembles Burkitt's lymphoma of man [9], and thus might serve as a model for that condition. The epizootic nature of the disease at the NCPB suggests the possibility of a viral etiology and that under certain circumstances a fairly sizable outbreak may occur, although other causes have by no means been excluded. Currently, while it has been reported that at least two herpes-type viruses of New World monkeys induce lymphosarcoma in monkeys of other species [6, 7], no agent has been reported which will induce lymphosarcoma in members of its own species. Other spontaneous primate tumors have had viruses associated with them. These include a

Table I. Attempted transmission of spontaneous lymphosarcoma of rhesus monkey MMU 6029

Monkey	Age at inoculation	Inoculum/route	Other treatment	Results
MM[1] 7068	34 days	4.3×10^7 viable, fresh tumor cells, s.c.	none	died 113 days post-inoculation, no tumor
SS[2] 80	1 day	1.6×10^7 viable, 8-day cultured tumor cells, s.c.	imuran	no tumor > 310 days postinoculation
CA[3] 302	2 days	1.6×10^7 viable, 9-day cultured tumor cells, s.c.	imuran	no tumor > 310 days postinoculation
MM[1] 7094	1 day	1 gram-equivalent differentially centri-fuged tumor extract, s.c.	imuran	died 28 days post-inoculation, no tumor
MS[4] 291	26 days	1 gram-equivalent differentially centri-fuged tumor extract, s.c.	none	died 253 days post-inoculation, no tumor
MM[1] B4084	2 years	3.4×10^7 (1% viable) frozen tumor cells, i.v.	bone marrow re-placement and ALS[5]	no tumor > 80 days postinoculation
MM[1] B4080	2 years	3.4×10^7 (1% viable) frozen tumor cells, i.v.	none	no tumor > 80 days postinoculation

1 *Macaca mulatta,* rhesus monkey.
2 *Saimiri sciureus,* squirrel monkey.
3 *Cercopithecus aethiops,* African green monkey.
4 *Macaca spesiosa,* stump-tailed macaque.
5 Antilymphocyte serum.

fibrosarcoma of a woolly monkey (*Lagothrix* sp.) [10], a mammary carcinoma of a rhesus monkey [2], and lymphosarcoma of a gibbon (*Hylobates* sp.) [5]. Of these viruses, the isolate from the woolly monkey tumor has been shown to be oncogenic for marmosets (*Saguinus* sp.) [11].

Furthermore, it would be of direct research value to have either a transmissible or transplantable neoplasm of a highly evolved Old World monkey, especially of a well-studied and readily propagated species such as rhesus, available for experimental purposes.

Acknowledgements

We should like to acknowledge the co-operation and assistance of Dr. H. C. CHOPRA, Dr. R. L. HEBERLING, Dr. S. S. KALTER, Dr. R. A. GRIESEMER, Dr. C. C. DARROW, Dr. E. W. KINGSBURY, Mr. E. E. CALLAWAY, and Mrs. JUANITA BROWN in various aspects of this study.

References

1 CHOPRA, H. C.; HOOKS, J. J.; WALLING, M. J., and GIBBS, C. J., jr.: Morphology of simian foamyviruses, with particular reference to virus isolated from spontaneous tumor of a rhesus monkey. J. nat. Cancer Inst. *48:* 451–463 (1972).

2 CHOPRA, H. C. and MASON, M. M.: A new virus in a spontaneous mammary tumor of a rhesus monkey. Cancer Res. *30:* 2081–2086 (1970).

3 HSU, T. C. and BENIRSCHKE, K.: An atlas of mammalian chromosomes, vol. 3, p. 147 (Springer, New York 1969).

4 JOHNSTON, P. B.: Taxonomic features of seven serotypes of simian and ape foamy-viruses. Infect. Immun. *3:* 793–799 (1971).

5 KAWAKAMI, T. G.; HUFF, S. D.; BUCKLEY, P. M.; DUNGWORTH, D. L., and SNYDER, S. P.: C-type virus associated with gibbon lymphosarcoma. Nature New Biol. *235:* 170–171 (1972).

6 MELENDEZ, L. V.; HUNT, R. D.; DANIEL, M. D.; GARCIA, F. G., and FRASER, C. E. O.: *Herpesvirus saimiri.* II. Experimentally-induced malignant lymphoma in primates. Lab. Anim. Care *19:* 378–386 (1969).

7 MELENDEZ, L. V.; HUNT, R. D.; KING, N. W.; BARAHONA, H. H.; DANIEL, M. D.; FRASER, C. E. O., and GARCIA, F. G.: *Herpesvirus ateles,* a new lymphoma virus of monkeys. Nature New Biol. *235:* 182–184 (1972).

8 MOLONEY, J. B.: Biological studies on a lymphoid-leukemia virus extract from sarcoma 37. I. Origin and introductory studies. J. nat. Cancer Inst. *24:* 933–951 (1960).

9 STOWELL, R. E.; SMITH, E. K.; ESPANA, C., and NELSON, V. G.: Outbreak of malignant lymphoma in rhesus monkeys. Lab. Invest. *25:* 476–479 (1971).

10 THEILEN, G. H.; GOULD, D.; FOWLER, M., and DUNGWORTH, D. L.: C-type virus in tumor tissues of a woolly monkey (*Lagothrix* spp.) fibrosarcoma. J. nat. Cancer Inst. *47:* 881–889 (1971).

11 WOLFE, L. G.; DEINHARDT, F.; THEILEN, G. H.; RABIN, H.; KAWAKAMI, T. G., and BUSTAD, L. K.: Induction of tumors in marmoset monkeys by simian sarcoma virus, type 1 *(Lagothrix).* A preliminary report. J. nat. Cancer Inst. *47:* 1115–1120 (1971).

Authors' addresses: HARVEY RABIN, PhD, Department of Virology and Cell Biology, Litton Bionetics, Inc., 5510 Nicholson Lane, *Kensington, MD 20795;* GORDON H. THEILEN, DVM, Department of Clinical Sciences, School of Veterinary Medicine and VICKI G. NELSON, DVM, CARLOS ESPANA, PhD and E. KAYE SMITH, DVM, National Center for Primate Biology, University of California, *Davis, CA 95616* (USA)

Medical Primatology 1972. Proc. 3rd Conf. exp. Med. Surg. Primates, Lyon 1972, part III, pp. 176–196 (Karger, Basel 1972)

Oncornaviruses Associated with Spontaneous and Experimentally Induced Neoplasia in Nonhuman Primates[1]

A Review

L. G. Wolfe and F. Deinhardt

Departments of Microbiology, Rush-Presbyterian-St. Luke's and University of Illinois Medical Centers, Chicago, Ill.

Introduction

The potential usefulness of nonhuman primates as experimental animal models for tumors induced by RNA viruses was first suggested in 1963 [44] by the report of tumor induction in rhesus monkeys *(Macaca mulatta)* by Rous sarcoma virus (RSV). During the past decade the susceptibility of nonhuman primates to RSV was confirmed and greatly expanded [2, 3, 9, 10, 13, 35, 42, 43, 45, 46, 49, 51–53, 71, 73–77] and the oncogenicity of several other oncogenic RNA viruses (oncornaviruses) was evaluated. Feline fibrosarcoma virus (FeSV) was oncogenic in several species of nonhuman primates [12, 13, 66, 72] whereas oncogenicity of avian leukosis viruses, murine leukemia and sarcoma viruses, and feline leukemia viruses has not been demonstrated in nonhuman primates as yet [71].

Within the past three years, oncornaviruses also were isolated from three naturally-occurring tumors of nonhuman primates. The Mason-Pfizer monkey virus (M-PMV) [4] was isolated from a mammary carcinoma of a rhesus monkey, simian sarcoma virus, type 1 *(Lagothrix)* (SSV-1) from a fibrosarcoma of a woolly monkey (*Lagothrix* sp.) [65] and a 'gibbon isolate' (GL) from a lymphosarcoma of a gibbon ape *(Hylobates lar)* [32]. All three isolates have structural and biochemical properties characteristic of oncornaviruses [48], including 60–70S single stranded RNA and RNA-dependent DNA

1 Conducted under contract No. 71–2032, Special Virus Cancer Program, NCI, and supported in part by grant RR-05477, General Research Support Branch, DRFR, NIH, USPHS.

polymerase but, so far, oncogenic activity has been demonstrated only for SSV-1 [70].

The principal objectives of this report are: (1) to review the role of nonhuman primates as experimental models for RSV and FeSV; (2) to discuss the oncogenicity of SSV-1; and (3) to discuss briefly M-PMV and GL, both of which will be discussed in more detail by other speakers at this symposium.

Rous Sarcoma Virus

A discussion of the susceptibility of nonhuman primates to RSV will be limited to general considerations in lieu of an excellent comprehensive review of the subject recently published by RABIN [51]. Strains of RSV oncogenic for nonhuman primates [51] include Schmidt-Ruppin (SR-RSV), Carr-Zilber (CZ-RSV), Bryan high titer (Br-RSV) and CT 559 (a strain representative of the RSV used by Dr. BRYAN to develop Br-RSV), with oncogenicity of the SR-RSV and CZ-RSV strains being more thoroughly studied. Tumors have been induced, by one or more of these strains, in one species of prosimian *(Galago crassicaudatus)* [53, 71], in two genera of marmoset monkeys *(Saguinus, Callithrix)* [9, 10, 13, 35, 49, 71], in squirrel monkeys *(Saimiri sciureus)* [51, 52, 71], in several species of Old World monkeys *(Macaca mulatta* [2, 3, 42–46, 53, 75–77], *M. fascicularis* [53, 73, 74, 77], *M. nemestrina* [75–77], *Cercopithecus aethiops* [53, 75–77], *C. pygerthyrus* [71], *C. talapoin* [51]) and in baboons *(Papio hamadryas)* [30, 75–77]. Of this group, marmosets (genus *Saguinus)* and rhesus monkeys were the most thoroughly studied. Based on incidence, latent period and behavior of the tumors, marmoset monkeys *(S. fuscicollis, S. nigricollis, S. oedipus)* were the most susceptible followed in descending order of susceptibility by squirrel monkeys and marmosets of the genus *Callithrix*, by Old World monkeys and baboons, and finally, by galagos.

In our laboratory, all 34 marmosets of genus *Saguinus* inoculated with $\geq 10^5$ FFU of SR-RSV before five months of age and without immunosuppressive conditioning developed progressive sarcomas (fibrosarcomas, undifferentiated sarcomas) after latent periods of 23 days (arithmetic mean time) and died approximately five weeks postinoculation (arithmetic mean time) [13, 71]. Marmosets inoculated when one year old or older were still susceptible [13, 49, 71] but, in our experience, the tumor incidence dropped from 100 to 83%, the percentage of progressive tumors decreased from 100 to 70, and the latent periods and clinical courses were significantly longer than in those animals inoculated before five months of age. Serial transmission of RSV-induced tumors was successful between chimeric twin or unrelated marmosets without immunosuppressive conditioning [13, 38, 71]. In addition to fibrosarcomas and undifferentiated sarcomas, Levy *et al.* [35] reported the induction of rhabdomyosarcomas in genus *Saguinus* and rhabdomyosarcomas and osteosarcomas in genus *Callithrix*. Although the data are limited, marmosets appeared more susceptible to SR-RSV than to CZ-RSV [14] or Br-RSV [13].

Squirrel monkeys inoculated up to ten months old were consistently susceptible to tumor induction by RSV and 45% of these animals developed locally progressive sarcomas (no distant metastases) whereas animals older than four years were refractory to RSV inoculation [51]. Old World monkeys and baboons inoculated as newborns or neonates also developed local fibromas or fibrosarcomas at the inoculation sites but nearly all of these tumors spontaneously regressed [2, 3, 42–45, 53, 71, 74–77]. Berman *et al.* [2], comparing prenatal *versus* newborn inoculation of rhesus monkeys, found no appreciable differences in tumor behavior or susceptibility to tumor induction. However, juvenile and adult Old World monkeys, normally completely refractory to RSV inoculation, were made as susceptible as newborns, or more so, by immunosuppressive or progesterone conditioning [43, 45, 46]. Tumor induction by serial passage of homologous tumor cells of rhesus monkeys was only successful in immunosuppressed recipients [43]. Pregnant rhesus monkeys inoculated in late gestation also were susceptible to RSV [43, 45], much like progesterone-conditioned adults. In addition, enhanced susceptibility in older animals was achieved in baboons by cortisone treatment [30] and in a squirrel monkey by treatment with caprine antisquirrel monkey thymocyte globulin [51].

C-type virus particles have not been found in RSV-induced tumors of nonhuman primates [13, 42, 46, 71, 74], with the exception of a few extracellular virus-like particles observed in two tumors of squirrel monkeys [71]. Intracytoplasmic membranous structures previously described in RSV-induced marmoset tumor cells [62] might have represented sites of viral activity, but they were not specific for RSV-infected cells; identical structures were found in marmoset cells infected with FeSV and SSV-1. In addition to absence of complete virions in RSV-induced tumors, avian group specific (GS) antigen also was not detected by complement-fixation tests in tumor extracts from marmoset [13, 71] and rhesus monkeys [3], except for a single observation reported by Rabotti *et al.* [53] in a rhesus monkey. However, the RSV genome was recovered from RSV-induced tumors either by back-passage of minced neoplastic tissue into susceptible chickens with subsequent tumor development and virus reisolation [2, 42, 43, 73–77], or by cocultivating tumor cells grown *in vitro* with susceptible chick embryo fibroblasts (CEF) [13, 71]. Despite the apparent absence of C-type virus particles and GS antigen in most RSV-induced tumors, neutralizing and/or complement fixing avian leukosis (COFAL) (GS) antibodies were demonstrated in many tumor-bearing animals [2, 3, 13, 42, 71, 74, 77]. Casey *et al.* [3] found COFAL antibodies but no neutralizing antibodies in two of two rhesus monkeys, whereas Berman *et al.* [2] detected both COFAL and neutralizing antibodies in two of four rhesus monkeys and reported that the appearance of neutralizing antibody preceded the demonstration of COFAL antibody. In all four antibody-positive animals, the antibody responses paralleled tumor growth, i.e., antibody titers were highest when the tumors were largest, and then decreased to undetectable levels after tumor regression. In our laboratory serum neutralizing antibodies to RSV were detected in seven of 13 marmosets tested [13] whereas COFAL antibodies were demonstrated in three other animals not tested for neutralizing antibodies. The apparent inconsistency of production of neutralizing and COFAL antibodies in tumor-bearing animals without expression of complete virus or GS antigens in the tumors is not presently understood.

Several simian cell lines have been transformed *in vitro* by RSV. Marmoset kidney, skin, and muscle cell lines transformed by SR-RSV [37, 39] contained small amounts of avian GS antigen, detected by indirect immunofluorescence, but did not produce infectious virus. In contrast to marmoset tumor cells grown *in vitro,* virus was not recovered after cocultivation of the transformed marmoset cells with highly susceptible CEF, and the transformed cells were not tumorigenic in quail. Similar results were reported for RSV-infected African green monkey kidney cells [24]. However, the marmoset cells that were transformed *in vitro,* from which no virus was rescued, produced tumors (progressive or regressive) in autologous hosts and the RSV genome was rescued from the tumor cells by cocultivating them *in vitro* with CEF [13, 37, 39]. Similar experiments are in progress to determine the reproducibility of this finding, i.e., the inability to rescue the RSV genome after transformation of marmoset cells *in vitro* but rescue of complete virus after these cells have grown *in vivo.* Rhesus leptomeningeal and brain cells also have been transformed *in vitro* by SR-RSV and these transformed cells contained GS antigen but produced no infectious virus [53], comparable to the RSV-transformed marmoset and African green monkey cells. The transformed rhesus cells induced tumors in chickens, from which infectious SR-RSV was recovered, and grew in newborn rhesus monkeys as progressive tumors, seemingly more malignant than tumors induced in rhesus monkeys either by cell-free virus or by tumor cells grown *in vitro*.

Marker chromosomes were not found in marmoset cells transformed *in vitro* by RSV or in cell lines established from RSV-induced marmoset tumors [13, 37, 71]. Random changes including chromatid breaks, secondary constrictions, and dicentric or ring chromosomes were observed in a variable percentage of diploid and aneuploid cells from both RSV-infected and uninfected cell cultures.

Feline Sarcoma Virus

The transmissibility of naturally-occurring fibrosarcomas of cats was first described in 1969 [64] and was confirmed in later reports [19, 41, 63, 66]. All transmissible sarcomas contained C-type virus particles and cell-free virus preparations of the spontaneous tumors were oncogenic in cats. Oncogenicity of two strains of FeSV, Snyder-Theilen (ST-FeSV) and Gardner-Arnstein (GA-FeSV), was demonstrated in nonhuman primates. Marmoset monkeys *(S.fuscicollis, S.nigricollis, S.oedipus)* were highly susceptible to both strains of FeSV [13, 72]; macaques *(M.mulatta, M.radiata, M.fascicularis)* [66] and squirrel monkeys *(S.sciureus)* [51] were susceptible to ST-FeSV. All 11 marmoset monkeys $\leq$ one month old inoculated i.p. or i.m. with $\geq 2.0 \times 10^3$ focus forming units of virus [40] developed sarcomas after latent periods of two to four weeks and died from their progressive neoplastic disease one to four months after inoculation. Animals inoculated when two months old were less susceptible than newborns or neonates; two of three animals developed tumors at the i.m. inoculation sites, one progressive and one regressive. Of marmosets inoculated when four months old or older, only an aged marmoset ($>$ nine years old) developed a tumor (regressive) during an observation period of two years. Although only a single observation, the latter finding suggested that aged marmosets might be more susceptible, perhaps comparable to animals approximately two months old. All six squirrel monkeys inoculated s.c. with cell-free preparations of ST-FeSV developed tumors after latent periods of two to five weeks [51]. Two animals inoculated as newborns developed rapidly-growing sarcomas whereas the tumors regressed four to six weeks after inoculation in one animal inoculated when two days old and in three inoculated as juveniles or adults. Five of six macaques inoculated s.c. when five to ten days old with ST-FeSV also developed local tumors 15–17 days after inoculation, but they completely regressed within 50 days [66].

Tumor induction by transplantation of viable tumor cells was studied in squirrel [51] and marmoset [13, 72] monkeys. Allotransplantation and autotransplantation in squirrel monkeys produced only local nodules that regressed. In contrast, ten serial passages, with both strains of FeSV, were accomplished in marmosets by serial i.m. inoculation of minced neoplastic tissue into animals of opposite sex. All 36 marmosets inoculated when two days to three years old with intact cells developed sarcomas after latent periods of only four days to two weeks. Except for the tumors in three animals, all tumors progressively enlarged, attaining sizes of 3–6 cm in diameter, and the tumor-bearing animals became debilitated and died one to two months and one to six months, respectively, after inoculation with ST-FeSV or GA-FeSV. Of the tumors in the three other animals, two tumors are presently regressing, 18 months after inoculation, and the tumor in the third animal had completely regressed by one year postinoculation. Cytogenetic studies were done on cell cultures (after one to nine subpassages *in vitro)* established from 16 of these marmosets; 11 cultures were composed entirely of recipient cells, four cultures were composed of both recipient (36–93%) and donor (7–46%) cells and only one culture (fifth passage *in vivo* of ST-FeSV) was composed entirely of donor cells. Cultures containing the larger numbers of donor cells were established from tissues explanted *in vitro* 21 days or less after inoculation, suggesting that donor cells contributed to the early proliferative response but were later rejected and overgrown by recipient cells.

Pathologic studies have been performed on one or more tumors from all susceptible genera of nonhuman primates. The experimentally-induced tumors in macaques (biopsy specimens) were classified as fibrosarcomas [66] and the two progressive tumors in squirrel monkeys as undifferentiated sarcomas [51]. In marmosets the morphologic appearance of the 53 tumors studied [72] was not affected by the type of inoculum (cell-free or mince), route of inoculation or location of the tumor; there were some histologic differences, however, related to the virus strain. ST-FeSV induced undifferentiated sarcomas, poorly-differentiated fibrosarcomas or well-differentiated fibrosarcomas whereas GA-FeSV consistently induced only well-differentiated fibrosarcomas. The morphology of marmoset tumor cells grown *in vitro* closely resembled the respective tumor morphology and the two virus strains also induced morphologically-distinct foci in cat [57] and marmoset cells, suggesting that the differences in morphologic appearance of the tumors induced by ST- and GA-FeSV reflected differences in the virus genomes rather than selective affinity of the two virus strains for different cells. Metastatic lesions were found in the lungs of 11 % and in regional lymph nodes of 19 % of the tumor-bearing marmosets. Multinucleated giant cells, identical to those commonly found in the regional lymph nodes of marmosets inoculated with RSV [13, 49, 71], also were observed in regional lymph nodes of 45 % of the tumor-bearing marmosets.

C-type virus particles were not found by electron microscopy in any tumors induced by cell-free FeSV preparations, namely those induced in Old World, squirrel and marmoset monkeys [13, 51, 66, 72]. However, the serially-transmitted marmoset tumors contained budding and extracellular C-type virus particles, 110–120 nm in diameter, at all passage levels examined (first, third, fifth and tenth) [72]. Based on a study of the sequential development of marmoset tumors and on the presence or absence of virus, the development of the tumors induced by cell-free preparations was best explained by clonal proliferation of the originally-transformed cells, whereas infection and transformation of contiguous mesenchymal cells probably contributed to the development of the virus-producing, serially-transmitted tumors. Virus produced by the transplanted tumors transformed marmoset and cat cells *in vitro* although its oncogenicity *in vivo* has not been demonstrated as yet [72]. Of cell cultures established from FeSV-induced tumors, C-type virus was not found in two cell lines derived from squirrel monkey tumors [51], but was produced by 11 of 16 cell lines established from marmoset tumors, including four of six cell lines established from tumors induced by cell-free ST-FeSV in which no virus was detected in the neoplastic tissue. Therefore, although marmoset tumor cells induced by cell-free virus did not produce detectable virus in the original host, transfer of these cells to other marmosets or the growth of these cells *in vitro* resulted in complete virus expression. The virus produced by the tumor cell lines was oncogenic in marmosets and cats and transformed marmoset and cat cells *in vitro*.

GS antigen was demonstrated by microcomplement-fixation tests [56] in marmoset tumors, marmoset tumor cell lines [72] and a squirrel monkey tumor cell line [51]. GS antigen was present in marmoset tumors induced either by cell-free virus preparations or minced neoplastic tissue, irrespective of demonstration of virus particles by electron microscopy, indicating at least partial expression of the virus genome in all of the tumors. Serums of tumor-bearing marmosets were tested for GS antibodies by counterimmunoelectrophoresis (CIEP) [22] and immunodiffusion tests. GS antibodies were demonstrated in 17 of 50 tumor-bearing marmosets; both species-specific and interspecies [59] GS antibodies were demonstrated by gel diffusion, using murine leukemia virus and feline leukemia virus GS antigens. The time interval between initial detection of tumors and the detection of GS antibodies was usually six weeks or longer. One animal, for example, developed antibodies detectable by CIEP six weeks after inoculation, and by five months postinoculation had a titer of 1:512. Of the 37 tumor-bearing marmosets without demonstrable GS antibodies, only seven of 37 had postinoculation courses of six weeks or longer.

Marmosets in the serial-transmission series also developed antibody to feline oncornavirus-associated cell membrane antigen (FOCMA) [16], demonstrated by indirect immunofluorescence using viable feline and human lymphoblastoid cell lines infected with feline leukemia virus [17]. In preliminary studies, a correlation between the progressive or regressive behavior of marmoset tumors and the titers of FOCMA-specific antibody was not evident in the seven animals tested, in contrast to cats and dogs with FeSV-induced tumors. Little or no detectable antibody was found in cats and dogs with progressive tumors, whereas those with regressive tumors developed a substantial rise in membrane-reactive antibody [15, 16]. In addition to GS and FOCMA antibodies, serum neutralizing antibodies also were demonstrated in several marmosets with serially-transmitted tumors, but these studies are still in progress.

Mason-Pfizer Monkey Virus

Mason-Pfizer monkey virus (M-PMV), the first RNA virus found associated with a spontaneous tumor in a nonhuman primate, was isolated from a spontaneous mammary adenocarcinoma of an eight-year-old rhesus monkey [4, 25]. The virus had a buoyant density of 1.14–1.16 g/ml in potassium citrate and sucrose gradients [25, 60], possessed an RNA-instructed DNA polymerase [60, 61] and contained a species of RNA with a sedimentation coefficient of 60–70 S [47, 60]. Polyacrylamide gel electrophoresis of the viral RNA indicated a molecular weight of approximately 7×10^6 daltons [36]. Replication of the virus was inhibited by actinomycin D [36, 47]. Cross-reactivity between M-PMV and simian foamy viruses [5, 47], visna, murine leukemia virus, hamster sarcoma virus, feline leukemia virus or mouse mammary tumor virus [47] was not demonstrated by immunodiffusion [47], indirect immunofluorescence [5] and neutralization tests [5].

M-PMV infected and replicated in rhesus monkey, chimpanzee, and human cell lines [6, 7, 18, 25]. One laboratory [18] reported the appearance of multinucleated giant cells in fetal rhesus-monkey lung and foreskin and human foreskin cell lines as early as 24 h after infection with M-PMV whereas other laboratories reported no apparent cytopathic changes in rhesus embryo and fetal lung, chimpanzee lung, and human embryo and lymphocyte (NC-37) cell cultures [6, 7, 25]. Electron microscopic studies of the original neoplastic tissue [4, 7] and of infected cell cultures [5–7, 25, 34, 36] revealed two types of particles, i.e., an intracytoplasmic, electron-dense, ring-shaped particle measuring about 70 nm in diameter and an extracellular particle about 110 nm in diameter, characterized by a centric dense nucleoid bounded by an intermediate membrane and an outer unit membrane without surface projections. The extracellular particles apparently were produced by budding of pre-assembled intracytoplasmic particles from the plasma membrane. Oncogenicity of M-PMV has not been demonstrated as yet, either with marmosets in our laboratory or with other species of nonhuman primates [7]. Marmosets inoculated with cell-free virus or infected human cells have not developed tumors during observation periods of 12–18 months.

Gibbon Lymphoma Isolate

C-type virus particles were present in lymph nodes, liver, spleen and bone marrow of a gibbon ape *(Hylobates lar)* with naturally-occurring lymphoma and were produced in cell cultures established from the neoplastic tissue [32]. GL had a buoyant density of 1.16 g/ml in sucrose gradients [32] and possessed an RNA-dependent DNA polymerase [32, 61]. It lacked the species-specific GS antigen of feline, murine and hamster oncornaviruses but contained the interspecies GS antigen common to known mammalian oncornaviruses [32, 61]. So far, oncogenicity of GL has not been demonstrated; marmosets inoculated with concentrated virions produced *in vitro* and supplied to us by Drs. KAWAKAMI and BUSTAD (University of California, Davis) have not developed any abnormalities during an observation period of one year.

GL infected and replicated in normal bovine, simian and human cells without producing morphologic transformation or a cytopathic effect [32]. We recently found that a fetal marmoset lung cell line also was susceptible to GL and that the mixed culture cytopathogenicity reaction (MC) [33, 55] could be used as an indicator system for infection. Marmoset lung cells infected with GL were seeded into 60-mm plastic Petri dishes (3.0×10^5 cells/dish), incubated at 37 °C for 16–24 h and then overlaid with XC cells (1.0 ×

10^6 cells/dish). The XC cell line, first used in a MC test by KLEMENT *et al.* [33] for detection of cells producing murine leukemia virus, was established from a rat tumor induced by RSV. Within 24–48 h after the XC cells were added to the GL-infected marmoset cells, large multinucleated syncytial cells formed throughout the cell sheet, representing a simple and rapid indicator system. SCOLNICK *et al.* [61] demonstrated 'helper activity' with GL wherein GL and murine leukemia virus rescued comparable titers of focus forming mouse virus from an nonproducer rat cell line transformed by Kirsten sarcoma virus.

Simian Sarcoma Virus, Type 1 (Lagothrix)

The C-type RNA virus isolated from a spontaneous fibrosarcoma of a three-year-old male woolly monkey (*Lagothrix* sp.) [65] was designated SSV-1 based on its origin and on the probability that additional C-type sarcoma viruses will be isolated from nonhuman primate tumors [70]. Virions present in the neoplastic tissue and bone marrow of this animal [65] were similar morphologically to the C-type viruses associated with leukemias and sarcomas in chickens, mice and cats. The virus had a buoyant density of 1.14–1.15 g/ml in sucrose gradients [26, 31], possessed an RNA-directed DNA polymerase [26, 31, 61], and contained the interspecies GS antigen [11, 31, 61]. Oncogenicity of SSV-1 was demonstrated in white-lipped *(S.nigricollis, S.fuscicollis)* and cotton-topped *(S.oedipus)* marmosets [11, 13, 70], a white-moustached *(S.mystax)* marmoset [51], and squirrel monkeys [51].

Tumors developed at the inoculation sites in two of four squirrel monkeys and in one of one white-moustached marmoset that were inoculated when one to five days old or *in utero* with homogenates or cell-free preparations of the original woolly monkey sarcoma [51]. However, these tumors 'could not be classified unequivocally as sarcomas' and no virus particles were found by electron microscopy. The susceptibility of marmosets, genus *Saguinus,* to SSV-1 is summarized in table I. The marmoset tumors were classified as fibromas or well-differentiated fibrosarcomas, with either slowly progressive or regressive behavior, and C-type virus particles were observed in five of six tumors studied. Of the 17 tumor-bearing animals presented in table I, only the animal with a postinoculation course of one year (group A) developed tumor metastases. C-type virus was present in a metastatic tumor and in regional lymph nodes, spleen and bone marrow of this animal. Serial transmission to unrelated marmosets was accomplished using minced neoplastic tissue and the tumors in the recipients were composed of recipient

Table I. Induction of tumors in newborn and neonatal marmosets[1] with SSV-1 preparations.

Group	Inoculum		Inoculation		Number inoculated	Tumors developed	Tumor			
	source	amount[2]	age, days	route			latent period weeks	behavior[3]	course months	C-type virus[4]
A	woolly monkey tumor (cell-free extract)	0.4 gte	1	i.m.	1	1	4	progressor	12	yes
B	marmoset lung cells transformed by inoculum used in group A	5.0×10⁶ cells	1–5	i.m.	4	3	1–2	progressor (1) ND (2)	4.5 –	NE yes
C	tumor mince (group A or B tumors)	<0.1 gms	1–90	i.m.	4	4	1–2	progressor (1) regressor (3)	2.5 3–5	NE yes
D	marmoset tumor cell lines (derived from group A, B or C tumors)	5.0–6.0 ×10⁶ cells	3–7	i.m.	6	6	1–6	progressor (1) regressor (5)	4.5 3–6	NE NE
E	cell-free supernatant (group B tumor cell cultures)	1.0–6.0 ×10³ FFU	1–9	i.m. or i.p.	5	0	–	–	–	–
		4.0–8.0 ×10⁴ FFU	2–5	i.m.	3	2	4, 6	progressor (1) regressor (1)	4.5 4	yes NE
F	human fetal lung cells transformed by group E inoculum	5.0×10⁶ cells	5	i.m.	1	1	3	progressor	2	yes

1 *Saguinus fuscicollis, S. nigricollis, S. oedipus.*
2 gte = gram tumor equivalents; FFU = focus forming units on marmoset lung indicator cells.
3 ND = not determined: One tumor-bearing animal died of pneumonia two weeks after inoculation; tumor from one animal was excised *in toto* three weeks after inoculation; number of animals with progressor or regressor tumors in parenthesis.
4 NE = not evaluated.

cells as determined by sex chromosomal analyses. The tumor-bearing marmosets developed serum neutralizing antibody titers up to 1:64, the highest titer demonstrated in the animal with the longest clinical course (group A, table I). Attempts to demonstrate serum GS antibodies in the tumor-bearing marmosets are in progress. Five marmoset tumor cell lines studied so far all produced C-type virus which transformed marmoset, human and cat cells *in vitro* and was oncogenic *in vivo*.

The effect of neonatal thymectomy [27] and administration of rabbit antimarmoset thymocyte serum (ATS) on latent period, clinical course and behavior of SSV-1 induced tumors in marmosets also was evaluated, using viable tumor cells cultured *in vitro* as inocula [28]. Neonatal thymectomy had no significant effect on the susceptibility of six marmosets studied. Marmosets treated with ATS (1.0 ml daily; 15 mg γ-globulin/ml) for two to three weeks after inoculation developed tumors that usually grew more rapidly than those of untreated controls but regressed when the ATS therapy was discontinued. In contrast an animal pretreated with ATS for four days prior to inoculation and continued on ATS therapy throughout a six-week clinical course developed a massive tumor at the i.m. inoculation site and widespread metastases to subcutaneous tissues, lung and kidney, representing an increased severity of the malignant disease caused by immunosuppressive conditioning.

SSV-1 was characterized by a broad host range *in vitro,* with transformation of rat [61], cat, marmoset and human cells [68] reported so far. Focus assay of SSV-1, routinely performed in our laboratory on fetal marmoset lung cells [68], was highly reproducible and quantitative without need for an agar overlay. Foci of piled-up, spindle-shaped cells appeared as early as four days postinfection, and final counts were made 14–21 days postinfection. Pretreatment of the indicator cells with DEAE-dextran (20 μg/ml) for 60 min before inoculation increased the sensitivity of the assay 10–50 times (mean: 25.6) [68]. Unconcentrated supernatants collected from marmoset tumor cell lines contained titers of SSV-1 ranging between 1.0×10^3 and 1.5×10^4 focus forming units/ml. The number of focus forming units in each preparation was proportional to the virus dilution factor (one-hit titration pattern). The SSV-1 produced by cells transformed *in vitro* retained its oncogenicity for marmosets (table I) [68].

All SSV-1 stocks tested so far contained a nontransforming associated virus (SSAV-1), similar to previous findings with avian, murine and feline sarcoma viruses. Interference tests performed in cell cultures infected with SSV-1 stock preparations beyond the endpoint of focus induction and subsequently challenged with SSV-1 after three or four subcultures indicated a 10- to 100-fold excess of an interfering agent. The presence or absence of C-type virus demonstrated by electron microscopy in unchallenged parallel cultures correlated with the presence or absence of interference [11, 13, 68]. Cell lines established from marmoset cells infected with SSV-1 beyond the focus endpoint (producing SSAV-1 but no detectable SSV-1) grew as monolayer cultures indistinguishable from uninfected cells [68]. SCOLNICK *et al.* [61] used SSAV-1 produced by rat kidney cells to rescue focus-forming, mouse sarcoma virus from a nonproducer rat cell line transformed by Kirsten sarcoma virus, thereby demonstrating 'helper activity' of SSAV-1. In addition to rescue, interference, electron microscopic, and immunologic (indirect immunofluorescence or complement-fixation) methods for demonstration of SSAV-1, the MC test [33, 55], briefly described in the preceding section, also was used as an indicator system for SSAV-1 infections in cell culture. RANGAN *et al.* [54] described a positive MC reaction in canine embryo fibroblast and canine fibrosarcoma cell lines infected with SSV-1 stock preparations (preparations containing both SSV-1 and SSAV-1), and we confirmed their observations using canine fibrosarcoma and fetal marmoset lung cell lines infected only with SSAV-1. Numerous multinucleated giant cells developed within 24 h after adding XC cells to the SSAV-1 infected cells.

Discussion

Several species of nonhuman primates were susceptible to tumor induction by avian, feline and simian sarcoma viruses. Of the species evaluated, marmoset monkeys, genus *Saguinus,* were the most susceptible based on tumor incidence and on the malignant behavior of the tumors, even without immunosuppressive conditioning. MUNROE and his colleagues [43, 45, 46] demonstrated that immunosuppressive and hormonal conditioning of rhesus monkeys greatly increased their susceptibility to tumor induction by RSV, perhaps equaling the susceptibility of marmosets, but the effect of similar conditioning on the susceptibility of rhesus monkeys to other oncogenic viruses has been either ineffective or not studied. In single observations, conditioning of squirrel and marmoset monkeys with ATS also enhanced their susceptibility to RSV and SSV-1, respectively. Based on information presently available, attempts to develop other sarcoma model systems in nonhuman primates with potentially oncogenic materials, e.g., human tumor materials, should include inoculation of newborn marmosets, with and without ATS conditioning, and as second choices dependent on availability, immunosuppressed or hormonally-treated squirrel and/or Old World monkeys.

Universal susceptibility to all avian and mammalian oncornaviruses has not been demonstrated in any nonhuman primate species so far. For unexplained reason(s), oncogenicity of murine sarcoma viruses has not been demonstrated in nonhuman primates, including marmosets [71], and no nonhuman primates have proven susceptible to avian, murine and feline leukemia viruses, despite broad host ranges of infectivity *in vitro*. Marmosets inoculated with Rauscher murine leukemia [71] and feline leukemia viruses have not developed abnormalities during observation periods of one to three years although none of the animals have been evaluated for virus replication *in vivo*. In contrast marmoset lymphoreticular cells are highly susceptible to malignant transformation *in vivo* by *Herpesvirus saimiri* [23, 67].

An explanation for the difference in susceptibility to oncornaviruses among species of nonhuman primates is presently unknown. Two major considerations are the inherent, relative susceptibility of target cells to different oncogenic viruses and the maturity of the immune system. Meaningful comparisons of target-cell susceptibility in different species of nonhuman primates have not been made, and even so, such information obtained *in vitro* might be impossible to extrapolate to conditions *in vivo*. Many studies in other species have suggested that the stage of immunologic maturity in the experimental host is the principal regulator of susceptibility or resistance to tumor induction by oncogenic viruses, which theoretically could explain the difference in susceptibility among some or all of the nonhuman primates. Fetal rhesus monkeys, for example, soon after midgestation can produce antibodies in response to certain antigens and can reject skin homografts [8]. The observations of BERMAN *et al.* [2] that RSV-induced tumors regressed in rhesus monkeys whether induced in fetuses during midgestation or in neonates might indicate that rhesus monkeys have a degree of immunologic competence to tumor-associated antigens very early in fetal life. The marked effect of immunosuppressive conditioning on susceptibility of rhesus monkeys also favors an immunologic basis for resistance. If the hypothesis is correct that immunologic competence regulates susceptibility and resistance to experimental tumor induction, the immune mechanism of the highly susceptible marmoset must be impaired or immunologic maturity at least considerably delayed, compared to other nonhuman primates. Unfortunately, the humoral and cell-mediated immune responses have not been thoroughly investigated in marmosets of any age group so detailed data to support or reject this hypothesis are unavailable. A major difference between marmosets and other species of nonhuman primates lies in the fact that fraternal twinning regularly occurs [14, 21, 69] and the twins are hematopoietic chimeras [1, 20], a state that may impair their immunologic responses. In support of immunologic impairment, PORTER and GENGOZIAN [50] found that rejection of skin allografts is delayed in adult marmosets, compared to other species. However, evidence suggesting that marmosets already have at least some measure of immunologic maturity during the early neonatal period or at birth includes: (1) inability of neonatal thymectomy to alter the clinical course of SSV-1 induced tumors in contrast to enhanced malignant behavior after treatment with ATS [28]; (2) peripheral lymphocytes of marmosets at various ages (two weeks, two months, six months, adults) respond similarly to stimulation with phytohemagglutinin-P [29]; and (3) the presence of small lymphocytes in lymphoid tissues at birth.

Age-related susceptibility was demonstrated in rhesus monkeys to RSV-induced tumors and in marmoset monkeys to RSV- and FeSV-induced tumors. Rhesus monkeys one month old or less were consistently susceptible to local tumor induction by RSV (although the tumors usually spontaneously regressed), but complete resistance was established by six months; little is known about their susceptibility to RSV when one to six months old. Marmoset monkeys inoculated with RSV when eight months old or less consistently developed progressive sarcomas; 80–85% of adult animals also were susceptible to tumor induction by RSV although approximately 30% of tumors in adults spontaneously regressed. In contrast, marmosets became relatively resistant to tumor induction by cell-free FeSV at a much younger age, sometime between 1 and 4 months of age, suggesting that they were immunologically competent to eliminate FeSV-transformed cells at a younger age than RSV-transformed cells. Differences in immunologic responsiveness of the marmoset host in these two systems were not related to complete virus production because both RSV and FeSV tumors induced by cell-free virus were nonproducers. The susceptibility of one aged marmoset (> nine years old) to tumor induction by FeSV, although only a single observation, suggested that the susceptibility of aged marmosets may be enhanced, perhaps a manifestation of depressed immune potential. Little information has been accumulated so far on relative susceptibility of aged nonhuman primates to oncogenic viruses, primarily because of the limited availability of appropriate experimental hosts, but such information would be of interest in lieu of the increased incidence of spontaneous neoplasia with advancing age in both animals and man. Age-independent susceptibility of target cells has been demonstrated *in vitro* wherein cell cultures established from muscle biopsies of marmosets of different ages (newborn, neonates, juveniles, adults) were equally susceptible to transformation by RSV, FeSV and SSV-1.

Spontaneous neoplasia has been reported in most genera of nonhuman primates although the incidence is considered low, perhaps because of the young age groups evaluated. With current development of large breeding colonies and with more emphasis on long-term experimental studies, larger numbers of nonhuman primates will reach their natural life span and eventually the true incidence of neoplasia in simians will become apparent. A large percentage of spontaneous neoplasms reported so far have been in rhesus monkeys, probably reflecting the fact that they are the most widely used simian in research. During the past three years in our marmoset colony, we have observed spontaneous neoplasms in five of 994 animals studied: two of 402 white-lipped and one of 47 cotton-topped, colony-born animals and two of 479 white-lipped and zero of 66 cotton-topped marmosets imported as adults. Of these five neoplasms, two were lymphomas, reticulum cell type, that developed in parent-reared, fraternal twins (cross: *S. nigricollis* × *S. f. illigeri*) and killed the animals when ten and 11 months old, respectively. Virus particles were not found in the neoplastic tissues or in cell cultures established from the tumors. A bronchogenic carcinoma killed one imported animal (*S. f. illigeri*), maintained in our colony for six years, and bronchiolar adenocarcinomas were found in a 28-month-old, colony-born animal (*S. oedipus*) and in an imported white-lipped marmoset, maintained in our colony for seven years. Oncornaviruses were isolated from three spontaneous tumors of nonhuman primates during the past three years and more will probably be isolated in the future.

A thorough understanding of oncogenic virus-host cell interrelationships in infected cells of nonhuman primates, including the study of isolates both from simian and heterologous species, hopefully will result in a better understanding of potentially similar interactions involved in human neoplasia. The tumor models described in this report and similar models established with oncogenic herpesviruses also provide experimental systems for therapeutic trials that may yield valuable information for similar conditions in man.

References

1 Benirschke, K.; Anderson, J.M., and Brownhill, L.E.: Marrow chimerism in marmosets. Science *138:* 513–515 (1962).

2 Berman, L.D.; Cotes, P.M., and Simons, P.J.: Tumors and immunological response in rhesus monkeys born after *in utero* inoculation with Rous sarcoma virus. J.nat. Cancer Inst. *39:* 119–134 (1967).

3 Casey, M.J.; Turner, H.C.; Huebner R.J.; Sarma, P.S., and Miller, R.L.: Complement-fixing antibodies in monkeys bearing tumors induced by Rous sarcoma virus. Nature, Lond. *211:* 1417–1418 (1966).

4 Chopra, H.C. and Mason, M.M.: A new virus in a spontaneous mammary tumor of a rhesus monkey. Cancer Res. *30:* 2081–2086 (1970).

5 Chopra, H.C.; Hooks, J.J.; Walling, M.J., and Gibbs, C.J., jr.: Morphology of simian foamy viruses, with particular reference to virus isolated from spontaneous tumor of a rhesus monkey. J.nat.Cancer Inst. *48:* 451–463 (1972).

6 Chopra, H.C.; Zelljadt, I.; Jensen, E.M.; Mason, M.M., and Woodside, N.J.: Infectivity of cell cultures by a virus isolated from a mammary carcinoma of a rhesus monkey. J.nat.Cancer Inst. *46:* 127–137 (1971).

7 Chopra, H.C.; Zelljadt, I.; Woodside, N., and Walling, M.J.: Studies on virus particles resembling oncogenic RNA viruses in monkey breast carcinoma. Cancer *28:* 1406–1414 (1971).

8 Cotes, P.M.; Hobbs, K.R., and Bangham, D.R.: Development of the immune response in the fetal and newborn rhesus monkey. I. Response to bovine serum albumin. Immunology *11:* 185–198 (1966).

9 Deinhardt, F.: Neoplasms induced by Rous sarcoma virus in New World monkeys. Nature, Lond. *210:* 443 (1966).

10 Deinhardt, F.: Rous sarcoma virus-induced neoplasms in New World nonhuman primates. Perspectives in virology, vol.5, pp.183–197 (Academic Press, New York 1967).

11 Deinhardt, F.; Wolfe, L.; Massey, R.; Hoekstra, J., and McDonald, R.: Simian sarcoma virus. Oncogenicity, focus assay, presence of associated virus, and comparison with avian and feline sarcoma virus-induced neoplasia in marmoset monkeys; in Chieco-Bianchi and Dutcher Proc. 5th Int.Symp. on Comparative Leukemia Research, Padova 1971. Bibl.haemat., vol.39 (Karger, Basel, in press).

12 Deinhardt, F.; Wolfe, L.G.; Theilen, G.H., and Snyder, S.P.: ST-feline fibrosarcoma virus. Induction of tumors in marmoset monkeys. Science *167:* 881 (1970).

13 Deinhardt, F.; Wolfe, L.; Northrop, R.; Marczynska, B.; Odgen, J.; McDonald R.; Falk, L.; Shramek, G.; Smith, R., and Deinhardt, J.: Induction of neoplasms by viruses in marmoset monkeys. J.med.Prim. *1:* 29–50 (1972).

14 Epple, G.: Maintenance, breeding, and development of marmoset monkeys *(Callithricidae)* in captivity. Folia primat. *12:* 56–76 (1970).

15 Essex, M.; Snyder, S.P., and Klein, G.: Relationship between humoral antibodies and the failure to develop progressive tumors in cats injected with feline sarcoma virus (FSV); in Chieco-Bianchi and Dutcher Proc.5th Int.Symp. on Comparative Leukemia Research, Padova 1971. Bibl.haemat., vol.39 (Karger, Basel, in press).

16 Essex, M.; Klein, G.; Snyder, S.P., and Harrold, J.B.: Feline sarcoma virus induced tumors. Correlation between humoral antibody and tumor regression. Nature, Lond. *233:* 195–196 (1971).

17 Essex, M.; Klein, G.; Deinhardt, F.; Wolfe, L.G.; Hardy, W.D., jr.; Theilen,

G.H., and PEARSON, L.D.: Induction of the feline oncornavirus associated cell membrane antigen in human cells. Nature New Biology *238:* 187–189 (1972).

18 FINE, D.L.; LANDON, J.C., and KUBICEK, M.T.: Simian tumor virus isolate. Demonstration of cytopathic effects *in vitro.* Science *174:* 420–421 (1971).

19 GARDNER, M.B.; ARNSTEIN, P.; RONGEY, R.W.; ESTES, J.D.; SARMA, P.S.; RICKARD, C.G., and HUEBNER, R.J.: Experimental transmission of feline fibrosarcoma to cats and dogs. Nature, Lond. *226:* 807–809 (1970).

20 GENGOZIAN, N.; BATSON, S.; GREENE, C.T., and GOSSLEE, D.G.: Hemopoietic chimerism in imported and laboratory-bred marmosets. Transplantation *8:* 633–652 (1969).

21 HAMPTON, J.K., jr.; HAMPTON, S.H., and LEVY, B.M.: Reproductive physiology and pregnancy in marmosets; in GOLDSMITH and MOOR-JANKOWSKI Medical primatology 1970, pp. 527–535 (Karger, Basel 1971).

22 HOEKSTRA, J. and DEINHARDT, F.: Counterimmunoelectrophoresis-rapid method for detecting gs antigen and antibodies associated with oncogenic RNA viruses. Appl. Microbiol. *22:* 1172–1173 (1971).

23 HUNT, R.D.; MELENDEZ, L.V.; KING, N.W.; GILMORE, C.E.; DANIEL, M.D.; WILLIAMSON, M.E., and JONES, T.C.: Morphology of a disease with features of malignant lymphoma in marmosets and owl monkeys inoculated with *Herpesvirus saimiri.* J. nat. Cancer Inst. *44:* 447–465 (1970).

24 JENSEN, F.C.; GIRARDI, A.J.; GILDEN, R.V., and KOPROWSKI, H.: Infection of human and simian tissue cultures with Rous sarcoma virus. Proc. nat. Acad. Sci., Wash. *52:* 53–59 (1964).

25 JENSEN, E.M.; ZELLJADT, I.; CHOPRA, H.C., and MASON, M.M.: Isolation and propagation of a virus from a spontaneous mammary carcinoma of a rhesus monkey. Cancer Res. *30:* 2388–2393 (1970).

26 JENSIK, S.; NORTHROP, R.L., and DEINHARDT, F.: Unpubl. data.

27 JOHNSON, D. and STRAUS, A.: Personal commun.

28 JOHNSON, D.; WOLFE, L.G., and DEINHARDT, F.: Unpubl. data.

29 JOHNSON, T.R.: *In vitro* response of marmoset lymphocytes to phytohemagglutinin; thesis Chicago, Ill. (1970).

30 KALTER, S.S.; EUGSTER, A.K.; VICE, T.E.; KIM, C.S., and RATNER, I.A.: Rous sarcoma in baboons. Bact. Proc. *68:* 175 (1968).

31 KAWAKAMI, T.: Personal commun.

32 KAWAKAMI, T.G.; HUFF, S.D.; BUCKLEY, P.M.; DUNGWORTH, D.L., and SNYDER, S.P.: C-type virus associated with gibbon lymphosarcoma. Nature New Biol. *235:* 170–171 (1972).

33 KLEMENT, V.; ROWE, W.P.; HARTLEY, J.W., and PUGH, W.E.: Mixed culture cytopathogenicity. A new test for growth of murine leukemia viruses in tissue culture. Proc. nat. Acad. Sci., Wash. *63:* 753–758 (1969).

34 KRAMARSKY, B.; SARKAR, N.H., and MOORE, D.H.: Ultrastructural comparison of a virus from a rhesus-monkey mammary carcinoma with four oncogenic RNA viruses. Proc. nat. Acad. Sci., Wash. *68:* 1603–1607 (1971).

35 LEVY, B.M.; TAYLOR, A.C.; HAMPTON, S., and THOMA, G.W.: Tumors of the marmoset produced by Rous sarcoma virus. Cancer Res. *29:* 2237–2248 (1969).

36 MANNING, J.S. and HACKETT, A.J.: Morphological and biophysical properties of the Mason-Pfizer monkey virus. J. nat. Cancer Inst. *48:* 417–422 (1972).

37 MARCZYNSKA, B.; TREU-SARNAT, G., and DEINHARDT, F.: Characteristics of long-term marmoset cell cultures spontaneously altered or transformed by Rous sarcoma virus. J.nat.Cancer Inst. *44:* 545–572 (1970).

38 MARCZYNSKA, B.: Personal commun.

39 MASSEY, R.: Rous sarcoma virus induced transformation of marmoset cells; thesis Chicago, Ill. (1972).

40 MCDONALD, R.; WOLFE, L.G., and DEINHARDT, F.: Feline fibrosarcoma virus. Quantitative focus assay, focus morphology and evidence for a 'helper virus'. Int. J.Cancer *9:* 57–65 (1972).

41 MCDONOUGH, S.K.; LARSEN, S.; BRODEY, R.S.; STOCK, N.D., and HARDY, W.D., jr.: A transmissible feline fibrosarcoma of viral origin. Cancer Res. *31:* 953–956 (1971).

42 MUNROE, J.S.: Viral oncogenesis in the rhesus monkey. Miscellaneous studies. Some recent developments in comparative medicine. Symp. Zool.Soc.London, vol.17, pp.229–249 (Academic Press, London 1966).

43 MUNROE, J.S.: Subhuman primates in experimental viral oncology. Ann.N.Y.Acad. Sci. *162:* 556–567 (1969).

44 MUNROE, J.S. and WINDLE, W.F.: Tumors induced in primates by chicken sarcoma virus. Science *140:* 1415–1416 (1963).

45 MUNROE, J.S. and WINDLE, W.F.: Tumors induced by chick sarcoma in monkeys conditioned with progesterone. Nature, Lond. *216:* 811–813 (1967).

46 MUNROE, J.S.; SHIPKEY, F.; ERLANDSON, R.A., and WINDLE, W.F.: Tumors induced in juvenile and adult primates by chicken sarcoma virus. International conference on avian tumor viruses. Nat.Cancer Inst.Monogr. *17:* 365–390 (1964).

47 NOWINSKI, R.C.; EDYNAK, E., and SARKAR, N.H.: Serological and structural properties of Mason-Pfizer monkey virus isolated from the mammary tumor of a rhesus monkey. Proc.nat.Acad.Sci., Wash. *68:* 1608–1612 (1971).

48 NOWINSKI, R.C.; OLD, L.J.; SARKAR, N.H., and MOORE, D.H.: Common properties of the oncogenic RNA viruses (oncornaviruses). Virology *42:* 1152–1157 (1970).

49 NOYES, W.F.: Tumors induced in the South American marmoset monkey by Rous sarcoma virus. J.nat.Cancer Inst. *45:* 579–587 (1970).

50 PORTER, R.P. and GENGOZIAN, N.: Immunological tolerance and rejection of skin allografts in the marmoset. Transplantation *8:* 653–665 (1969).

51 RABIN, H.: Assay and pathogenesis of oncogenic viruses in nonhuman primates. Lab. anim.Sci. *21:* 1032–1049 (1971).

52 RABIN, H. and COOPER, R.W.: Tumor production in squirrel monkeys *(Saimiri sciureus)* by Rous sarcoma virus. Lab. anim.Sci. *21:* 705–711 (1971).

53 RABOTTI, G.F.; LANDON, J.C.; PRY, T.W.; BEADLE, L.; DOLL, J.; FABRIZIO, D.P., and DALTON, A.J.: Tumors in rhesus monkeys inoculated at birth with homologous cells converted *in vitro* by Rous sarcoma virus, Schmidt-Ruppin strain. J.nat.Cancer Inst. *38:* 821–837 (1967).

54 RANGAN, S.R.S.; WONG, M.C.; UEBERHORST, P.J., and ABLASHI, D.V.: Mixed culture cytopathogenicity induced by virus preparations derived from simian sarcoma virus (SSV-1) infected cultures. J.nat.Cancer Inst. (in press).

55 RANGAN, S.R.S.; WONG, M.C.; MOYER, P.B., and JENSEN, E.M.: Cytopathogenic test for feline leukemia virus infections. Appl.Microbiol. *23:* 628–636 (1972).

56 SARMA, P.S.; GILDEN, R.V., and HUEBNER, R.J.: A complement-fixation test for detection of viral antigens and infective virus of feline leukemia and sarcoma. J.amer vet.med.Ass. *158:* 1055–1060 (1971).

57 SARMA, P.S.; LOG, T., and THEILEN, G.H.: ST-feline sarcoma virus. Biological characteristics and *in vitro* propagation. Proc.Soc.exp.Biol.Med. *137:* 1444–1448 (1971).

58 SARMA, P.S.; TURNER, H.C., and HUEBNER, R.J.: An avian leukosis group specific complement fixation reaction. Application for the detection and assay of non-cytopathogenic leukosis viruses. Virology *23:* 313–321 (1964).

59 SCHÄFER, W. and NORONHA, F.DE: A test system for identification of the antigen shared by leukemia viruses of the cat and other mammalian species. J.amer.vet.med. Ass. *158:* 1092–1098 (1971).

60 SCHLOM, J. and SPIEGELMAN, S.: DNA polymerase activities and nucleic acid components of virions isolated from a spontaneous mammary carcinoma from a rhesus monkey. Proc.nat.Acad.Sci., Wash. *68:* 1613–1617 (1971).

61 SCOLNICK, E.M.; PARKS, W.P.; TODARO, G.J., and AARONSON, S.A.: Immunological characterization of primate C-type virus reverse transcriptases. Nature New Biol. *235:* 35–40 (1972).

62 SMITH, R.D. and DEINHARDT, F.: Unique cytoplasmic membranes in Rous virus-induced tumors of a subhuman primate. J.Cell.Biol. *37:* 819–823 (1968).

63 SNYDER, S.P.: Spontaneous feline fibrosarcomas. Transmissibility and ultrastructure of associated virus-like particles. J.nat.Cancer Inst. *47:* 1079–1085 (1971).

64 SNYDER, S.P. and THEILEN, G.H.: Transmissible feline fibrosarcoma. Nature, Lond. *221:* 1074–1075 (1969).

65 THEILEN, G.H.; GOULD, D.; FOWLER, M., and DUNGWORTH, D.L.: C-type virus in tumor tissue of a woolly monkey *(Lagothrix spp.)* with fibrosarcoma. J.nat.Cancer Inst. *47:* 881–889 (1971).

66 THEILEN, G.H.; SNYDER, S.P.; WOLFE, L.G., and LANDON, J.C.: Biological studies with viral induced fibrosarcomas in cats, dogs, rabbits and nonhuman primates; in DUTCHER Comparative leukemia Research 1969. Bibl.haemat., vol.36, pp.393–400 (Karger, Basel 1970).

67 WOLFE, L.G.; FALK, L., and DEINHARDT, F.: Oncogenicity of *Herpesvirus saimiri* in marmoset monkeys. J.nat.Cancer Inst. *47:* 1145–1162 (1971).

68 WOLFE, L.G.; SMITH, R.K., and DEINHARDT, F.: Simian sarcoma virus, type 1 *(Lagothrix)*. Focus assay and demonstration of non-transforming associated virus. J.nat. Cancer Inst. *48:* 1905–1908 (1972).

69 WOLFE, L.G.; OGDEN, J.D.; DEINHARDT, J.B.; FISHER, L., and DEINHARDT, F.: Breedind and hand-rearing marmosets for viral oncogenesis studies; in BEVERIDGE Breeding primates. Proc.Int.Symp. on Breeding Non-Human Primates for Laboratory Use, Berne 1971 (Karger, Basel, in press).

70 WOLFE, L.G.; DEINHARDT, F.; THEILEN, G.H.; RABIN, H.; KAWAKAMI, T., and BUSTAD, L.K.: Induction of tumors in marmoset monkeys by simian sarcoma virus, type 1 *(Lagothrix)*. A preliminary report. J.nat.Cancer Inst. *47:* 1115–1120 (1971).

71 WOLFE, L.G.; MARCZYNSKA, B.; RABIN, H.; SMITH, R.; TISCHENDORF, P.; GAVITT, F., and DEINHARDT, F.: Viral oncogenesis in nonhuman primates; in GOLDSMITH and MOOR-JANKOWSKI Medical primatology 1970, pp.671–682 (Karger, Basel 1971).

72 WOLFE, L.G.; SMITH, R.D.; HOEKSTRA, J.; MARCZYNSKA, B.; SMITH, R.K.; MCDO-

NALD, R.; NORTHROP, R.L., and DEINHARDT, F.: Oncogenicity of feline fibrosarcoma viruses in marmoset monkeys. Pathologic, virologic and immunologic findings. J. nat. Cancer Inst. (in press).

73 YAMANOUCHI, K.: Role of newborn monkeys in the study of viral oncogenesis. Jap. J. med. Sci. Biol. *19:* 226–227 (1966).

74 YAMANOUCHI, K.; FUKUDA, A.; KOBUNE, F.; UCHIDA, N., and TSURUHARA, T.: Oncogenicity of SR-strain of Rous sarcoma virus in cynomolgus monkeys. Jap. J. med. Sci. Biol. *20:* 443–446 (1967).

75 ZILBER, L.A.: Pathogenicity and oncogenicity of Rous sarcoma virus for mammals; in HOMBURGER Progr. exp. Tum. Res., vol. 7, pp. 23–27 (Karger, Basel 1965).

76 ZILBER, L.A.; LAPIN, B.A., and ADGIGHYTOV, F.I.: Pathogenicity of Rous sarcoma virus for monkeys. Nature, Lond. *205:* 1123–1124 (1965).

77 ZILBER, L.A.; LAPIN, B.A.; ADGIGHYTOV, F.I.; SHEVLJAGHYN, V.JA., and JAKOVLEVA, L.A.: Rous tumors in monkeys. Int. J. Cancer *1:* 395–407 (1966).

Author's address: Dr. L.G. WOLFE, Department of Microbiology, Rush-Presbyterian-St. Luke's Medical Center, *Chicago, IL 60612* (USA)

Medical Primatology 1972. Proc. 3rd Conf. exp. Med. Surg. Primates, Lyon 1972, part III, pp. 197–214 (Karger, Basel 1972)

Oncogenic DNA Viruses of Primates[1]

D. S. Yohn

Department of Veterinary Pathobiology,
Ohio State University, Columbus, O.

Introduction

This review is intended to summarize pertinent information on DNA viruses of primates which are oncogenic *in vivo*. Emphasis will be given to virus-host interactions at the host and cellular level. The latter information will be presented on the belief that understanding these areas are prerequisite to effective control and prevention of virus-induced tumors in man and animals. That is not to say that we must thoroughly understand the natural history of each oncogenic virus and the details of its oncogenic mechanism prior to attempting control measures. However, the more information available in each system the greater the probability of new approaches to understanding and control in another system. For example, Marek's disease of chickens is now effectively controlled by vaccination with a related live herpesvirus, yet oncogenesis in Marek's disease and how the vaccine prevents it is not totally understood. We know equally as little about the virus-host cell relationship of *Herpesvirus saimiri* and *H. ateles* in their natural hosts and the oncogenic process by these viruses in susceptible primates. These viruses are probably more important models of Epstein-Barr (EB) virus in man than is Marek's disease herpesvirus. Control of EB virus, particularly should it be proven to be the *sine qua non* of Burkitt's lymphoma, nasopharyngeal-carcinoma and perhaps other lymphomatous diseases, would become highly desirable. Means to control *H. saimiri* and *H. ateles* and to prevent or interrupt their oncogenesis should be pursued on the basis, in part, that developments within this system will be applicable to understanding and control of EB virus or other potentially oncogenic herpesviruses of man.

1 Supported in part by USPHS. NCI grants CA-07998 and CA-11613.

For the purposes of this review, an oncogenic virus will be defined as one that induces leukemia or neoplastic growth in a susceptible host. The tumor may be malignant or benign. The DNA containing viruses, which are indigenous to subhuman primates and are considered oncogenic, can be grouped in the following manner, shown in table I.

Those which are not known to be oncogenic in primates but are oncogenic in newborn rodents. This includes the simian papovavirus SV-40 and various human and simian adenoviruses.

Those which produce benign neoplasms in the natural simian host and other primates including man. This includes Yaba tumor and Tana poxviruses.

Those which are not known to be oncogenic in the natural simian host but are oncogenic when experimentally transmitted to other subhuman primates. This includes *H. saimiri* and *H. ateles*.

Other papers in this symposium will deal primarily with the last group of viruses. Because of the importance of the first two groups, historically and mechanistically, a description of them is warranted prior to a discussion of the oncogenic herpesviruses.

Viruses of Primates Oncogenic in Rodents but not in Primates

Papovavirus (SV-40)

The simian papovavirus, SV-40, at one time called vacuolating agent of monkeys [SWEET and HILLEMAN, 1960a and b] is indigenous to Asian monkeys. It was first found in kidney cell cultures derived from rhesus monkeys. Subsequently it was shown that newborn hamsters injected with cell-free fluids obtained from cultures containing this virus developed malignant fibrosarcomas [EDDY *et al.*, 1961]. This observation was of grave importance inasmuch as many humans had received polio vaccine containing SV-40 virus during the 1950's and early 1960's. Continuous monitoring of selected groups of individuals given these contaminated vaccines have shown the incidence of neoplasms not different from expected levels. Apparently, infection and immunization of humans with SV-40 has neither increased nor reduced the incidence of tumors in this species to date.

The virus has been shown, however, to transform human cells *in vitro* [SHEIN and ENDERS, 1962; KOPROWSKI *et al.*, 1962]. Isolation of antigenically-

Table I. Oncogenic DNA viruses of primates

Viruses oncogenic in rodents but not in primates
Papovavirus (SV-40)
Adenoviruses
Human-serotypes 4, 7, 12, 18, 31
Simian-SA-7, SV-11, SV-20, SV-33, SV-34, SV-37, SV-38
Viruses oncogenic (benign) in primates including natural hosts
Yaba tumor poxvirus
Tana poxvirus (OrTeCa)[1]
Viruses oncogenic (malignant) in primates other than natural host
Herpesvirus saimiri
Herpesvirus ateles

1 OrTeCa has been suggested by NICHOLAS [1970] to identify isolates of Tanapox from Oregon, Texas and California, USA.

related viruses from humans has been reported [GARDNER *et al.*, 1971; PADGETT *et al.*, 1971]. Serologic evidence for a SV-40-like infection in man has been documented [SHAH *et al.*, 1972].

The mechanism of SV-40 oncogenesis in hamsters has been extensively explored. It is clear that during malignant transformation, SV-40 DNA is integrated into host genetic material, probably into chromosomal DNA (SAMBROOK *et al.*, 1968; HIRAI *et al.*, 1971]. Transformation does not require intact virus as the process has been induced with SV-40 DNA *in vitro* [KIMOTO and GRACE, 1966] and *in vivo* [KIMOTO and GRACE, 1965]. The entire viral genome or portions thereof may be integrated. The minimum number of SV-40 viral DNA copies present in nonvirus producing transformed cells is probably one, although original estimates based on nucleic acid hybridization experiments were much higher. These estimates have been revised downward as such procedures became more reliable.

The presence of the entire viral genome in transformed cells has been demonstrated by other procedures. Cocultivation of nonvirus producing cells with highly susceptible cercopithecus monkey kidney cells has resulted in synthesis of SV-40 by the cercopithecus cells [KOPROWSKI *et al.*, 1967]. Others have induced virus synthesis in the tumor cells by mitomycin-C treatment [BURNS and BLACK, 1969]. The latter experiments followed the procedures used to induce lambda phage in *E. coli* [LEVINE, 1961].

Indirect evidence of viral DNA integration in tumor cells has been supplied by serologic procedures. The transformed tumor cells produce new antigens (neo-antigens) which are coded by the virus. A nuclear antigen, readily demonstrable by immunofluorescence using sera from tumor-bearing hamsters, is known as SV-40 T-antigen [RAPP *et al.,* 1964]. It is produced in cells of all species of animals which undergo productive, abortive or tansforming infection by SV-40. Its synthesis does not require viral or cellular DNA synthesis since several inhibitors of DNA synthesis do not block its synthesis [RAPP *et al.,* 1965]. The biologic function of T-antigen is not known.

Other antigens peculiar to SV-40 tumor or transformed cells reside in or on the cellular membranes. One such antigen, 'S', for surface antigen [TEVETHIA *et al.,* 1968; TING and HERBERMAN, 1971], has been demonstrated by immunofluorescence or by radiolabeled antibodies. There is evidence that S-antigen may be, or may contain, an embryonic antigen determinant that is expressed following derepression of the relevant genetic information during SV-40 oncogenesis [COGGIN *et al.,* 1971].

A second membrane antigen, called tumor specific transplantation antigen (TSTA), provides the same unique antigenic determinant to all cells transformed by SV-40 regardless of species of origin [GOLDNER *et al.,* 1964; GIRADI, 1965]. The antigen is clearly demonstrated by *in vivo* cross-protection transplantation tests [DEFENDI, 1963; HABEL and EDDY, 1963; AXLER and GIRADI, 1970].

Recent studies by HIRAI and DEFENDI [1972] indicated that SV-40 DNA can be integrated into the cellular DNA of permissive African green monkey kidney (CV-1) cells when they were infected at a low multiplicity in the presence of 15 μg of cytosine arabinoside, an inhibitor of DNA synthesis. Under these conditions, cellular and viral DNA synthesis did not occur and the viral DNA became associated with the nuclear cellular DNA within 20 h post-infection. Although it was not shown that intact SV-40 DNA was integrated, the authors believed that oligomers were not involved, since the latter develop only during viral DNA replication. Whether integration of SV-40 DNA into host DNA occurs *in vivo* in the natural host is not known. There is no evidence that the virus is oncogenic in primates.

Adenoviruses

To a large extent oncogenesis and transformation of nonpermissive cells by adenoviruses occurs in a manner similiar to SV-40. The distinguishing difference is that intact adenovirus DNA is not integrated in a form that can be rescued or activated [KOPROWSKI *et al.,* 1967; WEBER, *et al.,* 1970]. It appears that segments of adenovirus DNA are integrated and that integration of the total viral genome is not necessary to achieve transformation [SCHALLER and YOHN, 1972]. Evidence that adenovirus DNA is present in tumor cells has come from nucleic acid hybridization studies [FUJINAGA and GREEN, 1967a and b] that demonstrated viral specific messenger RNA in tumor cells [FUJINAGA and GREEN, 1968]. Specific viral-induced T [POPE and ROWE, 1964], S [VASCONCELOS-COSTA, 1970; MCCAMMON and YOHN, 1972], and TSTA [TRENTIN and BRYAN, 1966; SJÖGREN *et al.*, 1967] antigens are found in tumor cells. As yet there is no good evidence that simian adenoviruses are oncogenic in primates. Like SV-40 they are oncogenic *in vivo* only when injected in newborn or very young rodents.

Viruses Oncogenic (Benign) in Natural Simian Hosts and Other Primates Including Man

The known viruses in this category are all poxviruses.

Yaba Tumor Poxvirus

The first recognized oncogenic simian poxvirus was isolated in Yaba, Nigeria, in 1956 from an epizootic of subcutaneous tumors among rhesus monkeys housed in Africa. An African baboon was also involved [BEARCROFT and JAMIESON, 1958]. The virus has become known as Yaba tumor poxvirus [ANDREWS *et al.*, 1959]. Susceptible species include man, Asian primates and most African primates (table II). New World primates are generally resistant.

The pathogenesis of the tumors was investigated by SPROUL *et al.* [1963] and the tumors were identified as benign histiocytomas. Fibroblasts and epithelial cells are not generally involved in the neoplastic process. The tumors usually erode through the skin and occasionally epithelial cells become infected but not neoplastic. The tumors contain infected histiocytes with large cytoplasmic inclusions. The inclusions contain the areas of virus synthesis. Cells synthesizing virus are not capable of further cell division and eventually die. Within the tumor other histiocytes, apparently not infected with virus or at least not synthesizing virus, undergo mitosis.

The mechanism of tumor induction is not totally understood. There is no evidence that Yaba poxvirus DNA or even portions of it become integrated in the tumor cell genome as in the case of SV-40 and adenoviruses. Malignant

Table II. Response of primates to oncogenic DNA viruses of primates

Primates		Viruses		
		Yaba poxvirus	*H. saimiri*	*H. ateles*
Man	*Homo sapiens*	T	NK	NK
Baboon	*Papio papio*	T	NK	NK
Rhesus	*Macaca mulatta*	T	R	NK
Pigtail	*Macaca nemestrina*	T	NK	NK
Cynomologus	*Macaca fascicularis*	T	NK	NK
Stump-tail	*Macaca speciosa*	T	NK	NK
Mangabey	*Cerocebus fulginosis*[1]	T	NK	NK
Green	*Cercopithecus aethiops*[1]	T	FD	NK
Patas	*Erythrocebus patas*[1]	T	NK	NK
Baboon	*Papio anubis*[1]	T	NK	NK
Marmosets				
Cottontop	*Saguinus oedipus*	R	Ly/Leuk	Ly/Leuk
White-lipped	*Saguinus fuscicollis*	R	Ly/Leuk	NK
White-lipped	*Saguinus nigricollis*	R	Ly/Leuk	NK
White-eared	*Callithrix jacchus*	R	R	NK
Pigmy	*Cebuella pygmaea*	R	NK	NK
Squirrel	*Saimiri sciureus*	R	Host	NK
Owl	*Aotus trivirgatus*	NK	Ly/Leuk	NK
Cebus	*Cebus albrifrons*	NK	FD	NK
Galago	*Galago crassicaudatus*	NK	R	NK
Spider	*Ateles geoffroyi*	NK	Ly	Host

T = tumor produced.
R = resistant.
NK = not known.
FD = fatal disease.
Ly/Leuk = lymphoma and/or leukemia.
Host = natural animal host of the virus.
1 Results obtained by Dr. J. AMBRUS, Roswell Park Memorial Institute in American born primates. Results supersede those previously published by AMBRUS *et al.* [1963].

transformation does not occur. Neoplastic-like hyperplasia of histiocytes induced in response to the viral infection is the most likely mechanism. SPROUL *et al.* [1963] noted migration and proliferation of histiocytes within 48 h at the site of virus injection. Cells in mitosis at any stage of tumorigenesis did not contain viral antigen as evaluated by immunofluorescence. The virus synthetic cycle as studied *in vitro* by YOHN *et al.* [1970], although prolonged as compared to other primate poxviruses was short enough, about 20 h, for the initially-infected cells to have produced viral DNA, viral proteins and other associated macromolecules. One or more of these viral coded products released by the infected cell may serve to stimulate histiocytic migration to the infected area and induce mitosis. A second possibility is that the viral infection may induce the cell to produce chemotactic factors specific for histiocytes.

The possibility of induced hyperplasia has been partially explored *in vitro* [YOHN *et al.*, 1970; MILO and YOHN, 1972]. Infection of contact-inhibited monolayers of primary or low passage levels of susceptible primate kidney cells with limiting dilutions of Yaba virus results in the formation of a 'microtumor' [YOHN *et al.*, 1964] at the site of each infected cell. These microtumors, as studied in BSC-1 and CV-1 cell lines, begin with spread of infection to three or four cells before proliferative changes occur. The infected cells coalesce and neighboring cells migrate to the area. Adjacent cells undergo mitosis and then become involved in the focus. As more cells become infected, apparently by contiguous spread of the virus, they adhere to the developing 'microtumor'. These foci are sometime visible by light microscopy in 12–14 days [YOHN *et al.*, 1966a and b] but usually require 18–21 days. Secondary foci form after 28 days.

Soluble factors released by the infected cells *in vitro* which stimulate cell replication have been found. After five to seven days in parabiosis with chambers separated by 100-nm milipore filters, uninfected cells opposite an infected chamber developed significantly higher mitotic indices and greater rates of ^{3}H-thymidine incorporation than cells in control chambers (table III). Extracts of tumors and of infected CV-1 cells contain soluble materials of less than 50,000 molecular weight which induce similar responses. One such material, a glycoprotein, has been obtained from plasma cell membranes of infected CV-1 cells. It has a molecular weight of 20,000 or less and is not present in uninfected control cells. Whether it is virus coded or is induced by Yaba virus infection is under investigation. It is conceivable that the glycoprotein may function similarly to the 'colony stimulating factor' of METCALF [1971]. Whatever its nature, it is specific *in vivo* in that only histiocytes seem to proliferate and form the tumor. The specificity holds from species to species since essentially identical tumors form in various species of monkeys [AMBRUS *et al.*, 1963] and in man [GRACE and MIRAND, 1963]. A protein with physical and biologic properties similar to that in Yaba tumor has been isolated by NAIR and DE OME [1972] from mouse mammary tumors.

Table III. Effects of diffusable materials produced by Yaba poxvirus infected CV-1 cells on uninfected cells in parabiosis[1]

Days post-infection	Experiment 1 multiplicity = 10 infectious units/cell			Experiment 2 multiplicity = 135 infectious units/cell		
	cell count ratio[2]	mitotic index ratio[2]	nuclear thymidine ratio[2]	cell count ratio[2]	mitotic index ratio[2]	nuclear thymidine ratio[2]
1	0.98	0.64	0.66	1.99	1.49	0.84
2	0.94	0.71	0.90	1.02	0.89	0.69
4	0.92	0.98	NT	1.34	1.24	1.15
5	0.95	1.92	1.26	1.71	1.32	1.72
6	1.21	1.58	4.51	2.02	1.30	NT
8	1.80	2.06	1.93	2.80	2.93	3.11
10	2.26	3.60	3.29	2.65	1.11	0.91
13	2.88	3.50	3.62	NT	NT	NT

1 Parabiotic chambers (Bellco) contained confluent monolayers of CV-1 cells on cover-slips separated by 100-mm millipore filters. In each experiment virus was added to one side of one-half the chambers. Four cover slips were removed at each time and cell counts, mitotic indices, and ^{3}H-thymidine uptake determined for cells opposite infected chambers (test cells) and those opposite uninfected chambers (control cells).

2 Ratios represent test values divided by control values. Any ratio greater than 1.00 indicates higher values in tests than in controls. In general a ratio of 1.5 or higher exceded the mean minus 2 standard errors and was considered significant.

NT = not tested.

Synthesis of Yaba tumor poxvirus *in vitro* is temperature sensitive [YOHN *et al.*, 1970]. Upon primary isolation from tumors, virus replication occurs in cell cultures at 37 °C, but generally after several passages, replication ceases at that temperature. Passage at 33 °C is optimal. The temperature sensitive event appears to be associated with DNA synthesis. The role, if any, temperature sensitivity plays in oncogenesis is not known. It is conceivable that histiocytes infected with temperature sensitive virions do not replicate the virus until the defect is corrected by a cellular mechanism or by infection of the cell with additional virions which act in concert (multiplicity reactivation). This hypothesis would allow cells to enter mitosis if infected by incompetent virus. At this point there is no convincing evidence that this mechanism operates *in vivo*. Temperature shift experiments *in vitro* [YOHN *et al.*, 1970] have not resolved the question. The evidence to date favors the first proposed mechanism, namely that of induced neoplastic hyperplasia owing to release of stimulating factors from infected cells.

Another noteworthy aspect of Yaba tumors is that they regress. Tumors may become as large as 30–50 mm in diameter before they begin to regress. Antibodies develop to the many virus structural antigens and nonstructural associated antigens [OLSEN and YOHN, 1970]. Among the antibodies are virus neutralizing antibodies, complement-fixing antibodies, and noncomplement-fixing antibodies [HALL, 1972]. The antibody response undoubtably plays a major role in controlling virus spread, however, the appearance of neutralizing antibodies does not correlate with onset of tumor regression; the latter occurs much later than the development of neutralizing antibodies. The development of antibodies to the factor(s) responsible for stimulation of histiocyte proliferation may play a key controlling role. Studies are in progress on this important facet of Yaba poxvirus oncogenesis.

The role of cell mediated immunity in Yaba tumor regression has not been thoroughly studied. In tumors that ulcerate through the skin and become secondarily infected with bacteria, necrosis and massive leukocytic infiltration occur. The amount of infiltration in those that do not ulcerate is less marked. Nonetheless, SPROUL *et al.* [1963] detected cellular reactions at the periphery of the tumor late in the first week of growth. This circumscribed reaction contained plasma cells, lymphocytes, histiocytes and a few eosinophilic leukocytes which remained peripheral until regression was well advanced. These workers contributed regression in nonulcerating tumors to virus-induced cytolysis and degeneration of individual cells.

Monkeys develop delayed hypersensitivity to Yaba virus antigens during early convalescence. The hypersensitivity, as measured by skin tests, persists for approximately a year or more after recovery. The significance of delayed hypersensitivity to viral antigens in the immune control of Yaba tumor oncogenesis is not clearly delineated. It is more likely that this type of immunity to viral antigens plays a role in protection against viral reinfection. Delayed hypersensitivity to nonviral tumor specific antigens in this system has not been reported.

In summary, Yaba tumors, although not malignant, provide an important model primate tumor in which to study viral-induced neoplastic processes and the development of effective immunologic responses to the inducing agent, Yaba poxvirus, and the tumor itself. Once the oncogenic and controlling mechanisms are understood it is likely that the basic concepts will pertain to induction and control of neoplasms induced by other viruses and carcinogens.

Tana Poxvirus

The second group of poxviruses that induce benign lesions in primates have been identified under several names, including Yaba-like poxvirus [ESPAÑA, 1966] benign epidermal monkey poxvirus [CASEY *et al.*, 1967], OrTeCa [NICHOLAS, 1970] and Tanapox [DOWNIE *et al.*, 1971]. All isolates of the virus induce similar lesions. During early development the lesions superficially resemble Yaba tumor owing to the indurated proliferation in the skin. However, the lesion is clearly differentiated from Yaba tumor histologically by the involvement of epithelial cells and lack of neoplastic changes in histiocytes. There is doubt by some observers that the lesion qualifies as a neoplasm.

The lesions, according to DOWNIE *et al.* [1971], resemble closely the lesions of swinepox. According to KUPPER *et al.* [1970] the lesions could be mistaken for other pox infections such as variola or monkey pox, but not for Yaba tumors. Sections of lesions revealed hyperplasia of epidermal cells and of hair follicles at six days. The hyperplasia persisted through 21 days or longer. Degenerating infected celles were present early in the disease. Exudative processes and inflamatory cellular infiltration developed by the second week of the lesion. The latter processes were less marked than with variola or monkey pox, but distinguished these lesions from those of Yaba poxvirus [KUPPER *et al.*, 1970].

Epizootics with spread to animal handlers occurred in at least three different primate holding facilities in the United States during 1966. The first of these was among rhesus monkeys housed in the primate center at Davis, Calif. [ESPAÑA, 1966]. Other outbreaks occurred in Oregon [HALL and MCNULTY, 1967] and in Texas [CASEY *et al.*, 1967]. Subsequently, isolates from all three outbreaks proved identical and the name OrTeCa was suggested (NICHOLAS, 1970]. DOWNIE and ESPAÑA [1972] have recently shown that all are isolates of Tanapox [DOWNIE *et al.*, 1971]. Tanapox was responsible for epidemics of the disease in 1957 and 1962 among members of the Wapakomo tribe along the Tana river in Kenya [ALLISON, 1965]. The reservoir of the virus is African green monkeys. Inasmuch as the source of the virus introduced into the United States was African monkeys [DOWNIE and ESPAÑA, 1972], the name Tanapox is acceptable. (It would be well to accept this name in order to end the confusion on naming this virus.)

Tanapox appears to be enzootic in Kenya and, from time to time, may be transmitted to man under environmental conditions wherein mosquitos feed on infected monkeys and transmit the virus to man. Adequate quarantine of

African primates and safety precautions by handlers should prevent epizootics in primate facilities and their spread to man.

The virus is cytolytic in cell cultures of primate origin producing plaques which can be enumerated for quantitative assay. The apparent lack of proliferative changes *in vitro* has precluded analysis of hyperplasia induced by this virus.

Viruses Oncogenic (Malignant) in Other Primates but not Known to Be in Their Natural Host

At the present time this category includes two simian herpesviruses, *H. saimiri* and *H. ateles.*

H. ateles, indigenous to spider monkeys *(Ateles geoffroyi),* has been reported to produce lymphoma in cotton-topped marmosets [HUNT *et al.,* in press]. The virus is antigenically distinct from other mammalian herpesviruses as shown by *in vitro* neutralization tests. It is further distinguished from *H. saimiri* by a different spectrum of cell cultures which support its replication. Furthermore, it is not oncogenic in rabbits, whereas *H. saimiri* has been reported to induce lymphoma in this species.

The lymphoma induced by *H. ateles* in cotton-topped marmosets has a rapid onset with death in four to five weeks. Lymphoblastic leukemic changes occurred in the peripheral blood. Lymphoblastic infiltration was noted in major internal organs including the heart, kidney and bone marrow. Spleen, thymus and lymph nodes were all enlarged [HUNT *et al.,* in press].

The natural history of *H. ateles* has not been thoroughly described, nor has the cell-virus relationship in the spider monkey been determined. It is likely that the oncogenic process in marmosets will be similar to that induced by *H. saimiri.*

Herpesvirus saimiri

H. saimiri, a virus indigenous to squirrel monkeys *(Saimiri sciureus)* [MELENDEZ *et al.,* 1968] is highly oncogenic in a number of primates [MELENDEZ *et al.,* 1969a and b, 1970, 1971; HUNT *et al.,* 1970; ABLASHI *et al.,* 1971; WOLFE *et al.,* 1971; DEINHARDT *et al.,* 1972; and FALK *et al.,* 1972a und b]. The original studies by MELENDEZ and colleagues suggested that the virus did not produce overt disease in the natural host. In contrast, however, malignant fatal lymphomas and/or leukemia were induced in owl monkeys (*Aotus* sp.) and marmosets (*Saguinus* sp.). Other species shown to be susceptible (see table II) to date include cinnamon ringtail monkeys *(Cebus albifrons)*, three species of marmosets *(Saguinus oedipus, S. nigricollis* and *S. fusicicollis)* and rabbits [DANIEL *et al.,* 1970]. Galagos *(Galago crassicaudatus)* and rhesus monkeys are apparently not susceptible [WOLFE *et al.,* 1971].

The pathology of the lymphomas and leukemias induced in these species have been described in the papers cited above and will not be reviewed here. There is excellent agreement that the diseases are malignant in owl monkeys and marmosets. The disease in cebus monkeys and green monkeys has been described as a reticuloproliferative disorder [MELENDEZ *et al.,* 1970; for a detailed review see DEINHARDT, in press.]

In susceptible primates the virus apparently infects cells of the lymphocytic series which then transform, multiply rapidly and form the neoplastic disease. Such cells *in vivo* do not contain virus or viral antigens [WOLFE *et al.,* 1971]. However, leukemic lymphoblasts from marmosets cultured *in vitro* produce viral antigens in 24 h but no virus [FALK *et al.,* 1972b]. Cultures of these cells held for 120 h did not yield free virus nor could infectious virus be extracted from them. Cocultivation of lymphoblasts with susceptible Vero cells resulted in transfer of the *H. saimiri* genome to these cells within 24 h followed by synthesis of complete virus by 48 h. Previously, WOLFE *et al.* [1971] had shown that cultured tumor explants did release virus, presumably due to transfer of genome to normal cells in the explant. Transplantation of lymphoblasts of one sex to animals of the opposite sex induces lymphoma in the recipient animal cells [DEINHARDT, in press].

In the natural host, the squirrel monkey, the virus exists similarly. Adult animals have readily detectable levels of antibody to the virus as determined by neutralization and indirect immunofluorescence [DEINHARDT *et al.,* 1972]. The virus can be isolated from these apparently normal animals. MELENDEZ *et al.* [1968] reported out-growth of the virus in kidney cultures of six to ten different squirrel monkeys. FALK *et al.* [1972] reported isolation of *H. saimiri* from peripheral lymphocytes by cocultivation. Details will be reported by FALK in this symposium. Apparently the virus genome exists in lymphocytes that transfer the information to nonlymphocyte cells under *in vitro* conditions. Although it would be of interest to know if antibody interferes with this transfer *in vitro,* it is likely that the mechanism by which the virus remains repressed *in vivo* is highly complex.

Recent studies [FALK *et al.,* 1972b; DEINHARDT, in press; WOLFE and DEINHARDT, 1972] have shown that newborn and suckling squirrel monkeys have maternal antibody. This antibody disappears and the animals become seronegative. Infection and seroconversion occurs within one or two years of age without overt signs of disease. The pattern is not unlike the natural history of EB virus in man. Horizontal transmission is believed to occur with both viruses in the natural host. It would be of interest to know if *H. saimiri* is excreted, e.g. in the feces, urine or saliva of squirrel monkeys.

In marmosets, horizontal transmission of *H. saimiri* to cagemates exposed to diseased animals has not been observed [WOLFE *et al.*, 1971]. These contacts did not seroconvert. Antibodies to *H. saimiri* have not been detected in three species of normal marmosets, *S. oedipus, S. fuscicolis* and *S. nigricollis,* but two of 19 of a fourth species, *S. geoffroyi,* contained neutralizing antibodies [DEINHARDT *et al.*, 1972]. The latter species has not been tested for susceptibility to *H. saimiri.*

H. saimiri in squirrel monkeys may be the counterpart of EB virus in man. It is, therefore, of major interest and prime importance to define the mechanism that permits *H. saimiri* to infect squirrel monkey lymphocytes, not to produce disease and remain in an apparently repressed state *in vivo,* yet be transmitted horizontally without producing overt disease in the natural host, while in other unnatural primate hosts the apparently same cell-virus relationship leads to malignant transformation of the lymphocytes but no horizontal transmission of the virus. The availability of experimental animals with which to explore these mechanisms is assured. It should be anticipated that the next several years will provide insight into these intriguing cell-virus relationships. Once the differences in molecular environment under which one species of lymphocyte controls the virus genome while another is transformed by the same genetic information are known, it should be possible to predict the conditions under which EB virus might be oncogenic in man.

Conclusions

It is readily apparent from this brief review that oncogenic DNA viruses of primates will continue to add significantly to our understanding of viral oncogenesis. Even though it is clear the SV-40 DNA and adenovirus DNA is integrated into rodent cell genomes and initiates those events known as malignant transformation, the precise alterations in cellular control mechanisms are still to be clearly defined. Whether integration of DNA from these viruses occurs in primate cells *in vivo,* but transforming events are not initiated, is yet to be resolved.

Yaba tumor poxvirus continues to be of interest since the tumorigenic process is not initiated by integration of viral DNA into host DNA. Rather the process appears to involve induction of hyperplasia by materials released by infected cells. The induction of histiocytes and not of other cells indicates a specificity of action. Whether the material is a viral or host cell gene product is under study. If found to be of host cell origin it will be of major interest to determine whether similar materials play a role in the neoplastic process induced by other viruses or carcinogens.

Herpesvirus ateles and *H. saimiri* are the only DNA viruses to date proven to induce malignant disease in primates. The possibility that under certain environmental conditions they may be oncogenic in their respective natural hosts has not been totally eliminated. Understanding the nature of the interaction of the virus or virus genome with lymphocytes or their genetic material *in vivo* will represent a major contribution. Definition of the mechanism by which *H. saimiri* infected squirrel monkey lymphocytes fail to transform *in vivo* will be equally important. However, development of means to control transformation of marmoset or owl monkey lymphocytes by *H. saimiri in vivo* will be invaluable. Each of these areas bear directly on major questions concerning the counterpart herpesvirus in man, EB virus. Is EB virus etiologically involved with human lymphoma, or other malignant diseases? If so, what means to control spread of EB virus or the transformation process might be employed?

In conclusion, primate DNA oncogenic viruses offer special research opportunities that relate directly to the overall problems of viral oncogenesis and carcinogenesis. Among these, the oncogenic primate herpesviruses appear highly relevant to current problems in viral oncogenesis in man.

References

Ablashi, D.V.; Loeb, W.F.; Valerio, M.G.; Adamson, R.H.; Armstrong, G.R.; Bennett, D.G., and Heine, U.: Malignant lymphoma with lymphocytic leukemia induced in owl monkeys by *Herpesvirus saimiri*. J.nat.Cancer Inst. *47:* 837–845 (1971).

Allison, A.C.: in Rook and Walton Comparative physiology and pathology of the skin, pp.665–684 (Blackwell, Oxford 1965).

Ambrus, J.L.; Feltz, E.T.; Grace, J.T., jr., and Owens, G.: A virus induced tumor in primates. J.nat.Cancer Inst. *10:* 447–458 (1963).

Andrews, C.; Allison, A.C.; Armstrong, J.A.; Bearcroft, G.; Niven, J.S.F., and Pereira, H.G.: A virus disease of monkeys causing large superficial growths. Acta Un.int.Cancr. *15:* 760 (1959).

AXLER, D.A. and GIRARDI, A.J.: SV_{40} tumor specific-transplantation antigen (TSTA) in NDV lysates of SV_{40} transformed cells. Proc. amer. Ass. Cancer Res. *11:* 4 (1970).

BEARCROFT, W.C.C. and JAMIESON, M.F.: An outbreak of subcutaneous tumors in rhesus monkeys. Nature *182:* 195–196 (1958).

BURNS, W.H. and BLACK, P.H.: Analysis of SV_{40}-induced transformation of hamster kidney tissue *in vitro*. VI. Characteristics of mitomycin C induction. Virology *39:* 625–634 (1969).

CASEY, H.W.; WOODRUFF, J.M., and BUTCHER, W.I.: Electron microscopy of a benign epidermal pox disease of rhesus monkeys. Amer. J. Path. *51:* 431–446 (1967).

COGGIN, J.H.; AMBROSE, K.R.; BELLOMY, B.B., and ANDERSON, N.G.: Tumor immunity in hamsters immunized with fetal tissues. J. Immunol. *107:* 526–533 (1971).

DANIEL, M.D.; MELENDEZ, L.V.; HUNT, R.D.; KING, N.W., and WILLIAMSON, M.E.: Malignant lymphoma induced in rabbits by *Herpesvirus saimiri* strains. Bact. Proc. *271:* 195 (1970).

DEFENDI, V.: Effect of SV_{40} virus immunization on growth of transplantable SV_{40} and polyoma virus tumors in hamsters. Proc. Soc. exp. Biol. Med. *113:* 12 (1963).

DEINHARDT, F.: *Herpesvirus saimiri. The Herpesviruses* (Academic Press, New York, in press).

DEINHARDT, F.; WOLFE, L.; NORTHROP, R.; MARCZYNSKA, B.; OGDEN, J.; MCDONALD, R.; FALK, L.; SHRAMEK, G.; SMITH, R., and DEINHARDT, J.: Induction of neoplasms by viruses in marmoset monkeys. J. med. Prim. *1:* 29–50 (1972).

DOWNIE, A.W. and ESPAÑA, C.: Comparison of Tanapox virus and Yaba-like viruses causing epidemic disease in monkeys. J. Hyg. *70:* 23–32 (1972).

DOWNIE, A.W.; TAYLOR-ROBINSON, C.H.; CAUNT, A.E.; NELSON, G.S.; MANSON-BAHR, P.E.C., and MATTHEWS, T.C.H.: Tanapox: A new disease caused by a poxvirus. Brit. med. J. *i:* 363–368 (1971).

EDDY, B.E.; BORMAN, G.S.; BERKELEY, W.H., and YOUNG, R.D.: Tumors induced in hamsters by injection of rhesus monkey kidney cell extracts. Proc. Soc. exp. Biol. Med. *107:* 191–197 (1961).

ESPAÑA, C.: A Yaba-like disease in primates. 17th Ann. Meet. Animal Care Panel, Chicago; cit. Lab. Primate News Letter *5:* ii (1966).

FALK, L.A.; WOLFE, L.G., and DEINHARDT, F.: *Herpesvirus saimiri* (HVS). Incidence of latent infection in squirrel monkeys. Fed. Proc. (abstracts) *31:* 806 (1972a).

FALK, L.A.; WOLFE, L.G.; HOEKSTRA, J., and DEINHARDT, F.: Demonstration of *Herpesvirus saimiri*-associated antigens in peripheral lymphocytes from infected marmosets during *in vitro* cultivation. J. nat. Cancer Inst. *48:* 523–529 (1972b).

FUJINAGA, K. and GREEN, M.: Mechanism of viral carcinogenesis by DNA mammalian viruses. II. Viral-specific RNA in tumor cells induced by 'weakly' oncogenic human adenoviruses. Proc. nat. Acad. Sci., Wash. *57:* 806–812 (1967a).

FUJINAGA, K. and GREEN, M.: Mechanism of viral carcinogenesis by deoxyribonucleic acid mammalian viruses. IV. Related virus-specific ribonucleic acids in tumor cell induced by 'highly' oncogenic adenovirus types 12, 18, and 31. Virology *1:* 576–582 (1967b).

FUJINAGA K. and GREEN, M.: Mechanism of viral carcinogenesis by DNA mammalian viruses. V. Properties of purified viral-specific RNA from human adenovirus-induced tumor cells. J. molec. Biol. *31:* 63–73 (1968).

GARDNER, S.D.; FIELD, A.M.; COLEMAN, D.V. *et al.:* New human papovavirus (B.K.) isolated from urine after renal transplantation. Lancet *i:* 1253 (1971).

GIRARDI, A.J.: Prevention of SV_{40} virus oncogenesis in hamsters. I. Tumor resistance induced by human cells transformed by SV_{40}. Proc. nat. Acad. Sci., Wash. *54:* 445–451 (1965).

GOLDNER, H.; GIRARDI, A.J.; LARSON, V.M., and HILLEMAN, M.R.: Interruption of SV_{40} virus tumorigenesis using irradiated homologous tumor antigen. Proc. Soc. exp. Biol. Med. *117:* 851 (1964).

GRACE, J.T., jr. and MIRAND, E.A.: Human susceptibility to a simian tumor virus. Ann. N.Y. Acad. Sci. *108:* 1123–1128 (1963).

HABEL, K. and EDDY, B.E.: Specificity of resistance to tumor challenge of polyoma and SV_{40} virus-immune hamsters. Proc. Soc. exp. Biol. Med. *113:* 1 (1963).

HALL, R.D.: Humoral antibody response of rhesus monkeys *(Macaca mulatta)* to three simian pox viruses; Masters thesis Ohio State University (1972).

HALL, A.S. and MCNULTY, W.P., jr.: A contagious pox disease of monkeys. J. amer. vet. med. Ass. *151:* 833–838 (1967).

HIRAI, K. and DEFENDI, V.: Integration of simian virus 40 deoxyribonucleic acid into the deoxyribonucleic acid of permissive monkey kidney cells. J. Virol. *9:* 705–707 (1972).

HIRAI, K.; LEHMAN, J., and DEFENDI, V.: Integration of simian virus 40 deoxyribonucleic acid into the deoxyribonucleic-acid of primary infected Chinese hamster cells. J. Virol. *8:* 706–715 (1971).

HUNT, R.D.; MELENDEZ L.V., and TRUM, B.F.: *Herpesvirus ateles* lymphoma in cotton-topped marmosets. The virus, the disease, and evidence for horizontal transmission; in GOLDSMITH and MOOR-JANKOWSKI Medical primatology 1972, part III, pp. 159–162 (Karger, Basel 1972).

KIMOTO, T. and GRACE, J.T.: Oncogenic properties of nucleic acid derived from SV_{40} virus. Acta med. Okayama *20:* 1–27 (1965).

KIMOTO, T. and GRACE, J.T.: Cell transformation of established human cell line induced by SV_{40} DNA. Acta med. Okayama *20:* 215–227 (1966).

KOPROWSKI, H.; JENSEN, F.C., and STEPLEWSKI, Z.: Activation of production of infectious tumor virus SV_{40} in heterokaryon cultures. Proc. nat. Acad. Sci., Wash. *58:* 127–133 (1967).

KOPROWSKI, H.; PANTEN, J.A.; JENSEN, F.; RANDIN, R.G.; MOORHEAD, P., and SAKSELA, E.: Transformation of cultures of human tissue infected with simian virus SV_{40}. J. cell comp. Physiol. *59:* 281–292 (1962).

KUPPER, J.L.; CASEY, H.W., and JOHNSON, D.K.: Experimental Yaba and benign epidermal monkey pox in rhesus monkeys. Lab. anim. Care *20:* 979–988 (1970).

LEVINE, M.: Effect of mitomycin C on interactions between temperate phages and bacteria. Virology *13:* 493–499 (1961).

MCCAMMON, J.R. and YOHN, D.S.: Membrane antigens on adenovirus (Ad-12) infected cells. Proc. amer. Soc. Microbiol. *72:* 235 (1972).

MELENDEZ, L.V.; DANIEL, M.D.; HUNT, R.D., and GARCIA, F.G.: An apparently new herpesvirus from primary kidney cultures of the squirrel monkey *(Saimiri sciureus)*. Lab. anim. Care *18:* 374–381 (1968).

MELENDEZ, L.V.; DANIEL, M.D.; GARCIA, F.G.; FRASER, C.E.O.; HUNT, R.D., and KING, N.W.: *Herpes saimiri.* I. Further characterization studies of a new virus from the squirrel monkey. Lab. anim. Care *19:* 372–397 (1969b).

MELENDEZ, L.V.; HUNT, R.D.; DANIEL, M.D.; BLAKE, B.J., and GARCIA, F.G.: Acute lymphocytic leukemia in owl monkeys inoculated with *Herpesvirus saimiri*. Science *171:* 1161–1163 (1971).

MELENDEZ, L.V.; HUNT, R.D.; DANIEL, M.D.; GAR CIA, F.G., and FRASER, C.E.O.: *Herpes saimiri*. II. Experimentally induced malignant lymphoma in primates. Lab. anim. Care *19:* 378–386 (1969a).

MELENDEZ, L.V.; HUNT, R.D.; DANIEL, M.D.; FRASER, C.E.O.; GARCIA, F.G., and WILLIAMSON, M.E.: Lethal reticuloproliferative disease induced in *Cebus albifrons* monkeys by *Herpesvirus saimiri*. Int. J. Cancer *6:* 431–435 (1970).

METCALF, D.: Humoral regulators in the development and progression of leukemia; in KLEIN, WEINHOUSE and HADDOW Adv. Cancer Res., vol. 14, pp. 181–230 (Academic Press, New York 1971).

MILO, G.E. and YOHN, D.S.: Changes in enzyme activities associated with membranes and organelles of Yaba tumor poxvirus infected CV-1 cells during micro-tumor formation. Fed. Proc. *72:* 887 (3817) (1972).

NAIR, B.K. and DE OME, K.B.: Induction of DNA synthesis in population density-inhibited cultures of mouse embryo cells by a factor present in mouse mammary tumors. In Vitro *7:* 272 (1972).

NICHOLAS, A.H.: A poxvirus of primates. I. Growth of the virus *in vitro* and comparison with other poxviruses. II. Immunology. J. nat. Cancer Inst. *45:* 897–914 (1970).

OLSEN, R.G. and YOHN, D.S.: Immunodiffusion analysis of Yaba poxvirus structural and associated antigens. J. Virol. *5:* 212–220 (1970).

PADGETT, B.L.; WALKER, D.J.; ZU RHEIN, G.M., *et al.*: Cultivation of papova-like virus from human brain with progressive multifocal leucoencephalopathy. Lancet *i:* 1257 (1971).

POPE, J.H. and ROWE, W.P.: Immunofluorescent studies of adenovirus-12 tumors and of cells transformed or infected by adenoviruses. J. exp. Med. *120:* 577–588 (1964).

RAPP, F.; BUTEL, J.S., and MELNICK, J.L.: Virus-induced intranuclear antigen in cells transformed by papovavirus. Proc. Soc. exp. Biol. Med. *116:* 1131–1135 (1964).

RAPP, F.; BUTEL, J.S.; FELDMAN, L.A.; KITAHARA, T., and MELNICK, J.L.: Differential effects of inhibitors on the steps leading to the formation of SV_{40} tumor and virus antigens. J. exp. Med. *121:* 935 (1965).

SAMBROOK, J.; WESTPHAL, H., and SRINIVASAN, P.R.: The integrated state of viral DNA in SV_{40} transformed cells. Proc. nat. Acad. Sci., Wash. *60:* 1288–1295 (1968).

SCHALLER, J.P. and YOHN, D.S.: Isolation and transformation capacity of defective adenovirions. Proc. amer. Soc. Microbiol. *72:* 218 (1972).

SHAH, K.V.; MCCRUMB, F.R., jr.; DANIEL, R.W., and OZER, H.L.: Serologic evidence for a simian-virus-40-like infection of man. J. nat. Cancer Inst. *48:* 557–561 (1972).

SHEIN, H.M. and ENDERS, J.F.: Transformation induced by simian virus 40 in human renal cell cultures. I. Morphology and growth characteristics. Proc. nat. Acad. Sci., Wash. *48:* 1164–1172 (1962).

SJÖGREN, H.O.; MINOWADA, J., and ANKERST, J.: Specific transplantation antigens of mouse sarcomas induced by adenovirus type 12. J. exp. Med. *125:* 689 (1967).

SPROUL, E.E.; METZGAR, R.S., and GRACE, J.T., jr.: The pathogenesis of Yaba virus-induced histiocytomas in primates. Cancer Res. *23:* 671–675 (1963).

SWEET, B.H. and HILLEMAN, M.R.: Detection of a 'non-detectable' simian virus (vacuolating agent) present in rhesus and cynomologus monkey-kidney cell culture material.

Second Int. Conf. on Live Poliovirus Vaccines, Pan American Health Organization and WHO, Washington, D.C. 1960, pp. 79–85 (1960a).

SWEET, B.H. and HILLEMAN, M.R.: The vacuolating virus. SV_{40}. Proc. Soc. exp. Biol. Med. *105:* 420–427 (1960b).

TEVETHIA, S.S.; COUVILLION, L.A., and RAPP, F.: Development in hamsters of antibodies against surface antigens present in cells transformed by papovavirus SV_{40}. J. Immunol. *100:* 358–362 (1968).

TING, C.-C. and HERBERMANN, R.B.: Detection of tumor-specific cell surface antigen of simian virus-40-induced tumors by the isotopic antiglobulin technique. Int. J. Cancer *7:* 499–506 (1971).

TRENTIN, J.J. and BRYAN, E.: Virus-induced transplantation immunity to human adenovirus type 12 tumors of the hamster and mouse. Proc. Soc. exp. Biol. Med. *121:* 1216 (1966).

VASCONCELOS-COSTA, J.: Detection by immunofluorescence of surface antigens in cells from tumors induced in hamsters by adenovirus type 12. J. gen. Virol. *8:* 69–71 (1970).

WEBER, J.; MAK, S., and YOHN, D.S.: Synthesis of adenovirus type-12 (AD 12) by normally nonpermissive BHK_{21} cells after heterokaryon formation with permissive cells. Bact. Proc. *70:* 180 (1970).

WOLFE, L.G.; FALK, L.A., and DEINHARDT, F.: Oncogenicity of *Herpesvirus saimiri* in marmoset monkeys. J. nat. Cancer Inst. *47:* 1145–1162 (1971).

YOHN, D.S.; GRACE, J.T., jr., and HAENDIGES, V.A.: A quantitative cell culture assay for Yaba tumour virus. Nature, Lond. *202:* 881–883 (1964).

YOHN, D.S.; HAENDIGES, V.A., and GRACE, J.T., jr.: Yaba tumor poxvirus syntheses *in vitro*. I. Cytopathological, histochemical, and immunofluorescent studies. J. Bact. *91:* 1977–1985 (1966a).

YOHN, D.S., MARMOL, F.R., and OLSEN, R.G.: Growth kinetics of Yaba tumor proxvirus after *in vitro* adaptation to cercopithecus kidney cells. J. Virol. *5:* 205–211 (1970).

YOHN, D.S.; MARMOL, F.R.; HAENDIGES, V.A., and GRACE, J.T., jr.: Yaba tumor poxvirus syntheses *in vitro*. II. Adsorption, inactivation, and assay studies. J. Bact. *91:* 1953–1958 (1966b).

Author's address: D.S. YOHN, PhD, Department of Veterinary Pathobiology, Ohio State University, *Columbus, OH* (USA)

Pharmacology and Toxicology

Medical Primatology 1972. Proc. 3rd Conf. exp. Med. Surg. Primates, Lyon 1972, part III, pp. 216–225 (Karger, Basel 1972)

Long-Term Administration of Carcinogenic Agents to Primates[1]

R. H. Adamson

Laboratory of Chemical Pharmacology, National Cancer Institute, National Institutes of Health, Bethesda, Md.

Introduction

Eleven years ago a program was initiated at the National Cancer Institute to evaluate the effects of long-term administration of several chemical carcinogens in nonhuman primates. This program was designed not only to obtain comparative data on the response of primates to known rodent carcinogens but also to obtain model primate tumors for chemotherapeutic studies, to study biochemical and immunological changes which occur during tumor induction and to develop biological markers for detecting preneoplastic changes as well as for frank neoplasia [2, 3]. Three factors of prime importance for the success of this program include: a primate breeding colony so as to insure both newborn monkeys and a sufficient supply of animals, long-term financial support and a closed primate colony in order to minimize health hazards to the animals.

Material and Methods

Carcinogens

Carcinogens presently on study are 3-methylcholanthrene, 3,4,9,10-dibenzpyrene, N-2-fluorenylacetamide, N,N-2,7-fluorenylenebisacetamide, copper chelate of N-hydroxy-2-fluorenylacetamide, ethyl carbamate, N,N′-dimethyl-*p*-phenylazo-analine, N,N′-dimethyl-*p*-(*m*-tolylazo)-analine, methylnitrosourea, aflatoxin B_1, methylazoxymethanol acetate, cyclamate, saccharin, dichlorodiphenyltrichloroethane, N-methyl-N′-nitro-N-nitro-

1 Supported in part by USPHS, NCI contract PH – 43–66–84 to Hazleton Laboratories, Falls Church, Va.

soguanidine, N-isopropyl-α-(2-methylhydrazino)-*p*-toluamide (procarbazine), N-nitrosodiethylamine (DENA), N-nitrosodimethylamine, N-nitrosodipropylamine, and 1-nitrosopiperidine (PIP).

The carcinogens are administered s.c., i.v., i.p. or orally. Oral administration of the carcinogen to newborn monkeys is accomplished by adding the compound to the Similac formula at the time of feeding. When the monkey is six months old, carcinogens given orally are added to a vitamin mixture and fed as a vitamin sandwich on a half slice of bread. The carcinogens are generally fed at doses that are maximally tolerated without toxicity as evidenced by weight gain, blood chemistry and hematology as well as clinical observation.

Animals

The primate colony consists of approximately 600 animals and is composed of six species: *Macaca mulatta mulatta* (rhesus), *Macaca mulatta fascicularis* (cynamolgus), *Cercopithecus aethiops* (African green), *Aotus trivirgatus, Galago crassicaudatus,* and *Tupaia glis.* Currently we are breeding rhesus, cynamolgus, and African green monkeys. The breeding colony consists of 150 animals and the other 450 animals are experimental. Whenever possible animals are first administered carcinogens when newborn. Routinely, newborn rhesus, cynomolgus, or African green monkeys are separated from their mother a few hours *post partum,* placed in a nursery and put on a carcinogenic regime or, in the case of the nitrosamines, after the monkey has been negative for α-fetoprotein (AFP) two successive weeks. Generally a minimum of 30 animals are placed on each carcinogen. This size group allows us to detect a tumor incidence of 10% within 95% confidence limits. Newborn animals are being used with the hope that the newborn monkey may be more susceptible than the adult and that the time required for tumor development will be less. Currently the monkeys are on a minimum treatment period of five years with an additional holding period of five years.

A variety of clinical, chemical and hematological parameters are monitored daily or weekly to evaluate the general health of all animals in the colony and for evidence of neoplasia. Surgical procedures were done under phencyclidine hydrochloride (Sernylan®) or sodium pentobarbital anesthesia. All animals which died or were sacrificed were carefully necropsied and all tissues examined microscopically.

Serum of monkeys was tested for AFP by double diffusion in agar gel using absorbed anti-AFP antiserum and control serum.

Results and Discussion

The various carcinogens used in our program have been administered to nonhuman primates for periods of time from ten months (N-methyl-N′-nitro-N-nitrosoguanidine) to periods of five years (ethyl carbamate, azo compounds, fluorenylacetamides, and polycyclic hydrocarbons) with an additional observation period of five years. Thus far three compounds have consistently produced tumors in the higher primates – DENA, PIP and procarbazine, although we expect that several other compounds and all the nitrosamines will ultimately induce tumors.

A variety of lesions have been caused by the other carcinogens being administered but thus far no tumors. For example, aflatoxin B_1 given orally at 0.8 mg/kg weekly every other week or i.p. at doses of 0.25 mg/kg weekly has produced toxic hepatitis with bile plugs in small canaliculi, proliferation of pseudotubules, severe liver necrosis, pulmonary edema and congestion. Methylazoxymethanol acetate, the active carcinogen in cycad nuts, has produced pancreatitis with focal hyperplasia, toxic hepatitis, jaundice, and hyperplasia of the seminal vesicles and prostate, but no tumors. The polycyclic hydrocarbons used produce giant cell granulomas, papillomas and keratoacanthomas of skin, pancreatitis, and periarteritis and periarteriolitis of pulmonary ateries, but no tumors in the higher primates. However, tumors were induced in the lower primates, tree shrews and galagos, 12 months after a single injection of the polycyclic hydrocarbons [1]. Thus the prosimians (tree shrews, lemurs, lorises, and tarsiers) may be more closely related to the rodent than to higher primates in their reactions to polycyclic hydrocarbon carcinogens.

N-isopropyl-α-(2-methylhydrazino)-*p*-toluamide hydrochloride (procarbazine) has been administered to monkeys by the s.c. and oral route. This compound induces a high incidence of leukemia and pulmonary tumors in mice and mammary tumors in rats. It is used in the chemotherapy of Hodgkin's disease and related conditions. Procarbazine has induced myelogenous leukemia in two monkeys which received the compound for 17 months and 5½ years, respectively (fig. 1 and 2). In addition, while on this compound two monkeys have died with hyperplastic bone marrow, three with ulceration of the esophagus and three with hyperplasia of the urogenital tract.

Currently we are evaluating four nitrosamines (see Material and Methods) for their ability to induce tumors in nonhuman primates. However, since two of these compounds have been used in primates for only one year, results are reported only on PIP and DENA.

Five of ten monkeys receiving PIP orally at a dose of 400 mg/kg five

---

Fig. 1. Peripheral blood smear of monkey with acute myelogenous leukemia. Nucleated cells (immature myeloid series) in the peripheral blood rose to 352,000 on the day of death. Wrights stain. × 690.

Fig. 2. Leukemic infiltration of the liver in the same monkey as in figure 1. Residual hepatic cells are on the left and a residual bile duct and hepatic artery can be seen in the lower right. HE. × 430.

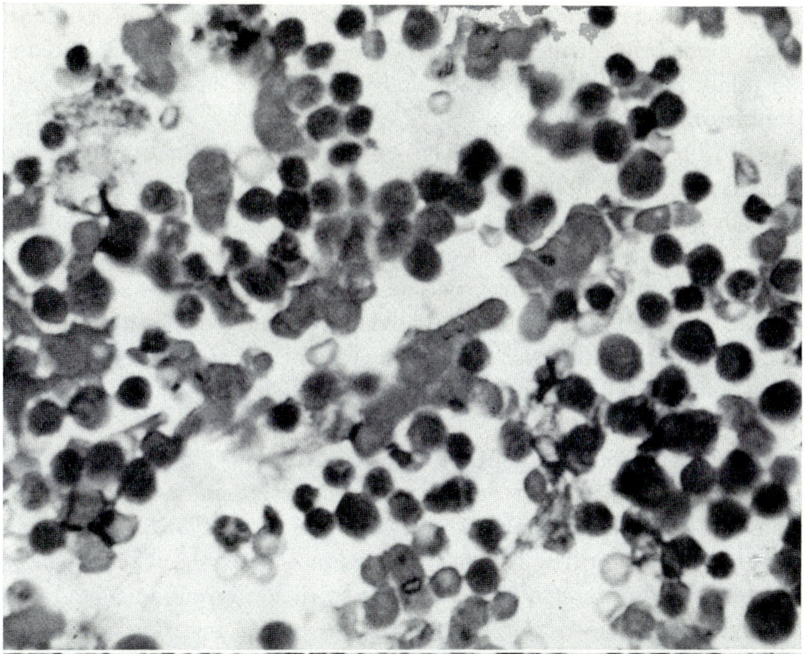

1

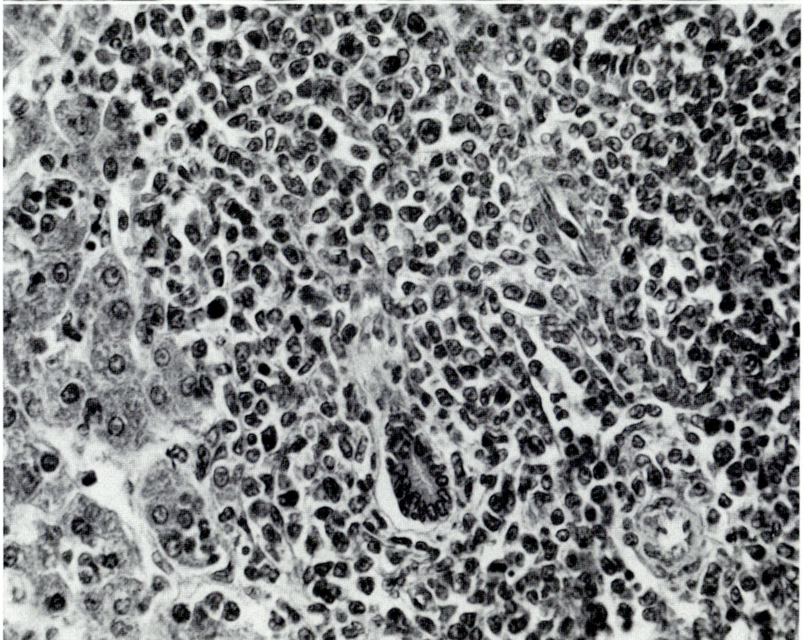

2

times a week have developed liver tumors after periods of 36–89 months on compound. Four of the five monkeys were tested for AFP, when diagnosed for tumor following biopsy, and two had a positive serum AFP as assayed by double diffusion technique.

During the past 11 years we have induced over 80 hepatomas and hepatic cell carcinomas [2–4] in four species of higher primates (rhesus, cynamolgus, African green and capuchin) after administration of DENA orally or i.p. (fig. 3–7). In addition several other tumors have been induced by DENA including two fibrosarcomas, two hemangioendotheliomas and one hemangioma. When DENA was incorporated into the diet via the vitamin sandwich, over 80% of the monkeys receiving the carcinogen at a dose of 40 mg/kg five times a week and surviving for two years developed hepatic cell neoplasms. When DENA was given by i.p. injection at a dose of 40 mg/kg once every two weeks 100% of the monkeys developed tumors. The earliest tumors were induced by i.p. injections (eight months); tumor induction by oral administration took at least 14 months. The lowest total dose of DENA which induced a hepatic cell tumor by i.p. administration was 0.54 g, whereas the lowest cumulative dose which induced a tumor by the oral route was six grams. The average time for induction was 17 months by i.p. injection and 22 months for oral administration. Liver tumors induced by i.p. injection had a greater frequency of metastases to lymph nodes and lung than did those induced by the oral route. In addition only 60% of the monkeys on oral treatment were AFP positive by the time liver tumors were diagnosed whereas all the i.p.-treated monkeys were positive for AFP by the time tumors were diagnosed. It should again be emphasized that AFP determinations were carried out by double diffusion techniques and it is likely that with the more sensitive radioimmunoassay we will observe levels above background (10–20 ng/ml) for all monkeys with liver tumors as well as all treated monkeys without tumors and precancerous monkeys. Indeed, using the relatively insensitive double diffusion technique which allows us to detect about 1 μg/ml of AFP we now are able to detect AFP six months before evidence of tumor in animals treated with i.p. DENA (table I). The DENA is injected with gradually-increasing doses 10, 20 then 40 mg/kg so that the monkey is receiving 40 mg/kg i.p. DENA every two weeks by three months of age. In addition, a number of monkeys when taken off DENA, upon becoming AFP positive (having no tumor at laparotomy) subsequently have developed hepatic cell carcinomas.

A positive serum AFP has not been detected in monkeys receiving carcinogens other than the nitrosamines and no hepatitis-associated antigen has been found in any monkeys in our colony. We are currently assaying our

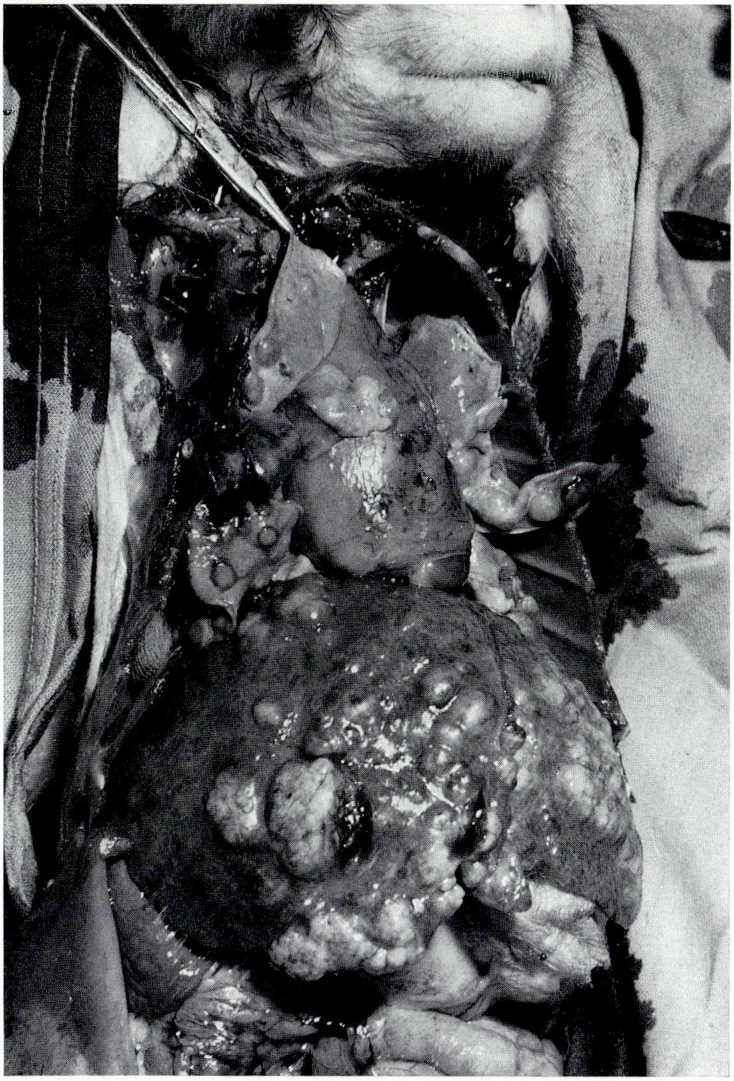

Fig. 3. Tumor induced by oral administration of DENA for 13 months. Liver contains numerous nodules of tumor and, in addition, metastatic tumor can be seen in the lungs.

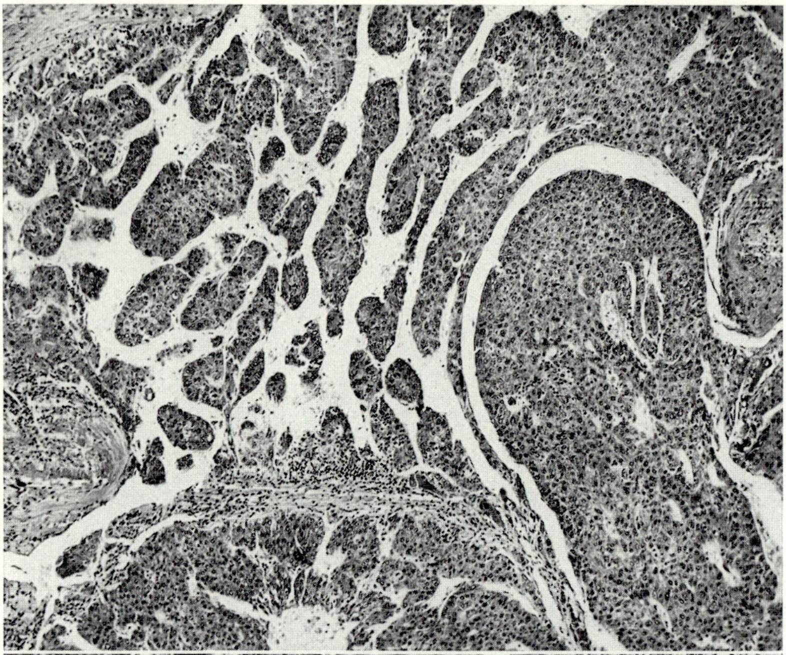

4

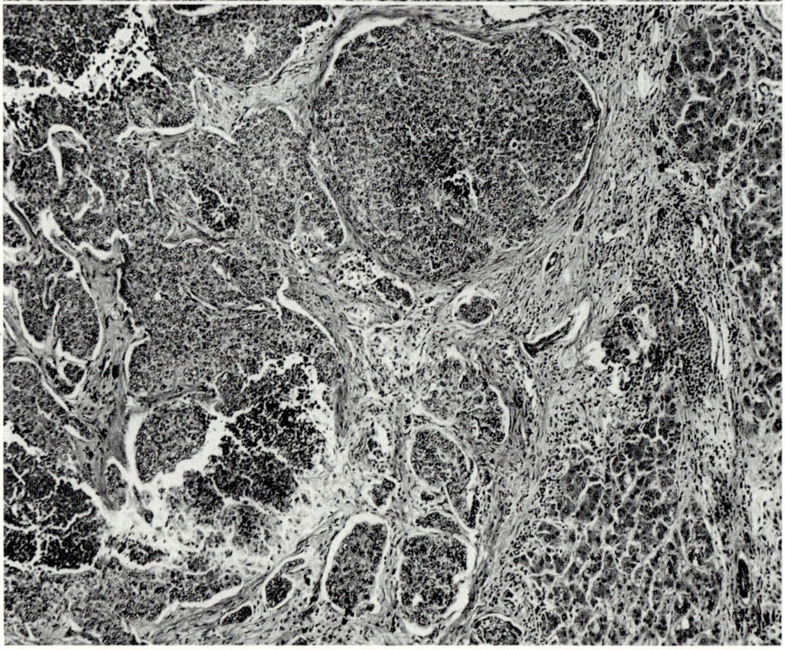

5

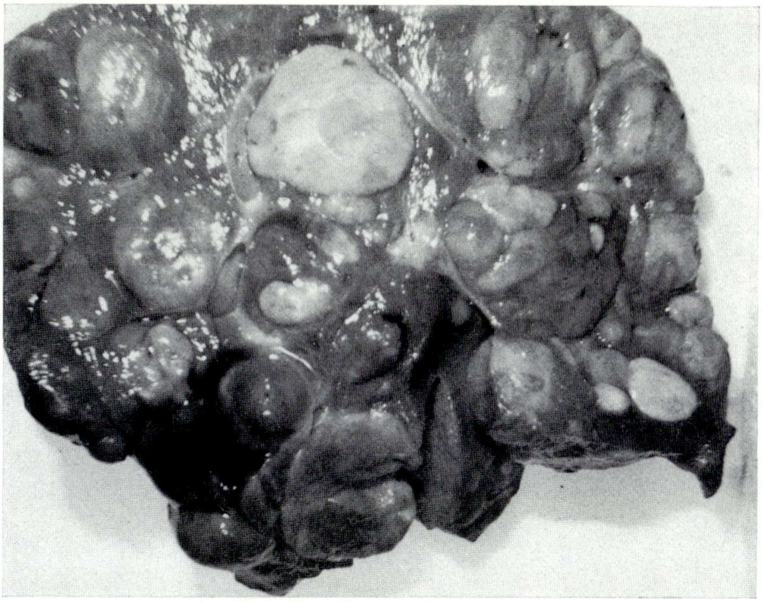

Fig. 6. Hepatic cell carcinoma of the liver induced by i.p. administration of DENA.

Table I. Monkeys AFP positive without tumor

Number of monkeys on DENA[1]	Number positive without tumor[2]	Average time for tumor after AFP positive[3]
30	30	6 months

1 Monkeys receiving 40 mg/kg i.p. every two weeks since originally AFP negative (generally at age of one month).
2 A laparotomy and biopsy was performed on all monkeys with positive serum AFP, in addition six monkeys were sacrificed and gross and microscopic serial sections performed on the liver without revealing tumor.
3 Tumor determined by laparotomy and biopsy.

Fig. 4. and 5. Photomicrograph of section of liver shown in figure 3. Areas of hepatoma cells arranged in trabeculae and areas of fibrosis can be seen. HE. × 84.

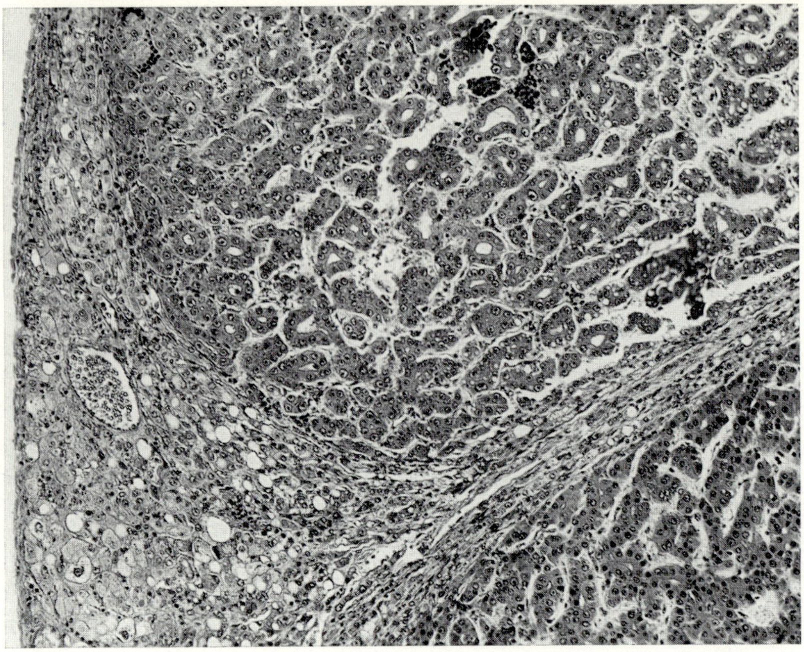

Fig. 7. Photomicrograph of section of tumor shown in figure 6. The tumor cells are arranged in trabeculae which are several cells thick and frequently contain a central channel. HE. × 135.

monkeys for AFP and carcinoembryonic antigen by radioimmunoassay and we believe our primate systems will be highly useful for quantitative and turnover studies on AFP, for studies of other biological markers, for studies of the immune system as tumor develops and attempts to reverse precancerous stages to normal.

Acknowledgements

For the care and maintenance of the breeding colony and the experimental monkeys, I am grateful to Dr. D. W. DALGARD, Mrs. JEANETTE REEVES, and the competent staff at Hazleton Laboratories.

References

1 Adamson, R.H.; Copper, R.W., and O'Gara, R.W.: Carcinogen-induced tumors in primitive primates. J.nat.Cancer Inst. *45:* 555–559 (1970).

2 Adamson, R.H.; Smith, C.F., and Dalgard, D.W.: Induction of neoplasms in non-human primates by chemical carcinogens. Correlation of serum alpha-fetoprotein and appearance of liver tumors; in Proc. 2nd Conf. and Workshop on Embryonic and Fetal Antigens in Cancer, Oak Ridge, Tenn. 1972 (in press).

3 Kelly, M.G.; O'Gara, R.W.; Adamson, R.H.; Gadekar, K.; Botkin, C.C.; Reese, W.H., and Kerber, W.T.: Induction of hepatic cell carcinomas in monkeys with N-nitrosodiethylamine. J.nat.Cancer Inst. *36:* 323–351 (1966).

4 O'Gara, R.W. and Adamson, R.H.: Spontaneous and induced neoplasms in non-human primates; in Fiennes Pathology of simian primates, pp. 190–238 (Karger, Basel 1972).

Author's address: Dr. Richard H. Adamson, Laboratory of Chemical Pharmacology, National Cancer Institute, National Institutes of Health, *Bethesda, MD 20014* (USA)

Medical Primatology 1972. Proc. 3rd Conf. exp. Med. Surg. Primates, Lyon 1972, part III, pp. 226–236 (Karger, Basel 1972)

The Baboon as an Experimental Animal for Metabolic Studies of Bone-Seeking Radionuclides in Man[1]

N. COHEN and M. E. WRENN

New York University Medical Center, Institute of Environmental Medicine, New York, N.Y.

The selection of an animal species to be used in the determination of metabolic parameters applicable to man is dependent on several considerations. These include: (1) similarity to man for the specific functions under investigation; (2) sample size and availability of whatever metabolic substance is analyzed; (3) normal variability of the specific function studied; (4) availability of the animal species; (5) cost; and (6) the simplicity of handling and maintenance procedures. The order of importance of these six factors may be determined for any specific program not only by scientific criteria but by practical considerations as well.

The choice of the adult female baboon, *Papio anubis,* as the experimental animal for the study of the retention and distribution of two bone-seeking radionuclides, ^{210}Pb and ^{241}Am, was based on the following characteristics imperative to this research: (1) bone and tooth metabolism analagous to that in man, i.e. remodeling rate, accretion and resorption, etc. [HENNEMAN, 1972; BRYANT and LOUTIT, 1964]; (2) bone surface to volume ratio similar to that in man (^{241}Am is known to deposit mainly on bone surfaces whereas ^{210}Pb can replace calcium in the hydroxyapatite matrix); (3) a life span of sufficient length for carrying out long-term retention studies; (4) anatomical characteristics similar to those of man for performing *in vivo* whole body, organ and skull measurements; (5) adequate animal size for obtaining blood volumes for routine hematology, clinical chemistry and sequential concentration measurements in plasma and red cell blood fractions; and (6) resilient consti-

1 This investigation was supported by grant No. AT (11-1) 3382 from the USAEC and is part of a center program supported by the National Institute of Environmental Health Sciences, grant No. ES 00260.

tution for withstanding sequential liver and bone biopsies for concentration measurements and autoradiography prior to sacrifice.

The studies now in progress at this laboratory, using the baboon as the experimental animal, are divided into three parts:

1. Metabolic Characteristics of ^{210}Pb [COHEN, 1970]

Using *in vivo* techniques, it is now possible to measure the ^{210}Pb body burdens of former uranium miners to estimate their cumulative occupational exposure to short-lived radon daughters [EISENBUD *et al.*, 1969; COHEN *et al.*, 1972a]. There are, however, several metabolic parameters necessary for this estimation which are not readily obtainable in man. These include the biological retention functions for ^{210}Pb in bone, the variation of ^{210}Pb concentrations among various bones of the skeleton, and the relationship between the ^{210}Pb body burden and concentrations in blood, urine, feces and hair as a function of time.

In this study the metabolic behavior of ^{210}Pb, injected i.v. as $^{210}PbCl_2$, has been observed in seven baboons by *in vivo* and bioassay techniques for various periods up to 3.5 years post injection. Retention of lead in the skeleton and in the total body was determined by *in vivo* measurements of the 47 keV γ-emission of ^{210}Pb over the skull and thorax area with a dual crystal NaICsI (Tl) scintillation detector operated in an anticoincidence mode. A typical photon spectrum obtained for ^{210}Pb in a massless configuration and in the baboon head is seen in figure 1. Positioning of the detector in relation to the baboon is illustrated in figure 2 with the major measurement sites indicated on the diagram. It was initially determined that more than 95% of the ^{210}Pb activity measured in the baboon head (after one month postinjection) is present in the bones of the skull and that there is no significant change in calibration factor over a 15.5-month period postinjection. Thus, it is with reasonable certainty that measurements of the ^{210}Pb content in the head have provided suitable data for the measurement of ^{210}Pb in the skull bones, i.e. the measurement site used for the determination of ^{210}Pb in uranium miners. A representative curve illustrating this measurement over a one-year period for four baboons is seen in figure 3.

As predicted by the power function model for the retention of bone-seeking isotopes, the effective half time for ^{210}Pb in bone has continued to increase as a function of the time elapsed postinjection. As of the most recent measurements, the retention of ^{210}Pb in the skull of two animals under test for

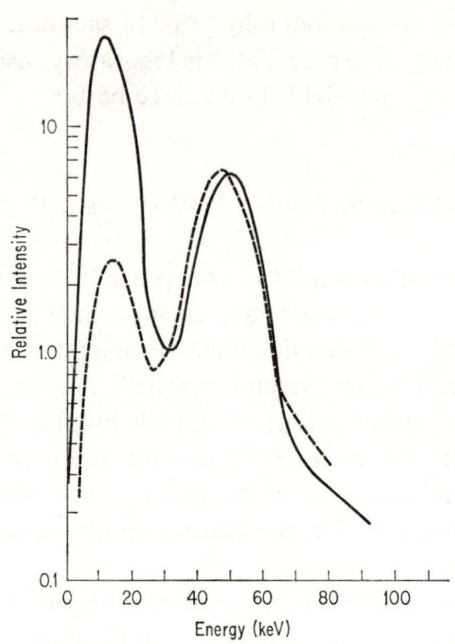

Fig. 1. ^{210}Pb photon spectrum for massless source (–) and in baboon skull (---) configurations. NaI-CsI 8″ diameter detector.

approximately three years can be approximated by a sum of two exponential components with half lives of 0.26 ± 0.04 and 1.96 ± 0.13 years.

In addition to *in vivo* measurements, sequential bioassay determinations of ^{210}Pb in urine, feces, blood and hair were performed for all baboons as an additional measure of whole body retention. Half times determined from these results were in good agreement with those obtained from *in vivo* measurements. Analysis of individual urine and fecal samples has established the fecal route as an important mode of lead loss from the body with 24-hour urine to fecal concentration ratios increasing from 1.25 to 1.80 at three years postinjection. Distribution of ^{210}Pb among soft tissues and bones was determined after autopsy at various times postinjection. Liver, kidney and spleen

---

Fig. 3. ^{210}Pb *in vivo* retention measurements over the skull for four baboons (□ = B-100; ○ = B-106; △ = B-358; × = B-394). $\gamma = 0.686e^{-1.81 \times 10^{-3}}$ (+ in days). t ½ = 1.05 ± 0.08 years, $\varrho = 0.94$.

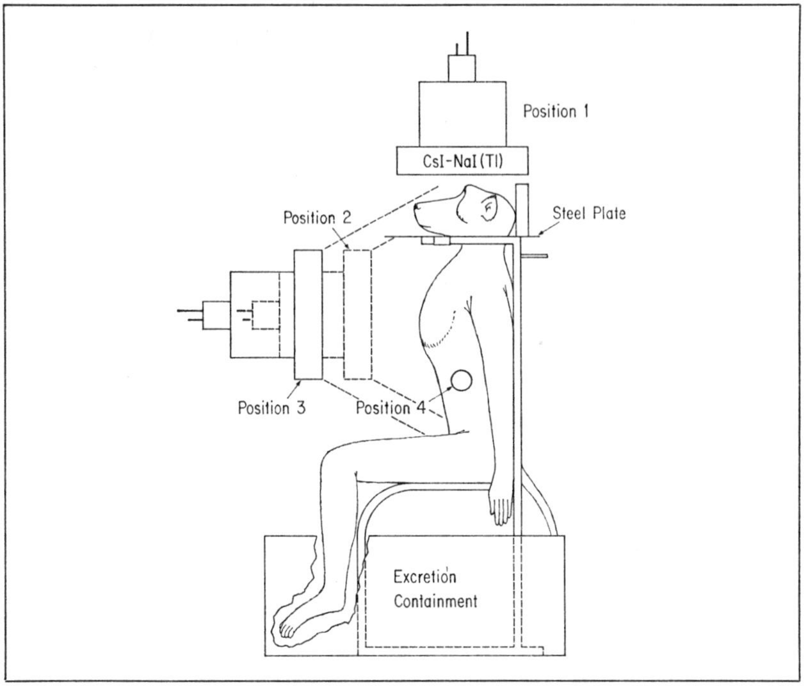

Fig. 2. Detector configurations for ^{210}Pb measurements in the adult baboon. Positions: 1 = head measurement; 2 = thorax measurement; 3 = effective whole body count; 4 = kidney measurement.

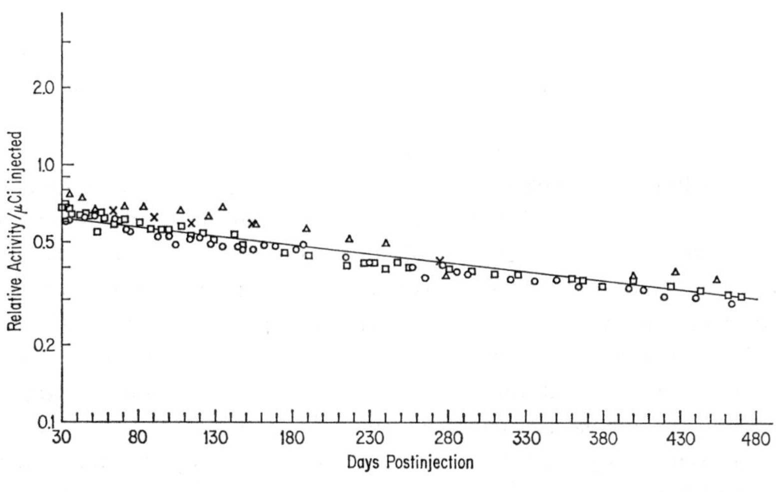

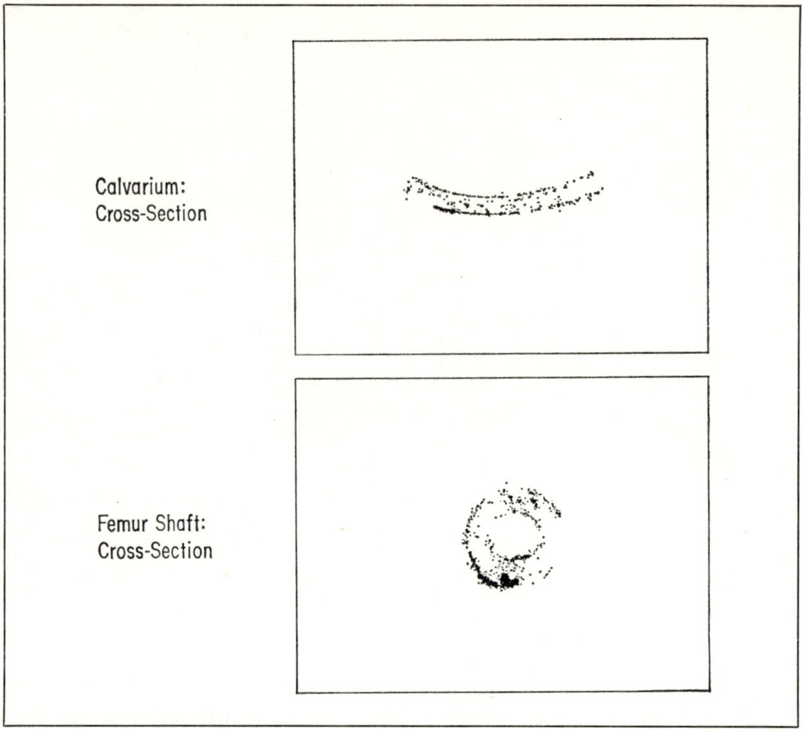

Fig. 4. Distribution of ^{210}Pb in bone determined by α-autoradiographic techniques. B-158 (two months postinjection; five-day exposure, enlarged).

were found to represent major soft tissue uptake sites with the liver predominating at 12.8, 4.7 and 2.3% of the injection dose at one day, one and two months postinjection. For the same time periods the skeleton contained 8.6, 52.2 and 71.3% of the body burden.

Distribution of ^{210}Pb among various bones of the skull and of the skeleton indicated that the mandible and maxilla are consistently a factor of 1.5 and 2 times greater in activity than in all other bones measured. Furthermore, the concentration of ^{210}Pb in teeth was only 40% of the average bone concentration. In addition to the concentration distribution of ^{210}Pb among the various bones, semimicrodistribution of ^{210}Pb within sections of calvarium and femur were determined by autoradiography of undecalcified bone and by sequential thick source α-emission measurements using controlled physical abrasion and standard α-ray proportional counter measurements. Both techniques led to the generalized conclusions that within an initial one- to-two month period after injection, the nuclide is primarily localized in the bone trabeculae with the distribution becoming more diffuse as a function of time (fig. 4).

2. *Short-Term Metabolism of* ^{241}*Am* [ROSEN *et al.*, 1972]

^{241}Am, a transuranium α-emitting nuclide with a radiological half life of 458 years, is a source of considerable concern as a potential contamination problem to man. Experience with ^{241}Am contamination to date has been mainly with workers accidently exposed via inhalation, cuts or puncture wounds. As a result of the greater production and use of the transuranic elements, the probability of such accidents occurring is expected to increase. It has been estimated, for example, that the production of ^{241}Am will be on the

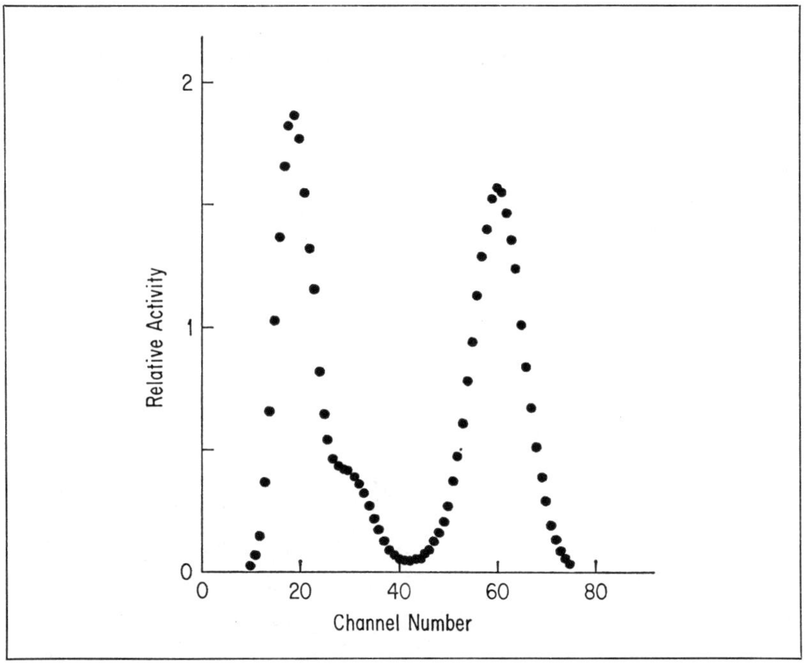

Fig. 5. ^{241}Am photon spectrum-massless source configuration. CsI-NaI 6″ diameter detector.

order of megacuries per year as breeder reactors become a major source of energy [WEINBERG and HAMMOND, 1970]. This laboratory has recently taken part in the measurement of ^{241}Am in several members of a family who became inadvertently contaminated [WRENN *et al.*, 1971]. Concurrent with this study, the distribution and retention of ^{241}Am has been measured in four adult female baboons after single i.v. injections of ^{241}Am citrate. Retention of ^{241}Am in the whole body, skeleton and liver has been determined by similar *in vivo* scintillation techniques as used for measuring ^{210}Pb, this time using the 60 keV γ-ray emission of ^{241}Am. A typical photon spectrum obtained for ^{241}Am and the positioning characteristics of the detector in relation to the baboon is given in figures 5 and 6.

The estimate of effective half time of ^{241}Am in the total body from excreta analysis and from *in vivo* measurements was approximately 270 days (fig. 7). *In vivo* measurements over the head showed no detectable clearance from the skull during the same period.

In addition to specific site *in vivo* measurements, serial biopsy samples were obtained to determine the rate of clearance of ^{241}Am from the liver (fig. 8).

Clearance of ^{241}Am from the blood was rapid with less than 1 % of the

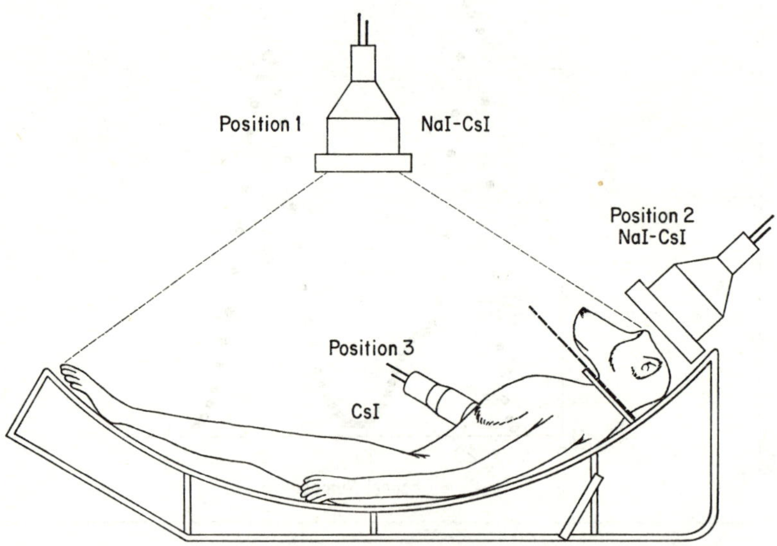

Fig. 6. Detector configuration for ^{241}Am-measurements in the adult baboon. Positions: 1 = whole body count; 2 = head count; 3 = liver area scan.

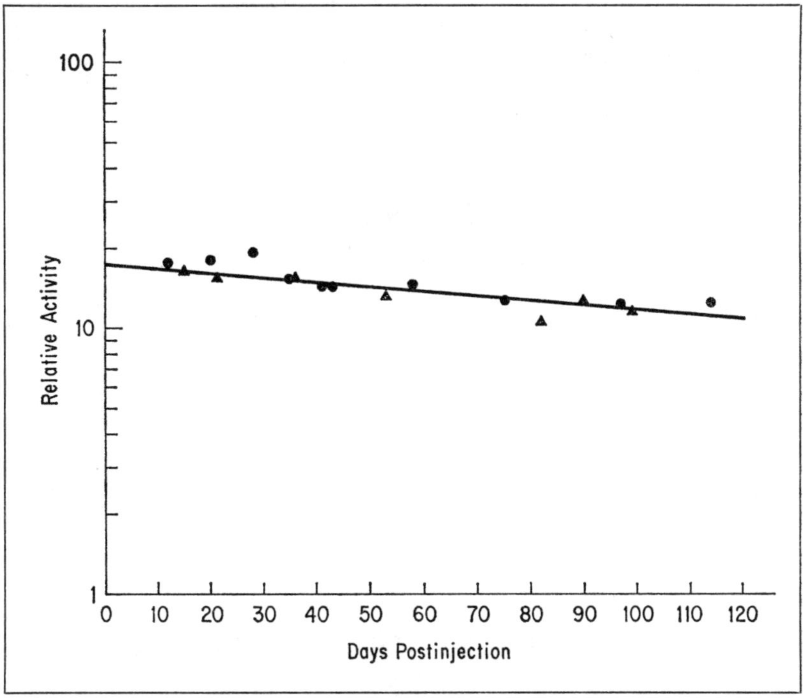

Fig. 7. ^{241}Am *in vivo* whole body retention measurements for two baboons (● = B-458; ▲ = B-460).

injected dose remaining at 48 h and less than 0.05% remaining one month postinjection. Greater than 90% of the activity was associated with the plasma fraction.

Two animals were sacrified at one and three months postinjection. In order of decreasing total activity, the major loci were the skeleton, liver, lungs and kidney, all accounting for approximately 85% of the retained ^{241}Am. At the end of one month, the highest concentration of activity was found in the liver with concentrations decreasing in the order of bone, lung, aorta, kidney and spleen. Among various bones, the concentration of ^{241}Am varied within a factor of four, with highest concentrations in the vertebrae. The concentration in the ends of long bone was two to three times higher than in the shafts.

There are no biopsy samples available from the accidentally-exposed humans under study. Based on *in vivo* counting, bone and liver appear to be

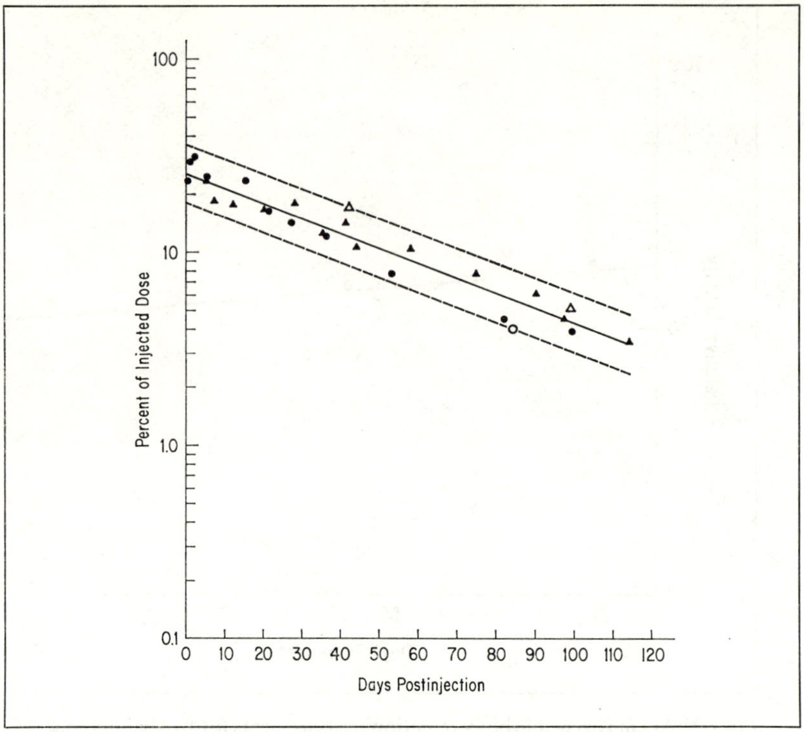

Fig. 8. In vivo and biopsy measurements of ^{241}Am in the livers of two baboons (B-460: ● = *in vivo;* ○ = biopsy. B-458: ▲ = *in vivo;* △ = biopsy). ---- = 95% prediction limits. $\gamma = 2.54 \times 10^4 e^{177 \times 10^{-2} t}$, where t is in days. $t^1/_2$ eff. = 39.1 days. Correlation coefficient = 0.97.

the major loci of deposition. This is consistent with the distribution observed in the baboon.

3. Lead Toxicity Studies

In addition to the two investigations described above, pilot studies of stable lead toxicity in the juvenile baboon, using ^{210}Pb as an isotopic tracer, have been initiated [COHEN *et al.*, 1972b]. To date this work has demonstrated the susceptibility of the baboon to the toxic effects of lead absorption (fig. 9). The symptoms and progress of the induced toxicity appear to duplicate those described for acute cases of pediatric lead poisoning, thereby making the baboon an ideal experimental animal in which to perform this research.

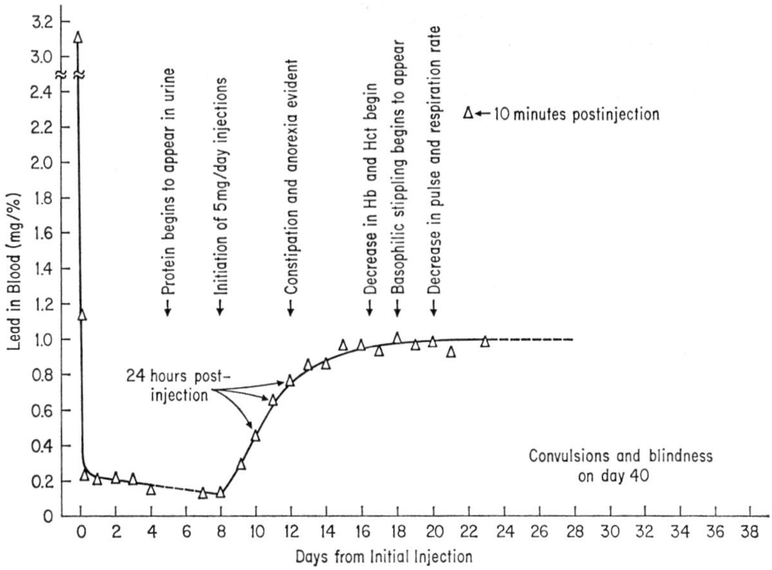

Fig. 9. Concentration of stable lead in blood and clinical symptomatology as a function of time. Five mg lead/day i.v. route.

Acknowledgements

The authors would like to thank Ms. Lynn Ayres and the staff of the LEMSIP Laboratory for their helpful advice and technical assistance in all phases of these studies.

References

Bryant, F.J. and Loutit, J.F.: The entry of Sr-90 into human bone. Proc. roy. Soc. B. *159:* 449–465 (1964).

Cohen, N.: The retention and distribution of lead-210 in the adult baboon. NYO-3086-10 (1970).

Cohen, N.; Jaakkola, T., and Wrenn, M.E.: Lead-210 concentrations in the bone, blood and excreta of a former uranium miner (to be publ. in Health Phys., 1972a).

Cohen, N.; Kneip, T.J.; Goldstein, D.H., and Muchmore, E.A.S.: The juvenile baboon as a model for studies of lead poisoning in children. J. med. Prim. *1:* 142–155 (1972b).

Eisenbud, M.; Laurer, G.R.; Rosen, J.C.; Cohen, N.; Thomas, J., and Hazle, A.J.: *In vivo* measurement of Pb-210 as an indicator of cumulative radon daughter exposure in uranium miners. Health Phys. *16:* 637–646 (1969).

HENNEMAN, D.H.: Comparative solubility of bone and skin collagen in primates including man. J.med.Prim. *1:* 58–67 (1972).

ROSEN, J.C.; COHEN, N., and WRENN, M.E.: Short term metabolism of Am-241 in the adult baboon (to be publ. in Health Phys., 1972).

WEINBERG, A.M. and HAMMOND, R.P.: Limits to the use of energy. Amer. Scient. *58:* 412 (1970).

WRENN, M.E.; ROSEN, J.C., and COHEN, N.: *In vivo* measurement of Am-241 burdens in man. NYO-3086-11 (1971).

Authors' address: NORMAN COHEN and McDONALD E. WRENN, New York University Medical Center, Institute of Environmental Medicine, *New York, NY 10016* (USA)

Medical Primatology 1972. Proc. 3rd Conf. exp. Med. Surg. Primates, Lyon 1972, part III, pp. 237–240 (Karger, Basel 1972)

Ethanol Dependence in Rhesus Monkeys[1]

F. W. ELLIS and J. R. PICK

Department of Pharmacology and Division of Laboratory Animal Medicine, School of Medicine, University of North Carolina, Chapel Hill, N.C.

An animal model of physical dependence on ethanol has been produced in our laboratory by the technique of forced heavy alcohol intake through nasogastric intubation in rhesus monkeys *(Macaca mulatta)*. Details of this procedure have been published [ELLIS and PICK, 1970].

The purpose of this communication is to summarize the essential principles of the procedure and to succinctly describe the typical withdrawal reactions which emerge upon abrupt termination of ethanol administration as evidence of the induction of dependence.

Material and Methods

Ethanol administration. Animals are housed in individual cages. After removal from the cage, a small lubricated catheter is passed intranasally into the stomach and a measured amount of aqueous ethanol solution (25%, w/v) is injected from a syringe. The animal is then returned to his home-cage. Doses of ethanol in the range of 2–4 g/kg are given twice daily, morning and evening to maintain a tolerable, reproducible degree of intoxication on a bidaily fluctuating basis. The specific dose given on any particular occasion to a specific animal is ascertained by the prevailing blood-ethanol concentration (BEC) monitored by an automated analytical method developed in our laboratory [ELLIS and HILL, 1969], and by the observed level of intoxication just prior to the next scheduled administration.

1 Supported in part by USPHS grants GRS 5-S01 Fr-05406, 1 R02 MH 16064 and RR 00478.

Results and Discussion

A summary of the regimen of administration in five typical animals is shown in table I. It is seen that BEC may be rather low the first day or two, which is due, commonly, to vomiting. After this early reaction to intubation the animals tolerate fairly large doses of ethanol which fall in the mean daily range of 5–6 g/kg. Such doses produce BEC ranges within about 100–500 mg/100 ml. Also, it is seen that only 10–16 days of ethanol administration is necessary to induce dependence.

Table I. Ethanol administration by gastric intubation to rhesus monkeys

Monkey No.	Period of intubation days	Weight of animal kg	Mean daily dose g/kg	Mean range of BEC[1] mg/100 ml
1	1–2	4.1	7.5	224–350
	3–14	3.8	6.63	179–452
2	1–2	3.9	7.25	ND[2]
	3–10	3.5	6.44	152–457
3	1–2	3.8	7.5	16–83
	3–14	3.5	6.21	225–443
4	1–2	3.8	6.75	17–234
	3–15	4.0	5.75	241–462
5	1–2	4.3	6.25	35–355
	3–16	4.2	6.13	218–447

1 Blood-ethanol concentration.
2 Not determined.

Nature of Withdrawal Reactions

Upon sudden cessation of the described administration regimen a predictable series of reactions emerge in chronological order related to the elapsed time since the last intubation and the declining BEC. In table II the *tremulous, spastic* and *convulsive* stages, which emerge with progressive severity, are defined in relation to the interval of time since ethanol was given and the residual BEC range associated with the respective stages. It should be emphasized that definitive tremors begin at BEC as high as 200 mg/100 ml and that convulsions almost routinely emerge prior to the complete disappearance of ethanol from the blood stream.

Table II. Ethanol withdrawal syndrome in rhesus monkeys

Stages	Reactions	Postethanol interval, h	BEC range mg/100 ml
Tremulous	hyperreflexia	12–15	125–200
	muscle tremors		
	muscle fasciculations		
Spastic	muscle spasticity	15–18	50–150
	muscle rigidity		
	apparent fright		
	behavioral changes		
	'automatic' effects		
	salivation		
	mydriasis		
	retching/vomiting		
	urination		
	defecation		
	hyperthermia (rectal)		
Convulsive	clonic-tonic convulsions	18–24	0–85
	(1–6 fully sustained)		

The withdrawal reactions will be described as illustrated by three typical experimental results:

The first animal had received ethanol for 14 consecutive days and on the 15th day, 16 h beyond the last intubation, the BEC was 175 mg/100 ml. Two hours later marked generalized tremors were present at BEC of 103 mg/100 ml. As tremors progressed altered behavioral mannerisms such as 'watching' patterns, grabbing reactions and 'apprehensive' facial expressions occurred. Spastic muscle movements and pulling at rear legs coincided with BEC of 50 mg/100 ml, 20 h after the last dose of ethanol. The first convulsion in this animal emerged about 21 h following the previous intubation when BEC had declined to 20 mg/100 ml. Within less than an hour, five other convulsions occurred, after which the animal died.

The second monkey was withdrawn from ethanol administration after 15 days. The initial view on withdrawal day showed calmness at BEC of 289 mg/100 ml, 15½ h after ethanol was given. Extreme spasticity and gross body shaking occurred about 20 h after the last ethanol dose and with BEC at 120 mg/100 ml. Retching followed 30 min later. Onset of the first convulsion occurred 21 h from intubation at 85 mg/100 ml BEC. Following the second convulsion in this animal ethanol was given first by i.v. administration

(10%, w/v in saline) and subsequently by intubation which immediately suppressed all withdrawal reactions.

Ethanol administration was terminated in a third animal after 16 consecutive days of intoxication. A 'guarded' position was observed 15½ h after the last ethanol administration with BEC at 73 mg/100 ml, and then reactions rapidly progressed within 30 min through this spastic stage to a convulsion. After surviving four additional convulsions during a period of 1½ h, this monkey gradually recovered without treatment from the withdrawal syndrome and appeared normal on the third postconvulsive day (a film illustrating the three cases described was presented by authors at the 3rd Conference on Experimental Medicine in Primates).

References

Ellis, F.W. and Hill, J.B.: An automated fluorometric procedure for the enzymatic determination of ethanol in fingertip blood. Clin. Chem. *15:* 91–101 (1969).

Ellis, F.W. and Pick, J.R.: Experimentally induced ethanol dependence in rhesus monkeys. J. Pharmacol. exp. Ther. *175:* 88–93 (1970).

Authors' addresses: Dr. Fred W. Ellis, Department of Pharmacology, School of Medicine, University of North Carolina, *Chapel Hill, NC 27514* and Dr. James R. Pick, Division of Laboratory Animal Medicine, School of Medicine, University of North Carolina, *Chapel Hill, NC 27514* (USA)

Medical Primatology 1972. Proc. 3rd Conf. exp. Med. Surg. Primates, Lyon 1972, part III, pp. 241–249 (Karger, Basel 1972)

Methods of Study and the Effects of the Naturally Occurring Bracken Fern Carcinogen in a Nonhuman Primate, *Macaca fascicularis*

I. ANTICE EVANS, R. MAINWARING-BURTON, B. R. ALLPORT and NOELINE GREY

Department of Biochemistry and Soil Science, University College of North Wales, Bangor

Bracken fern *(Pteridium aquilinum)* is a rampant weed, widespread throughout the world and estimated to occupy a million acres in the British Isles alone. The fern and rhizome, both fresh and dried, and extracts of the plant, contain a toxin(s) which if administered in sufficient concentration can be acutely toxic to a wide variety of species including mice, quail and bovines [3, 5, 15–18, 22, 23, 30). Sub-lethal doses have pluripotent carcinogenic and mutagenic properties, producing a high rate of malignancy and dominant lethal mutations [1, 5–7, 10, 12, 13, 20, 23–25, 27, 30]. The acute lethal syndrome is radiomimetic in nature, being characterised by bone marrow aplasia, haemorrhage and severe gastrointestinal damage, together with other systemic changes common to both syndromes [4, 5, 8, 11, 21, 24, 28]. Isolation of the toxin(s) has been carried out in this department in parallel with the study of the biological properties and a final stage of thin layer chromatography separation has resulted in a fraction, the major component of which gives a molecular formula $C_7H_{10}O_5$ [1, 5, 17, 18, 22–24, 30]. This has recently been characterised chemically and the results of this concurrent investigation will be reported elsewhere by the workers concerned.

In some parts of the world, notably Japan, the fern is consumed directly by humans, either in a raw, cooked or canned condition. This is the young, unfurled crozier stage when the plant is most toxic, and it has been shown that neither method of treatment has removed the toxin [18, 20, 22, 30]. Of much wider significance is the fact that the contamination of milk is possible and could well constitute a hazard for human health in many areas throughout the world of marginal and upland farming where cattle are known to consume bracken [9, 14]. The presence of a carcinogen in the urine of such animals has also been reported [19, 26]. The danger accruing from the consumption of contaminated milk is accentuated by the demonstration of age dependence in bracken-induced tumours, where it is the young animal which is at risk [12, 30].

Although it is not yet known if the causative agent is the same as the carcinogen, it is of interest that bracken has been shown experimentally to produce irreversible eye damage in sheep known as 'wall eye' or 'bright blindness', and characterised by stenosis of the blood vessels and progressive degeneration of the neuro-epithelium of the retina [2, 29]. Apart from the short and long-term effects of radiation already mentioned, it is well known that it can have a deleterious influence on vision, notably by the production of cataracts.

There are still many types of human cancer with a marked regional incidence which is largely unexplained, such as the high rate of stomach cancer in Japan and North Wales, or oesophageal and bladder tumours in other areas. It is quite likely that more than one factor is involved, but it is important to know if a naturally occurring carcinogen, with possible human hazard, can produce malignancies in primates as it does in so many other species and, if so, what is their nature. Even though one cannot extrapolate from non-human primates to man or, for that matter, from one individual to another, this is the nearest experimental approach to an evaluation of the human response. As this will in all probability entail a protracted wait during the latent period, the present paper is concerned with the immediate response and reactivity of *Macaca fascicularis* to oral administration of the bracken carcinogen. Young monkeys (two males and six females, during late puberty and early sexual maturity) have received concentrated extracts of the toxin, while at the same time infants (three males and five females, under 12 months at the beginning of the experiment) have been fed daily with a supplement of fresh milk from cows consuming a sub-lethal amount of bracken in their diet. This latter part of the investigation is an attempt, as nearly as possible, to reproduce the situation of human infants consuming daily amounts of fresh milk (i.e. unbulked, unprocessed) from cows grazing bracken contaminated pastures anywhere in the world.

Methods

If the bracken toxin has activity in *Macaca fascicularis*, this should result in changes in the bone marrow and peripheral haematological picture. Adequate monitoring entails the collection of frequent blood samples (every two to three days) for extended periods. Only a small volume (about nine drops) is needed at any one time, but for platelet counts it must be used immediately without an anticoagulant, and the smears for leucocyte differentials are also better if made from fresh drawn blood. It is also necessary to minimise disturbance, since monkeys are particularly prone to misleading physiological leucocytosis. It was, therefore, desirable to avoid catching and undue restraint, anaesthesia, or repeated entry into large veins such as the cephalic or saphenous. Caudal bleeding was adopted, and, after more than a year's usage, has proved successful with both fully grown and baby monkeys. Full details will be given in an extended publication.

The following parameters were recorded using the methods described in our previous publications: total leucocytes, thrombocytes and erythrocytes; differential leucocytes and packed cell volume. Variability in the degree of erythrocyte lysis, which tended to obscure thrombocyte enumeration, was overcome by addition of one drop of $^{1}/_{10}$ Coulter Zaponin per 1.0 ml modified Rees-Ecker diluting fluid.

Fractionation of the bracken toxin was taken to the post-Sephadex stage [22, 23], which is unpalatable for monkeys but was accepted without wastage when mixed with thick fruit-flavoured sauces marketed by the HP Company. During the periods of dosing the six female monkeys were given extract twice weekly and the total amount per week was extracted from 240 g dried bracken (240 g ≡). For monkeys averaging 3 kg this gives a rate of dosage of approximately 11.0 g ≡ dried bracken per kilogram body weight per day. (In rats a dose of 10–15 g ≡ per kilogram body weight per day was found to be carcinogenic.) The two larger male monkeys (4 kg) were dosed at the rate of 19 g ≡ dried bracken per kilogram body weight, for 24 days. As this was tolerated, the dose was doubled for a fortnight.

To produce the bracken milk for the baby monkeys, two Friesians and an Ayrshire cow have been fed bracken twice daily at a sub-lethal rate of 1–2.8 g dried bracken per kilogram body weight daily, being given as a supplement to their normal diet by pelleting into reconstituted nuts. The morning and afternoon milk is fed fresh to the young monkeys every day as a substitute for water. On average, they drink 0.75–1.0 l each a week.

In order to take weights, rectal temperatures and carry out regular ophthalmic studies and eye photography we constrict the monkeys by wrapping in a net. Photographic records are obtained by use of a Kowa R.C-2 Fundus Camera. A mydriatic is necessary, and one drop of 1% Lachesine has been found satisfactory.

Results

The following figures for normal blood counts for young adult *Macaca fascicularis* have been compiled from records collected over 14 months for eight animals, prior to bracken administration. Normal total leucocyte counts fall between 7,000–16,000 mm^3, with the majority between 8,000–13,000 mm^3. The normal variation in counts for an individual monkey can be up to 3,500. Physiological leucocytosis results in figures of 19,000–21,000 mm^3, and these are discounted. The differential leucocyte counts are as follows: lymphocytes 6,000–9,000 mm^3 (55–70%), neutrophils 1,600–4,400 mm^3 (15–40%), monocytes 160–540 mm³ (1.5–5.0%), eosinophils 120–410 mm³ (1.1–3.7%), basophils 0–130 mm³ (0–1.2%).

Platelet counts are as usual very steady, with normal values ranging from 200,000–700,000 mm³, the majority between 300,000–400,000 mm³, with individual variation up to 100,000. Erythrocyte counts vary from 4,5 to 7.0 million/mm³. The majority fall between 5.0–6.0 million/mm³ and the normal variation in an animal can be up to 1 million. There does not seem to be a sex difference as in humans; the female counts can be as high as, or higher than, the males. Normal microhaematocrit readings range from 35 to 50%, with a standard 40-percent, and the normal variation does not exceed 5%.

Normal blood counts for *M. fascicularis* six to 12 months old are found to be in the same range as the adults for leucocytes and thrombocytes, but erythrocytes are high and come between 6.0 and 7.0 million/mm³.

The adult female monkeys were dosed for three and a half weeks and the males for five weeks; the graphs (fig. 1–4) are typical for the results obtained. The leucocyte and platelet figures did not fall dramatically as would occur in bovines at a similar dose level (a total of 300 g dried bracken per kilogram body weight is sufficient to produce a fatal outcome in a calf after four to six weeks). However, analysis of the monkey results showed that the average fluctuations in all the counts were approximately twice as large during the bracken period when compared with control figures, and would indicate bone marrow response and reparative overcompensation. Myeloid impairment was confirmed in some monkeys in which neutrophil counts fell at times below

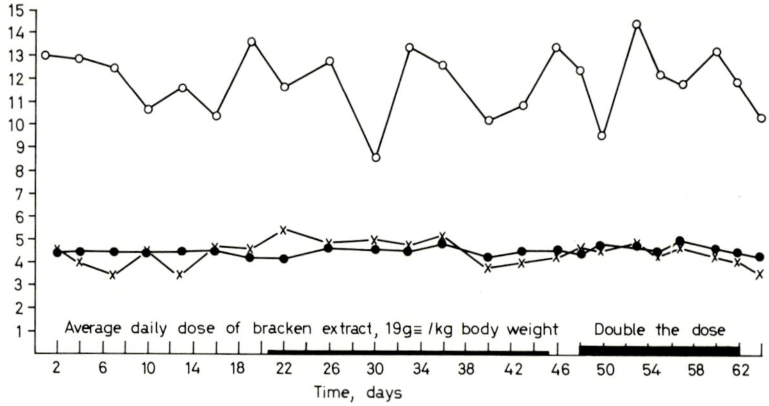

Fig. 1. Macaca fascicularis, 'George' (male). Haematological response to bracken extract. × = Platelets × 10⁵/mm³; ○ = total leucocytes × 10³/mm³; ● = microhaematocrit erythrocytes volume %.

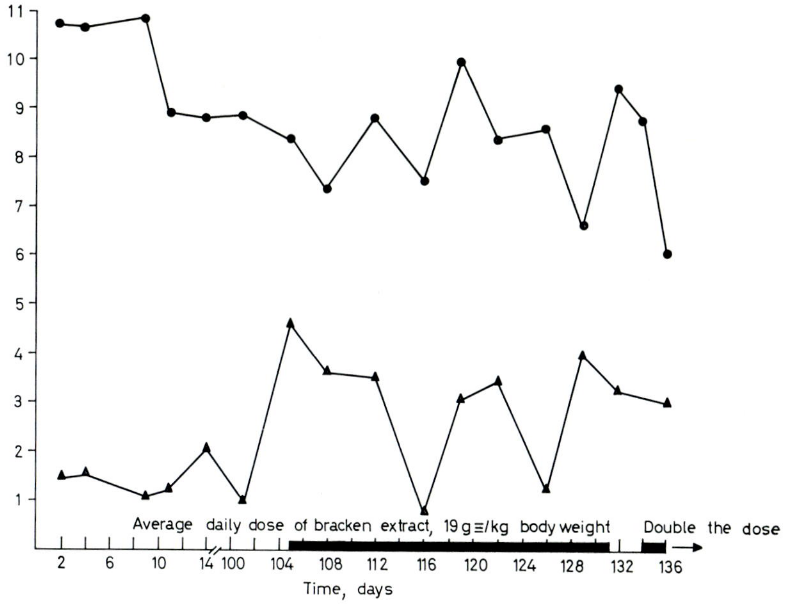

Fig. 2. Macaca fascicularis, 'George' (male). Haematological response to bracken extract. Differential leucocyte count. ▲ = Neutrophils $\times 10^3/mm^3$; ● = lymphocytes $\times 10^3/mm^3$ (average of 1,000 cells per count).

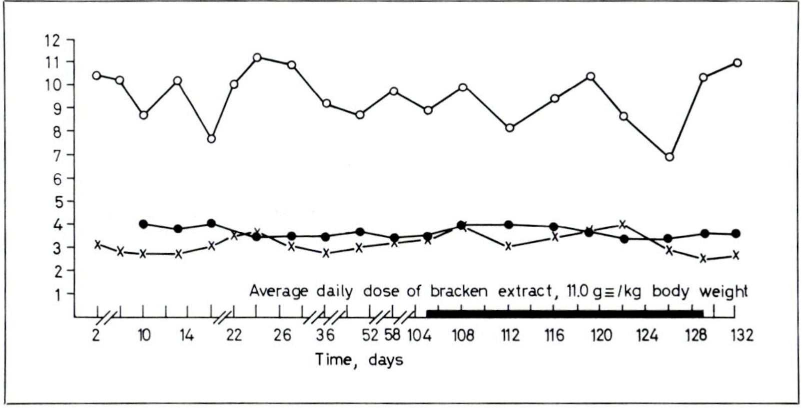

Fig. 3. Macaca fascicularis, 'Whiskas' (female). Haematological response to bracken extract. × = Platelets $\times 10^5/mm^3$; ○ = total leucocytes $\times 10^3/mm^3$; ● = microhaematocrit erythrocytes volume %.

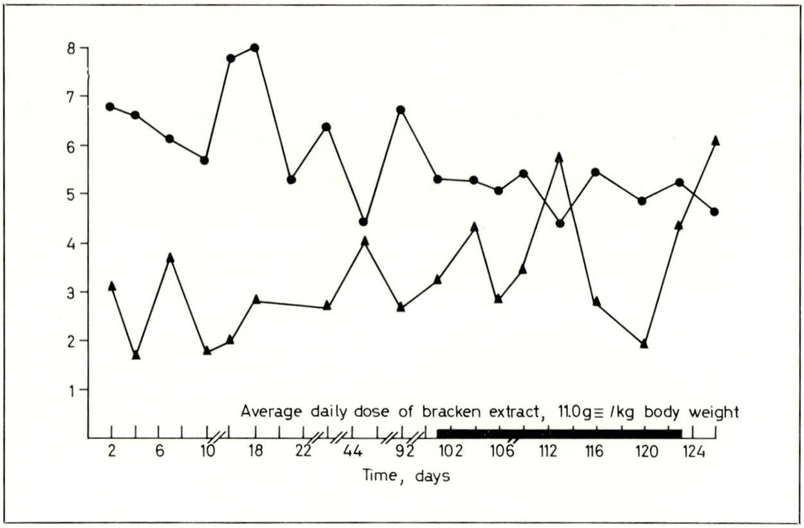

Fig. 4. Macaca fascicularis, 'Whiskas' (female). Haematological response to bracken extract. Differential leucocyte count. ▲ = Neutrophils $\times 10^3/mm^3$; ● = lymphocytes $\times 10^3/mm^3$ (average of 1,000 cells per count).

10 %, significantly outside the normal range, and very reminiscent of the calf picture.

Owing to their small size, the baby monkeys have been bled much less frequently than the adults and so far the counts are normal, although recently the thrombocyte figures have shown a slight fall which will be of interest if maintained.

The majority of monkeys appeared to be normal and healthy with regard to the condition of their eyes. Generally, the results of this examination showed that both infant and adult *M. fascicularis* can be expected to have an arcus temporally and nasally, which is sharply defined peripherally but tends to fade into the central cornea. In some, including the young, there is central lenticular nuclear haziness. Both these features are present prior to administration of bracken.

Discussion

It is clear from the results that *M. fascicularis,* like other simple-stomached animals, does not have an acute reaction to bracken toxin at a dose level which would be lethal in bovines. However, the production of the acutely fatal gastrointestinal and bone marrow syndrome in animals such as both bovines and mice depends only on the administration of a large enough dose and, so far, this experiment indicates that the same could be true for primates. It may be justifiably questioned that humans would ever consume bracken at the rate ingested by these different experimental animals. Nevertheless, basic susceptibility to the toxin is the important thing, since the fact remains that in mice we have produced malignancies by a single sub-lethal dose of toxin, given either orally by stomach tube, or by i.p. injection. If the latter route is used, the toxin extracted from only 3.5 g dried bracken is sufficient to furnish a carcinogenic dose. Further, we have results [as yet unpublished] which show that significant numbers of tumours, including gastric neoplasms, occur in mice which have suckled for only a three-week period from mother mice given bracken toxin supplement to their diet during lactation.

There is thus every reason for the continuation of this nonhuman primate experiment which will ultimately furnish information not only on the nature of possible bracken tumourigenesis in monkeys, but also indicate the reality or otherwise of the indirect hazard to human populations in bracken lands.

Acknowledgements

We wish to thank the following for their generous financial support: The Cancer Research Campaign, The Wellcome Foundation, Rank Hovis Ltd., The Medical Research Council, Monsanto Chemicals Ltd. We are most grateful to the following for their time, help and interest: Prof. W. C. Evans, Mr. R. F. E. Axford, M. R. C. V. S., Mr. W. H. Lloyd, M. R. C. V. S., Mr. K. R. Hobbs, Prof. S. Cohen, Prof. J. T. Eayrs, Mrs. Angela Davey, the Pathology Laboratory, C. & A. Hospital and the Veterinary Investigation Centre, Bryn Adda. This project has only been made possible by the sustained hard work and support of Mr. E. Hughes and many members of the technical staff, to whom we ar most grateful.

References

1 Barber, G. D.: Mutagenic and other radiomimetic properties of bracken; PhD thesis Bangor (1969).

2 Barnett, K. C. and Watson, W. A.: Bright blindness in sheep. A primary retinopathy due to feeding bracken *(Pteris aquilina)*. Res. Vet. Sci. *11:* 289–290 (1970).

3 Evans, E. T. R.; Evans, W. C., and Hughes, L. E.: Developments in the investigation into 'bracken poisoning' in cattle. Vet. Rec. *63:* 444 (1951).

4 EVANS, I.A.: The radiomimetic nature of bracken toxin. Cancer Res. *28:* 2252–2261 (1968).

5 EVANS, I.A.: Bracken fern toxin. Oncology 1970. Proc. 10th Int. Cancer Congress, vol.5. Part A: Environmental cancer (Year Book, Chicago 1972).

6 EVANS, I.A.; BARBER, G.D.; JONES, R.S., and LEACH, H.: Carcinogenic activity of bracken. British Empire Cancer Campaign for Research, Annual Report, p.416 (1968).

7 EVANS, I.A.; BARBER, G.D.; JONES, R.S., and LEACH, H.: Carcinogenic activity of bracken. British Empire Cancer Campaign for Research, Annual Report, pp.446–447 (1969).

8 EVANS, I.A. and HOWELL, R.M.: Bovine bracken poisoning. Nature, Lond. *194:* 584 (1962).

9 EVANS, I.A.; JONES, R.S., and MAINWARING-BURTON, R.: Passage of bracken fern toxicity into milk. Nature, Lond. *237:* 107–108 (1972).

10 EVANS, I.A. and MASON, J.: Carcinogenic activity of bracken. Nature, Lond. *208:* 913–914 (1965).

11 EVANS, I.A.; THOMAS, A.J.; EVANS, W.C., and EDWARDS, C.M.: Studies on bracken poisoning in cattle. Brit.vet.J. *114:* 253–267 (1958).

12 EVANS, I.A. and WIDDOP, B.: Carcinogenic activity of bracken. British Empire Cancer Campaign for Research, Annual Report, p.377 (1966).

13 EVANS, I.A.; WIDDOP, B., and BARBER, G.D.: Carcinogenic activity of bracken. British Empire Cancer Campaign for Research, Annual Report, pp.411–412 (1967).

14 EVANS, I.A.; WIDDOP, B.; JONES, R.S.; BARBER, G.D.; LEACH, H.; JONES, D.L., and MAINWARING-BURTON, R.: The possible human hazard of the naturally occurring bracken carcinogen. Biochem.J. *124:* 28–29 (1971).

15 EVANS, W.C.; EVANS, E.T.R., and HUGHES, L.E.: Studies on bracken poisoning in cattle. Brit.vet.J. *110:* 295–306, 365–380, 426–444 (1954).

16 EVANS, W.C.; EVANS, I.A.; AXFORD, R.F.E.; THRELFALL, G.; HUMPHREYS, D.J., and THOMAS, A.J.: Studies on bracken poisoning in cattle. VII. The toxicity of bracken rhizomes. Vet.Rec. *35:* 852–853 (1961).

17 EVANS, W.C.; EVANS, I.A.; CHAMBERLAIN, A.G., and THOMAS, A.J.: Studies on bracken poisoning in cattle. Brit.vet.J. *115:* 83–85 (1959).

18 EVANS, W.C.; EVANS, I.A.; THOMAS, A.J.; WATKIN, J.E., and CHAMBERLAIN, A.G.: Studies on bracken poisoning in cattle. Brit.vet.J. *114:* 180–196 (1958).

19 GEORGIEV, R.; VRIGASOV, A.; ANTANOV, S., und DIMITROV, A.: Versuche zur Feststellung der Anwesenheit kanzerogener Stoffe im Harn der mit Heu aus Hämaturiegebieten gefütterten Kühe. Wien.tierärztl. Mschr. *50:* 589–595 (1963).

20 HIRONO, I.; SHIBUYA, C.; FUSHIMI, K., and HAGA, M.: Studies on carcinogenic properties of bracken, *Pteridium aquilinum.* J.nat.Cancer Inst. *45:* 179–188 (1970).

21 HOWELL, R.M. and EVANS, I.A.: Chromatographic characteristics of fibrinogen and seromucoid in bovine bracken poisoning. J.comp.Path. *77:* 117–128 (1967).

22 LEACH, H.: The chemical isolation of a toxic component of bracken; MSc thesis Bangor (1970).

23 LEACH, H.; BARBER, G.D.; EVANS, I.A., and EVANS, W.C.: Isolation of an active principle from the bracken fern that is mutagenic, carcinogenic and lethal to mice on intraperitoneal injection. Biochem.J. *124:* 13–14 (1971).

24 MASON, J.: Pathology of radiomimetic conditions; PhD thesis Bangor (1965).

25 PAMUKCU, A.M.; GÖKSOY, S.K., and PRICE, J.M.: Urinary bladder neoplasms induced by feeding bracken fern *(Pteris aquilina)* to cows. Cancer Res. *27:* 917–924 (1967).

26 PAMUKCU, A.M.; OLSON, C., and PRICE, J.M.: Assay of fractions of bovine urine for carcinogenic activity after feeding bracken fern *(Pteris aquilina)*. Cancer Res. *26:* 1745–1753 (1966).

27 PRICE, J.M. and PAMUKCU, A.M.: The induction of neoplasms of the urinary bladder of the cow and the small intestine of the rat by feeding bracken fern *(Pteris aquilina)*. Cancer Res. *28:* 2247–2251 (1968).

28 TONG, A.J.: Circulatory changes in bovine bracken poisoning; MSc thesis Bangor (1966).

29 WATSON, W.A.; BARLOW, R.M., and BARNETT, K.C.: Bright blindness. A condition prevalent in Yorkshire hill sheep. Vet. Rec. *77:* 1060–1069 (1965).

30 WIDDOP, B.: Separation and characterisation of various toxicological components of bracken; PhD thesis Bangor (1967).

Authors' address: Dr. I. A. EVANS, Dr. R. MAINWARING-BURTON, Dr. B. R. ALLPORT and Dr. NOELINE GREY, Department of Biochemistry and Soil Science, University College of North Wales, *Bangor, Caernarvonshire* (North Wales)

Medical Primatology 1972. Proc. 3rd Conf. exp. Med. Surg. Primates, Lyon 1972, part III, pp. 250–258 (Karger, Basel 1972)

Two Years' Experience with *Macaca arctoides* as an Experimental Animal for Teratologic Drug Testing

J. GRAUWILER and S. BRÜGGEMANN

Biological and Medical Research Division, Sandoz Ltd., Basel

Introduction

Requests for the use of nonhuman primates in teratological drug testing have intensified in the last few years but, in fact, rather few of the drug-testing toxicological laboratories are really performing teratological work in these animals. There is no doubt that simians are expensive experimental animals, and we feel it would be unwise to use them for extensive screening tests in primate teratology. On the other hand, teratological experimentation in simians can be indispensable in special cases when there are scientific reasons for testing a drug in a species the taxonomy of which is closely related to man. Looking for a suitable primate species, we came to the conclusion that macaques are very useful, in view of the results of the experiments by DELAHUNT and LASSEN [1964] in *Macaca irus philippinensis* and of WILSON and GAVAN [1967] and BARROW *et al.* [1969] in *Macaca mulatta*. In order to test the usefulness of another macaque species in teratology and to provide new information on an additional species, we established an experimental colony of *Macaca arctoides*. This paper is to report our two years' experience with this species and to show that this animal is at least as suitable for teratological testing of drugs as are other macaque species.

Maintenance of the Breeding Colony

The animals were obtained from the dealer in several lots. They were kept in quarantine for 12 weeks. During this time clinical observation, examinations for ecto- and endoparasites, and tuberculin testing were performed, as described elsewhere [WEBER and GRAUWILER, in press].

In June, 1970, a breeding colony was started with 36 females. Ten new females were added to the colony in January, 1971, and another 28 females were taken into experimentation in February, 1972. Up to the present day, seven females had to be eliminated on account of menstrual cycle disorders or amenorrhea and three died spontaneously. The cause of death was severe hepatic cirrhosis in one animal, postoperative suffocation in anesthesia after cesarean section in another, and duodenal ulceration with massive hemorrhage in the third. Today our colony comprises 64 females. In the first series (June, 1970), 11 males were kept, six of which are still in our breeding colony. Three males were eliminated because of poor breeding performance and azoospermia, and two were sacrificed because they had been in contact with a group of tuberculous rhesus monkeys. With the third series (February, 1972) another two males were added to the colony; one of them recently died with uremia following chronic nephritis. The actual number of males in the breeding colony is seven animals.

Cycle Determination and Mating Procedures

Precise evaluation of the reproductive cycle in the female monkey is considered the most important requirement for successfully-timed breeding in teratological experiments, for the exact day of conception must be known if the dam is to be treated during a specific phase of gestation. For this reason, the female should only be mated once during a menstrual cycle: thus it is important that the optimal day for successful conception should be carefully chosen.

The methods for follow-up of menstrual cycle, mating and pregnancy diagnosis as well as the data on fetal growth and duration are described in detail elsewhere [BRÜGGEMANN and GRAUWILER, 1972]. The menstrual cycle being normally 30 days approximately, with a span of 26–40 days, it was decided to have the females mated on day 11, 12 or 13 of the cycle, if possible using HENDRICKX's formula (midcycle minus 2 days) [HENDRICKX, 1971]. The male and female were left together for 30 min, and the day of mating was considered as day 0 *post copulationem* (p.c.).

Breeding Results

Pregnancy Rates

Until April 30, 1972, 81 pregnancies occurred in our colony. Forty-two females had one pregnancy, 23 had two, 12 had three and four had four pregnancies. The total number of matings was 418; this gives a rate of 19.4% of successful matings (thus every 5th mating was successful).

Abortions

Fifteen abortions occurred during the reported time span: one of 25 untreated controls aborted within the first 30 days of pregnancy. In 25 pregnancies 11 abortions occurred in the teratological experiment with thalidomide.

Fetuses and Infants

The development of the fetuses and infants is described in detail elsewhere [BRÜGGEMANN and GRAUWILER, 1972].

Teratology in M. arctoides

Thalidomide Experiment

Methods

In order to test – in comparison with other nonhuman primates – the suitability of *M. arctoides* for teratological experimentation, a positive control with thalidomide was performed. The aim was mainly to examine the susceptibility of this species to a teratogen in comparison with the well-known results obtained in *M. mulatta, M. irus, Papio cynocephalus* and other species [WILSON *et al.*, 1970; BARROW *et al.*, 1969; DELAHUNT and LASSEN, 1964; HENDRICKX *et al.*, 1966; HENDRICKX, 1971; TANIMURA *et al.*, 1971].

In all, 25 pregnant animals were used in this study. They were treated on four consecutive days, between day 21 and 33 p.c., at dose levels of 1.25, 2.5, 5, 10 and 20 mg/kg/day orally. The compound was given in edible oblates filled with melasses. In this form it was readily accepted by the animals at all dose levels when offered before feeding. The aforementioned fetuses of nonmedicated dams, examined at various developmental stages, served as controls.

The fetuses were delivered by cesarean section. Originally this operation had been scheduled for day 100 p.c., but as most abortions occurred earlier, it was preferred to terminate pregnancy between days 60 and 80. The fetuses were dissected, examined macroscopically, X-rayed and checked for skeletal malformations.

Results (table I)

Two dams from days 21 to 24, and three from days 24 to 27 p.c. were treated with 20 mg/kg. All, except one, aborted between days 40 and 60 p.c. From one dam, treated from day 21 to 24 p.c., a normal fetus was recovered on day 97 p.c. One dam treated on days 27–30 p.c. aborted on day 64 p.c., and another treated early from days 3 to 6 p.c. had a normal fetus by cesarean section on day 97 p.c.

One dam only was treated with 10 mg/kg, from day 27 to 30 p.c. She aborted on day 32 p.c.

5 mg/kg were given to three dams from day 24 to 27 p.c. Two of them

Table I. Teratogenicity of thalidomide in *Macaca arctoides*. Four-day treatments between days 24 and 33 p.c. led to typical limb malformations with a certain phase-specificity in the 2.5-mg/kg dose. The lowest teratogenic dose was 1.25 mg/kg

Dose mg/kg	Phase of treatment, days p.c.				
	3–6	21–24	24–27	27–30	33–33
20	N	N	A	A	
		A	A		
			A		
10				A	
5			A	A	
			A		
			M/CFI		
2.5			A?/M/C	DM/FH	M/H
			M/CF	M/FHI	M/G
			N	M/F	N
1.25			N	M/FI	
			A?N	M/CF	

N = normal fetus; M = malformed fetus; A = abortion; A? = threatening abortion; D = dead fetus; C = head; F = forelimbs; H = hindlimbs; G = genitalia; I = internal organs.

aborted on days 53 and 72 p.c., respectively. The third dam had a malformed fetus on day 68 p.c., with abnormalities of the forelimbs, to be described later. Another dam was treated with the same dose from day 27 to 30 p.c. and aborted before day 40 p.c.

Three groups of three dams each were given 2.5 mg/kg on days 24–27, 27–30 and 30–33 p.c., respectively. In the group treated from day 24 to 27 one dam had a normal fetus on day 52 p.c. Another was operated on day 66 p.c. after having shown signs of impending abortion. The fetus showed severe malformations of the forelimbs. The fetus of the third dam, recovered on day 77 p.c., showed abnormalities of the forelimbs also. From the three animals treated between days 27 and 30 p.c. and operated on days 61, 69 and 70 p.c., respectively, all fetuses were malformed, one of them on the forelimbs only, and the other two on both forelimbs and hindlimbs. One of the dams was operated when it was found that the uterus had stopped to increase. The fetus was in a distinct state of autolysis. It was at a developmental stage of 45 days approximately, with severe abnormalities of the forelimbs and hindlimbs.

Of the three dams treated from days 30 to 33 p.c., one had a fetus with hindlimb abnormalities only (fig. 1), and another had a fetus with severe displacement of the external genitalia. The third fetus did not reveal any morphological anomalies.

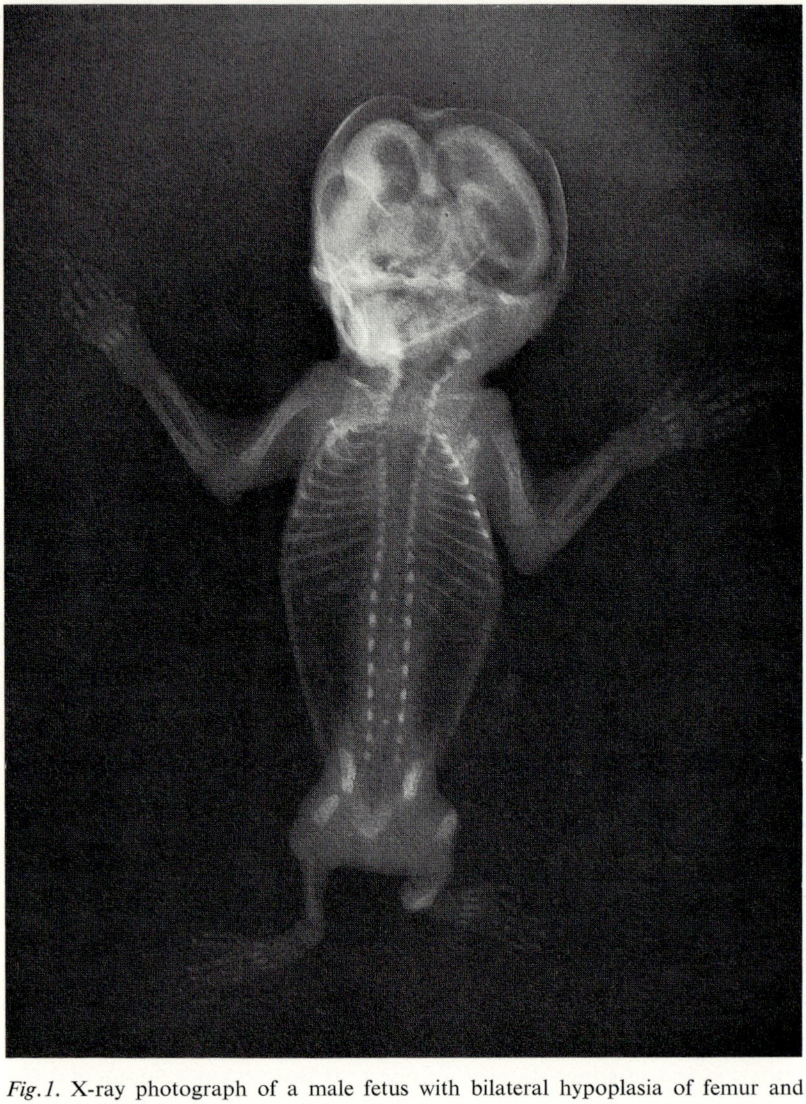

Fig. 1. X-ray photograph of a male fetus with bilateral hypoplasia of femur and aplasia of tibia, as well as aplasia of the right fibula. Cesarean section on day 69 p.c., dam treated with thalidomide, 2.5 mg/kg orally, from day 30 to 33 p.c.

A dose of 1.25 mg/kg was given to two groups of two animals each. One group was treated from day 24 to 27 p.c. and both its dams had normal fetuses at examination, although in one instance an emergency operation had to be performed on day 54 p.c., on account of impending abortion. The two dams from the other group were treated from day 27 to 30 p.c. and both had fetuses with malformations of the anterior extremities (fig. 2).

The predominant type of abnormality was aplasia and hypoplasia of the distal long bones of the extremities, i.e. radius/ulna and/or tibia/fibula. It was

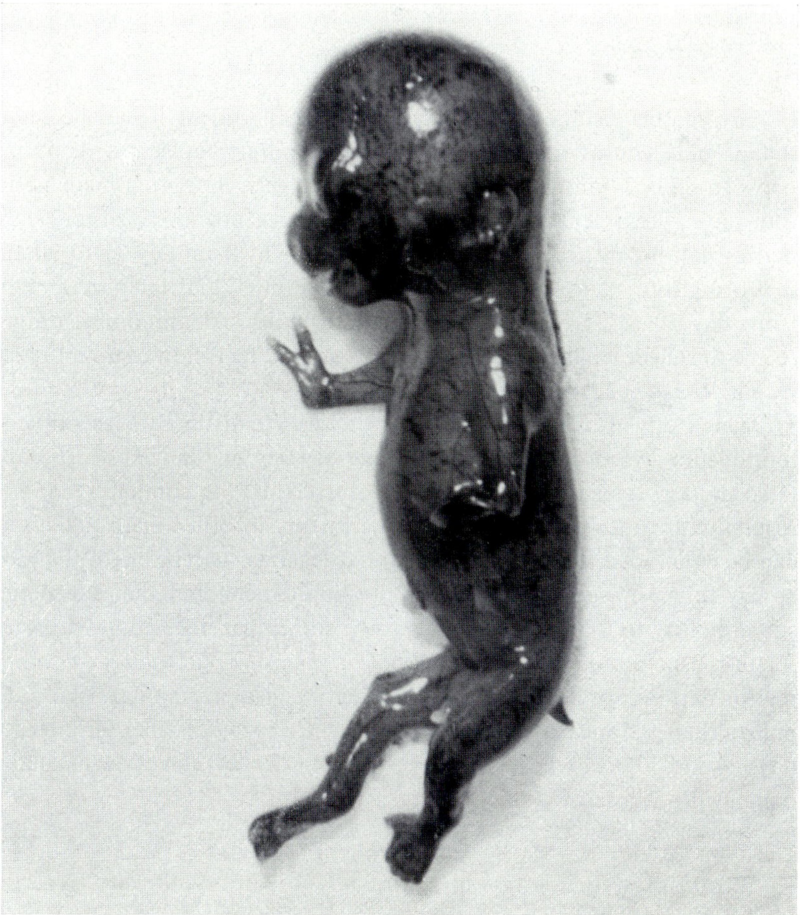

Fig. 2. Male fetus with severe malformations of both forelimbs. Cesarean section on day 69 p.c.; dam treated with thalidomide, 1.25 mg/kg orally from day 27 to 30 p.c.

always accompanied by extreme abnormal flexion of the carpal (or tarsal) joints. In some cases hypoplasia of the humerus or femur also occurred. One of the embryos showed aplasia of all fingers, and another unilateral polydactyly with thumb aplasia on the contralateral hand. Malformations of the internal organs were seen in several fetuses. Two, treated from day 27 to 30, and one from day 24 to 27, had hypoplasia or aplasia of one or both kidneys. This occurred in doses from 1.25 mg to 5 mg/kg. One fetus (2.5 mg/kg on day 24–27) had unilateral microphthalmia, and two (2.5 mg/kg on day 24–27) showed cleft lip, one of them in addition to forelimb malformations.

Discussion

From the results of this teratological experiment it can be seen that thalidomide causes malformations in *M. arctoides* fetuses of dams treated between days 24 and 33 p.c., during a relatively short treatment period of four days. Treatment during the earlier part, i.e. from day 24 to 27, caused malformations of head and forelimbs, treatment from day 27 to 30 elicited malformations of forelimbs as well as hindlimbs, and later treatment, i.e. from day 30 to 33, could result in abnormalities of hindlimbs only. This seems to reflect a phase-specificity which should be followed up more closely by single-day treatments.

Our study also revealed that *M. arctoides* are distinctly susceptible to the teratogenic action of thalidomide, since already at the lowest dose applied (1.25 mg/kg) typical malformations occurred. If one compares our present results with those of thalidomide experiments in other macaque species, it can be concluded that *M. arctoides* are at least as susceptible to thalidomide as are other macaques. Moreover, it should be noted that the period of susceptibility to thalidomide seems to be somewhat delayed in *M. arctoides;* for in rhesus monkeys [WILSON, 1968] or baboons [HENDRICKX *et al.,* 1966] malformations are not reported after treatment later than day 30 p.c. Doses higher than 2.5 mg/kg cause abortion in *M. arctoides* when given between days 24 and 30 p.c., whereas earlier treatment (21–24) can allow normal pregnancy with a dose of 20 mg/kg.

Proposition for the Use of *M. arctoides* in Embryotoxicity Experiments

Based on our results and propositions advanced by WILSON [1971] regarding embryotoxicity screening with rhesus monkeys, we should like to propose an administration schedule for the testing of drugs on embryotoxicity in *M. arctoides* (provided of course, that the embryological timetable of this species does not differ appreciably from that of rhesus monkeys).

Beginning with a long-term treatment of ten days (day 20–29 and 30–39), one should be able to ascertain any toxic effect on the embryo caused by prolonged application. If there is evidence of damage in late pregnancy, treatment from day 40 to 49 can be added. The initial dosage (X) should be chosen in relation to the anticipated dosage for clinical use in man (e.g. ten or 20 times the highest clinical dose).

If abortion or fetal damage occurs or is suspected, short-term (4 days) studies should be performed with the effective dose and with a higher dose. The times of administration should be chosen according to the time at which the suspected damage had occurred; two adjacent four-day periods (e.g. day 20–23 and 24–27 or day 24–27 and 28–31, etc.) could be covered (table II).

If three animals per dose and time group are used, a total number of 24–30 pregnancies would be required for testing a drug. Such an experiment should be sufficient to provide preliminary information regarding presence or absence of embryotoxicity.

Acknowledgements

The authors are gratefully indebted to Drs. H. WEBER and J. MESZAROS for performing the cesarean sections.

Table II. Time schedule proposal for testing drugs for embryotoxicity in *Macaca arctoides*. Test might be started with a long-term treatment of ten days' duration, followed by short-term application for four days during a phase to be tested more closely

	Long-term		Short-term		
Doses	2	nX, X, X/n	2	X, nX or X, X/n	
Duration	10 days	20–29	4 days[1]	20–23	36–39
		30–39		24–27	40–43
		(40–49)		28–31	44–47
				32–35	48–51
Animals	3 per group	12–18	3 per group		12

1 Two consecutive time groups.

References

BARROW, M.V.; STEFFEK, A.J., and KING, C.T.G.: Thalidomide syndrome in rhesus monkeys *(Macaca mulatta)*. Folia primat. *10:* 195–203 (1969).

BRÜGGEMANN, S. and GRAUWILER, J.: Breeding results from an experimental colony of *Macaca arctoides;* in GOLDSMITH and MOOR-JANKOWSKI Medical primatology 1972, part I, pp. 216–226 (Karger, Basel 1972).

DELAHUNT, C.S. and LASSEN, L.J.: Thalidomide syndrome in monkeys. Science *146:* 1300–1305 (1964).

HENDRICKX, A.G.: Teratogenicity of thalidomide in the baboon *(Papio cynocephalus)*, bonnet monkey *(Macaca radiata)* and cynomolgus monkey *(Macaca irus)*. Proc. 3rd Int. Congr. Primat., Zurich 1970, vol. 2, pp. 230–237 (Karger, Basel 1971).

HENDRICKX, A.G.; AXELROD, L.R., and CLAYBORN, L.D.: 'Thalidomide' syndrome in baboons. Nature, Lond. *210:* 958–959 (1966).

TANIMURA, T.; TANAKA, O., and NISHIMURA, H.: Effects of thalidomide and quinine hydrochloride on Japanese and rhesus monkey embryos. 11th Annu. Meet. Teratology Society, Williamsburg, Va. 1971. Teratology *4:* 247 (1971).

WEBER, H. and GRAUWILER, J.: Experience with a breeding colony of stumptail macaques for teratological testing of drugs. Proc. Int. Symp. Breeding Non-Human Primates for Laboratory Use, Bern 1971 (Karger, Basel, in press).

WILSON, J.G.: Teratological and reproductive studies in non-human primates; in NISHIMURA and MILLER Methods for teratological studies in experimental animals and in man, pp. 16–31 (Jgaku Shoin, Tokyo 1968).

WILSON, J.G.: Use of rhesus monkeys in teratological studies. Fed. Proc. *30:* 104–109 (1971).

WILSON, J.G. and GAVAN, J.A.: Congenital malformations in nonhuman primates. Spontaneous and experimentally induced. Anat. Rec. *158:* 99–109 (1967).

WILSON, J.G.; FRADKIN, R., and HARDMAN, A.: Breeding and pregnancy in rhesus monkeys used for teratological testing. Teratology *3:* 59–72 (1970).

Authors' address: Dr. JULES GRAUWILER and Dr. SIGRID BRÜGGEMANN, Biological and Medical Research Division, Sandoz Ltd., *CH-4000 Basel* (Switzerland)

Medical Primatology 1972. Proc. 3rd Conf. exp. Med. Surg. Primates, Lyon 1972, part III, pp. 259–269 (Karger, Basel 1972)

A Comparison of Temporal Factors in the Embryological Development of Man, Old World Monkeys and Galagos, and Craniofacial Malformations Induced by Thalidomide and Triamcinolone[1]

A. G. HENDRICKX

University of California Primate Research Center, Davis, Cal.

It is well established that the embryo must be at a susceptible stage in development in order to elicit a teratogenic response [WILSON, 1965]. This period of susceptibility usually coincides with organogenesis. The correlation of embryological events with some reproductive event such as menstruation or ovulation makes it possible to delineate the period of susceptibility in teratological studies. STREETER [1942, 1945, 1948, 1951] recognized the importance of cataloging embryos based on these parameters when he established his 'Developmental Horizons in Human Embryos'. His work with human embryos has provided the point of reference for further work with nonhuman primates [HENDRICKX *et al.*, 1971], and the work of NISHIMURA *et al.* [1968] provides another point of reference to compare embryological events, critical to teratological studies, in human and nonhuman embryonic development.

The results of preliminary experiments being presented here on the selective action of thalidomide on craniofacial development, and on the teratogenicity of triamcinolone relate to our interest in studying the action of known teratogens in the nonhuman primate species.

1 Supported by USPHS NIH grant RR00169.

Materials and Methods

Embryos

A total of 115 embryos were used in this study, including 67 baboon *(P. cynocephalus)*, 11 bonnet *(M. radiata)*, nine cynomolgus *(M. fascicularis)*, seven rhesus *(M. mulatta)*, 12 galago *(G. crassicaudatus)*, two stump-tailed *(M. arctoides)*, five green *(Cercopithecus* sp.) and two mangabeys *(C. atys)*. All of the embryos are not represented in the graphs; they were collected, processed and studied by the method described previously [HENDRICKX *et al.*, 1971].

Husbandry and Breeding

All Old World monkeys were housed individually in aluminum cages and fed Purina monkey chow and water *ad libitum*. Isoniazid, at an approximate dosage of 10 mg/kg/day, was incorporated in the diet. Menstruation was detected by daily visual examination of vaginal swabs. The females were bred once, usually two days before midcycle. The day of the two-hour mating was designated as day zero of pregnancy.

The adult galagos were housed either in pairs or singly in galvanized steel cages and fed as described above. Daily vaginal smears were obtained by lavage after the vulva opened during estrus. The first appearance of sperm in the lavage was considered as day zero of pregnancy. Parenthetically, sperm were rarely observed in the vaginal smear on more than three successive days.

Dosing

Thalidomide at doses of 10 and 30 mg/kg body weight was administered as a suspension in polyoxyethylene sorbitan (Tween 80, Sigma Chemical Co.) and tap water solution by gastric intubation, and triamcinolone at daily doses of 25, 75 and 250 mg was administered i.m. Thalidomide was administered on either day 24, 25, 26, 27, 28, or 29 of pregnancy and triamcinolone on days 37–40 or 41–44 of pregnancy.

Verification of Pregnancy

Prior to the collection of an embryo by hysterotomy or the administration of a drug, pregnancy was confirmed by bimanual palpation of the uterus *per rectum*.

Recovery and Examination of Fetuses

All fetuses were removed by hysterotomy on either day 70 or 100 of pregnancy. The fetuses were weighed, measured and photographed. After evisceration the skeleton was stained with alizarin Red S and the viscera were fixed in 10% formalin.

Results and Discussion

Crown-Rump Length in Relation to Age

In figure 1 the mean curves determined by NISHIMURA *et al.* [1968] for the human are compared with those determined for the baboon [HENDRICKX *et al.,* 1971], rhesus monkey, bonnet monkey and cynomolgus monkey. NISHIMURA's mean line is considerably more horizontally inclined than that compiled for the baboon and the three macaque species. This indicates that the mean length for human embryos at early ages (25–32 days) is greater than for baboon and macaque embryos but is lesser for the later stages (33–55 days). His data also show that the mean length increases more gradually with age in human than in baboon and macaque embryos (fig.2). On the other hand, green monkey embryos tend to increase in length at the same rate as human embryos, and galago embryos probably increase in length at even a slower rate (fig.2).

In figure 3 the crown-rump length of rhesus monkey embryos (broken line) compiled by HEUSER and STREETER [1941] are compared to baboon, rhesus monkey, bonnet monkey and cynomolgus monkey embryos studied in our laboratory. The similarity in length of all four species throughout the organogenic period is quite evident. However, the crown-rump length of the green monkey and galago is considerably shorter than either the rhesus monkey or the baboon (fig.3).

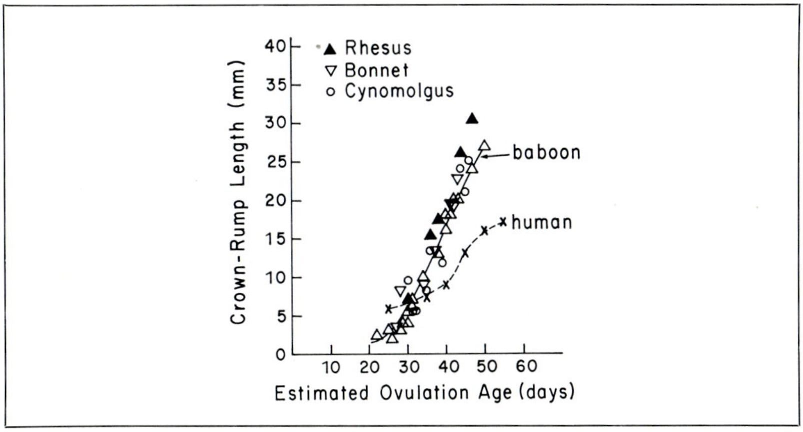

Fig. 1. Correlation of estimated ovulation age and crown-rump length in human (×), baboon (△), rhesus (▲), bonnet (▽) and cynomolgus (○) monkey embryos.

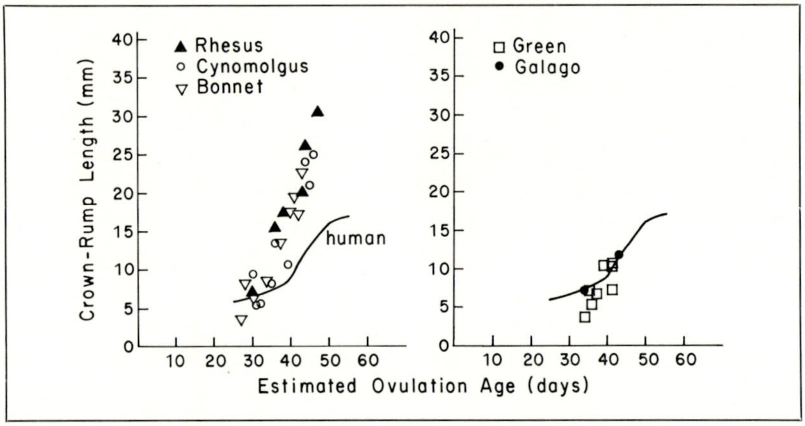

Fig. 2. Correlation of estimated ovulation age and crown-rump length in human (–), galago (●), green (□), bonnet (▽), cynomolgus (○) and rhesus monkey (▲) embryos.

Developmental Stage (Horizon) in Relation to Age

HENDRICKX [1972] has shown that baboon embryos are five days younger than human embryos [NISHIMURA *et al.,* 1968] for all of the developmental stages 12–23. Rhesus monkey, bonnet monkey and cynomolgus monkey embryos follow the same temporal developmental pattern as the baboon, but the galago and green monkey are more similar to the human embryo (fig. 4). Based on two embryos of each species, it appears that the stump-tailed monkey and the mangabey probably follow the developmental pattern of the baboon and macaques.

From a teratological viewpoint, the definition of the onset of organogenesis in the selected species is a prerequisite to any experimental protocol, and the recognition of species differences is essential to the accurate interpretation of drug screening. The developmental delay observed in the green monkey and galago embryos is unusual because of the shorter gestation periods. Our observations and thoserecorded by COOPER [personal commun.] indicate that the gestation period for *Galago crassicaudatus* is 133 ± 3 days; the gestation period for the green monkeys in our colony is 158 ± 3 days. Based on our preliminary observations in both these species the embryonic period is longer with a corresponding shortening of the fetal period. Since galagos and Old World monkeys achieve approximately the same degree of maturity at birth, fetal growth and development must be accelerated accordingly.

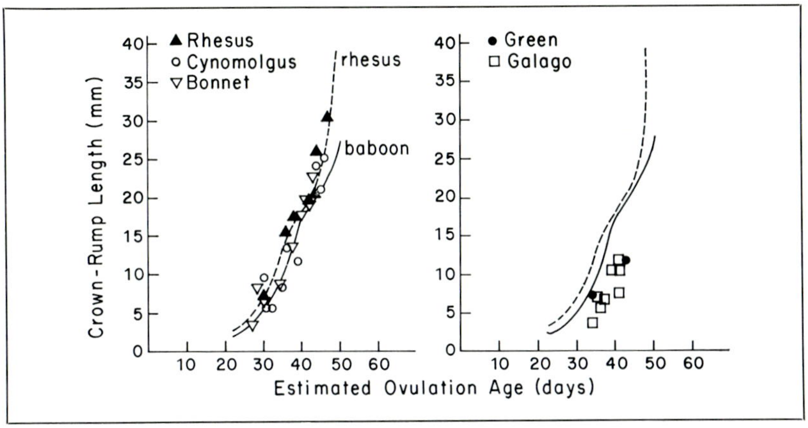

Fig. 3. Correlation of estimated ovulation age and crown-rump length in baboon, rhesus (▲), bonnet (▽), green (●), cynomolgus monkey (○) and galago (□) embryos. ---- = Data recorded by HEUSER and STREETER [1941] for rhesus embryos; ▲ = data collected in our laboratory.

The developmental delay in green monkeys in comparison to baboons and macaques has been confirmed by a corresponding delay in the teratogenic response to thalidomide (unpubl. observ.). The sensitive period for limbs in this species is between days 28 and 33 of pregnancy. In bonnet, cynomolgus, rhesus monkeys and baboons, the sensitive period falls between days 25 and 28 or 30 of pregnancy [HENDRICKX, 1971; WILSON and GAVAN, 1967].

Developmental Horizon in Relation to Crown-Rump Length

Considerable variation in length for any given stage (horizon) has been reported for the human embryo [NISHIMURA *et al.*, 1968]. The variation was found to be greater for human embryos than baboon embryos [HENDRICKX, 1972]. This might be expected because of the greater sample size of humans and the lack of opportunity to control conception. The crown-rump length in relation to developmental horizon is similar for human, baboon, green monkey and macaque embryos, but galago embryos are slightly shorter (fig. 5).

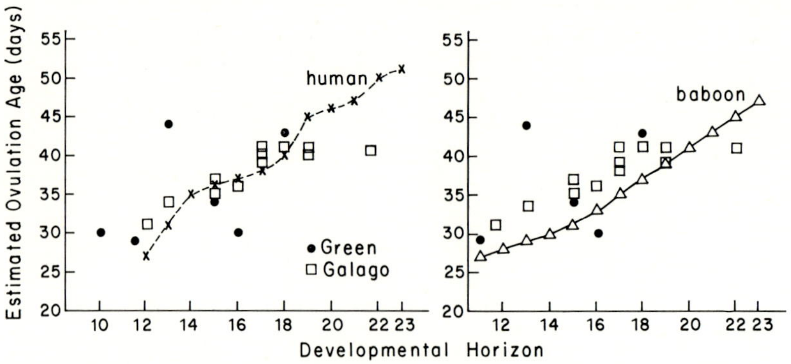

Fig. 4. Correlation of developmental horizon and estimated ovulation age in human (×), baboon (△), green monkey (●), and galago (□) embryos.

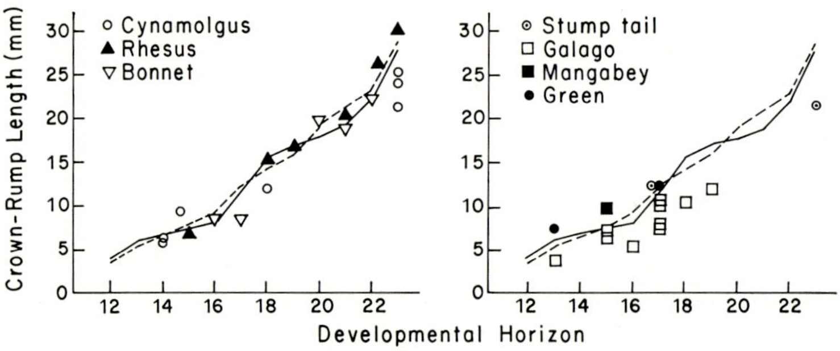

Fig. 5. Correlation of developmental horizon and crown-rump length in human (---), baboon (–), bonnet, (▽), rhesus (▲), cynomolgus (○), stump-tailed (△), galago (□), mangabey (■) and green monkey (●) embryos.

Thalidomide-Induced Craniofacial Anomalies

The teratogenic susceptibility of the developing limbs to thalidomide in nonhuman primates is well known [WILSON, 1972]; however, anomalies of the craniofacial region are less common, although they have been reported in at least two studies [HENDRICKX *et al.*, 1966; BARROW *et al.*, 1969]. We recently reexamined our specimens and found that approximately one-half

(11/24) of our bonnet monkey specimens had craniofacial malformations (table I). The most common defect was hyperplasia of the temporozygomatic region with an accompanying hyperplasia of the mandibular condyle and/or angular process. In the most severe cases the extensive exostosis resulted in fusion between the mandible and the temporozygomatic region (fig.6). Hypoplasia of the mandibular condyle and coronoid process was also common. The data suggest that treatment on days 28 and 29 of pregnancy is less likely to cause craniofacial malformations because only three of 11 fetuses were affected as compared to eight of 13 treated on either day 24, 25, 26 or 27 of pregnancy.

The craniofacial malformations in green monkeys are characterized by hypoplasia of the temporozygomatic region as compared to hyperplasia in the bonnet monkey (table II). The only explanation for this is that the treatment was several days earlier in organogenesis in the green monkey than it was in the bonnet, and this resulted in a more severe defect because of the increased sensitivity of the developing skeleton.

Table I. Thalidomide-induced craniofacial malformations in bonnet monkeys

Treatment		Number treated	Number[1] malformed	Malformations			
				temporo-zygomatic region	mandibular		
dose mg/kg	day(s) of pregnancy				condyle	coronoid process	angular process
10	24	5	2	+	−	−	
				+			
10	25	2	1	+	−	−	+
10	26	1	0				
10	27	2	2	+	+		
10	28	4	3	+	+	−	
				+	−	−	+
						−	
10	29	4	0				
30	25	3	3	+	−	−	
				+	−	−	
				+			
30	28	3	0				
Totals		24	11				

+ = Hyperplasia; − = hypoplasia.
1 All fetuses removed by hysterotomy at 70 or 100 days of gestation.

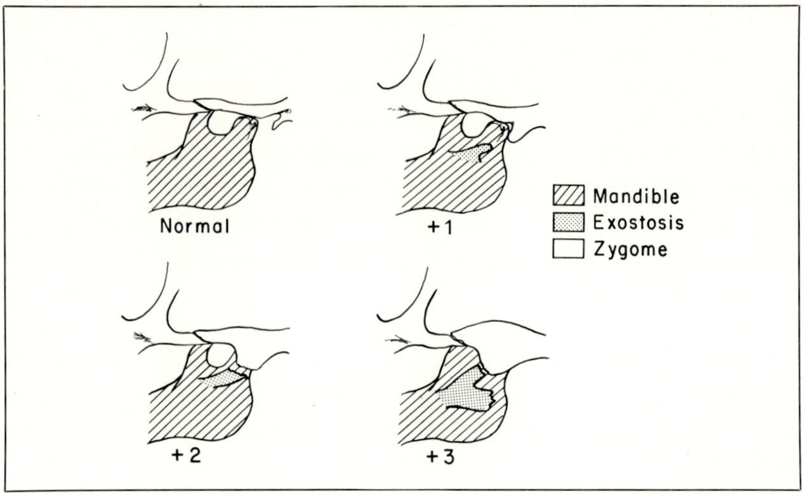

Fig. 6. Temporozygomatic and mandibular malformations produced by thalidomide in the bonnet monkey. The stippling shows the area of exostosis on the mandible and its area of fusion with the zygomatic process in slightly malformed (+1), moderately malformed (+2) and severely malformed (+3) fetuses.

Table II. Thalidomide-induced craniofacial malformations in green monkeys

Dose mg/kg	Day(s) of pregnancy	Number treated	Number malformed	Condition of malformed fetus
10	25	2	1	temporozygomatic hypoplasia
30	25	2	1	temporozygomatic hypoplasia
Totals		4	2	

Embryotoxicity of Triamcinolone

Based on our preliminary observations, the synthetic glucocorticoid, triamcinolone, appears to be both teratogenic and embryolethal in the baboon and bonnet monkey, and embryolethal in the rhesus monkey. Triamcinolone was selected because it departs radically from the ratio of teratogenic to therapeutic dosage found with other corticosteroids [WALKER, 1965]. In this study the target organ was the palate because of the high incidence of cleft palate produced with this drug in the mouse [WALKER, 1965]. Treatments were scheduled for the gestational period just prior to palate closure which occurs on days 45 and 46 in all three species [STEFFEK *et al.*, 1968; BOLLERT and HENDRICKX, 1971]. Median cleft palate was observed in one bonnet monkey fetus in association with hip dysplasia and adrenal hypoplasia (table III). The one case of facial dysmorphia in the baboon (table III) is characterized by asymmetry and mandibular underbite as well as a deformed nasal septum. Clinically, the nine-month-old infant still inhales nasally and exhales orally. The one case of adrenal insufficiency was characterized by clinical signs of weight loss progressing into acute adrenal crisis. Response to dexomethasone and electrolyte therapy was positive.

From these preliminary studies it appears that the palate and other organs are sensitive to triamcinolone; however, the teratogenic dose, the sensitive period and the incidence of malformations produced remain to be defined.

Table III. Embryotoxicity of triamcinolone in baboons, bonnet and rhesus monkeys

Species	Treatment			Number offspring studied	Condition of fetus
	day(s) of pregnancy	daily total	dose mg/kg		
Baboon	37–40	25	1	1	intrauterine death[1] 80 days
	41–44	25	1–2	3	2 – normal 1 – facial dysmorphia
Bonnet	41–44	75	14	1	cleft palate, hip dysplasia, adrenal hypoplasia
	41–44	250	75	1	abortion
Rhesus	37–40	25	6	1	abortion, 115 days
	41–44	25	3–5	4	2 – normal 1 – fetal resorption[2] 1 – normal at term, adrenal insufficiency at 3 months of age
	41–44	75	12–25	4	1 – resorption 3 – intrauterine death[3]

1 Hysterotomy on day 80 because of indication of treatened abortion.
2 Placenta and membranes delivered intact at 100 days of pregnancy.
3 Fetus dead and partially autolyzed at hysterotomy at 100 days of pregnancy.

Acknowledgements

Acknowledgements are due to Miss GERALDINE SANCHEZ, Miss LOIS NEWMAN, and Mr. S. SWAN for laboratory technical assistance, and to Mr. J. UTZ, Mr. J. BATCHELOR, Mr. J. CANO and Mr. D. WELTY for animal technical assistance.

References

BARROW, M.V.; STEFFEK, A.J., and KING, C.T.G.: Thalidomide syndrome in rhesus monkeys *(Macaca mulatta)*. Folia primat. *10:* 195–203 (1969).

BOLLERT, J.A. and HENDRICKX, A.G.: Morphogenesis of the palate in the baboon *(Papio cynocephalus)*. Teratology *4:* 343–354 (1971).

HENDRICKX, A.G.: Teratogenicity of thalidomide in the baboon *(Papio cynocephalus)*, bonnet monkey *(Macaca radiata)* and cynomolgus monkey *(Macaca irus)*. Proc. 3rd Int. Congr. Primat., Zurich 1970, vol. 2, pp. 230–237 (Karger, Basel 1971).

HENDRICKX, A.G.: Early development of the embryo in nonhuman primates and man. World Health Organization. Symp. on the Use of Nonhuman Primates for Research on Problems of Human Reproduction. Acta endocrin., Kbh., suppl. no. 166, pp. 103–130 (1972).

HENDRICKX, A.G.; AXELROD, L.R., and CLAYBORN, L.D.: Thalidomide syndrome in baboons. Nature, Lond. *210:* 958–959 (1966).

HENDRICKX, A.G.; HOUSTON, M.L.; KRAEMER, D.C.; GASSER, R.F., and BOLLERT, J.A.: Embryology of the baboon (University of Chicago Press, Chicago 1971).

HEUSER, C.H. and STREETER, G.L.: Development of the macaque embryo. Contrib. Embryol., Carneg. Inst. *29:* 15–55 (1941).

NISHIMURA, H.; TAKANO, K.; TANIMURA, T., and YASUDA, M.: Normal and abnormal development of human embryos. First report of the analysis of 1,213 intact embryos. Teratology *1:* 281–290 (1968).

STEFFEK, A.J.; VERRUSIO, A.C., and KING, C.T.G.: The histology of palate closure in the rhesus monkey *(Macaca mulatta)*. Teratology *1:* 425–429 (1968).

STREETER, G.L.: Developmental horizons in human embryos. Description of age group XI, 13 to 20 somites and age group XII, 21 to 29 somites. Contrib. Embryol., Carneg. Inst. *30:* 211–245 (1942).

STREETER, G.L.: Developmental horizons in human embryos. Description of age group XIII embryos about 4 or 5 millimeters long, and age group XIV, period of indentation of the lens vesicle. Contrib. Embryol., Carneg. Inst. *31:* 27–63 (1945).

STREETER, G.L.: Developmental horizons in human embryos. Description of age groups XV, XVI, XVII, and XVIII. Contrib. Embryol., Carneg. Inst. *32:* 133–203 (1948).

STREETER, G.L.: Developmental horizons in human embryos. Description of age groups XIX, XX, XXI, XXII, and XXIII. Contrib. Embryol., Carneg. Inst. *34:* 165–196 (1951).

WALKER, B.E.: Cleft palate produced in mice by human-equivalent dose with triamcinolone. Science *14:* 862–863 (1965).

WILSON, J.G.: Embryological considerations in teratology; in Teratology. Principles and techniques, chap. 10, pp. 251–261 (University of Chicago Press, Chicago 1965).

WILSON, J.G.: Abnormalities of intrauterine development in nonhuman primates. World Health Organization. Symp. on the Use of Nonhuman Primates for Research on Problems of Human Reproduction. Acta endocrin., Kbh., suppl. no. 166, pp. 261–292 (1972).

WILSON, J.G. and GAVAN, J.A.: Congenital malformations in nonhuman primates. Spontaneous and experimentally induced. Anat. Rec. *158:* 99–109 (1967).

Author's address: Dr. A.G. HENDRICKX, University of California Primate Research Center, University of California, *Davis, CA 95616* (USA)

Medical Primatology 1972. Proc. 3rd Conf. exp. Med. Surg. Primates, Lyon 1972, part III, pp. 270–278 (Karger, Basel 1972)

Hepatic Effects of Long-Term Ethanol Consumption in Primates[1, 2]

C. S. Lieber, L. M. DeCarli, H. Gang, G. Walker and E. Rubin

Section of Liver Disease and Nutrition, Veterans Administration Hospital, Bronx, New York, and the Departments of Medicine and Pathology, Mount Sinai School of Medicine of the City University of New York, New York

Introduction

We found previously that both in alcoholic and nonalcoholic individuals, ethanol consumption in a matter of weeks produces a fatty liver as shown by light microscopy [Lieber *et al.,* 1963 and 1965] with hepatic triglyceride accumulation [Lieber and Spritz, 1966; Lieber and Rubin, 1968; Rubin and Lieber, 1968a]. This was associated with striking ultrastructural changes, including distortion and disfiguration of the mitochondria and proliferation of the smooth endoplasmic reticulum (SER) [Lane and Lieber, 1966; Rubin and Lieber, 1967; Lieber and Rubin, 1968; Rubin and Lieber, 1968a]. The latter was accompanied by increased activities of microsomal drug detoxifying enzymes [Rubin and Lieber, 1968b]. Ethanol produced these effects whether added to an otherwise adequate diet or given as isocaloric substitution for carbohydrate in a variety of diets with either normal or low fat content [Lieber and Spritz, 1966]. These effects could not be prevented by supplementation with protein, vitamins, minerals and choline chloride [Lieber and Rubin, 1968; Rubin and Lieber, 1968a]. The question remained, however, whether these effects persist during long-term ethanol consumption and how they are affected by a restriction in dietary protein. Since these problems could not be studied in humans under controlled conditions, baboons were selected as experimental animals.

1 Presented, in part, at the Annual Meeting of the American Gastroenterological Association, Miami, Fla., May, 1971.

2 Supported in part by USPHS grants MH15558, AM12511, MH20067 and the Veterans Administration. The animal experimentation was performed at LEMSIP, New York.

Material and Methods

The baboons used for this study were either *Papio hamadryas* or *Papio anubis*. These animals were imported from Africa and were studied after prolonged quarantine periods. Their age was estimated at four to ten years. During the study period they were housed in individual cages. One group of animals received a custom made high protein biscuit diet with 34% of total calories as protein. Ethanol was added to the drinking water at a final concentration varying from 4.8 to 5.6 g/100 ml. Food and fluid intake was measured daily. The control animals received the same amount of biscuits but instead of ethanol they were given isocaloric amounts of a dextrin-maltose mixture in their drinking water. When the calories contained in the drinking water were added to those of the biscuits, the overall composition of the diet consisted of 20% of total calories as protein, 14% as fat, 30% as carbohydrates and 36% of calories either as ethanol or additional carbohydrates (controls). The animals also received daily a multivitamin preparation. The total amount of vitamins (including choline) ingested exceeded the recommendation of FOY *et al.* [1964] for the baboon.

A second group of baboons was treated in a similar fashion except that the protein content of the biscuits was decreased to achieve overall protein restriction amounting to 7% of total calories. The carbohydrate and fat content of the diet was 45 and 14% of calories, respectively, with, in addition, 33% of total calories either as ethanol or as supplementary carbohydrate (controls). After 15–19 months on this regimen, the protein intake was further reduced to approximately 4% of total calories by decreasing the protein content of the diet. Fat and carbohydrate content corresponded to 16 and 60–65% of calories, respectively, with an additional 25- to 30-percent of total calories as carbohydrates in the controls (in lieu of the ethanol).

Surgical biopsies of the liver were performed at regular intervals. Liver tissue specimens were taken for analysis of total lipids and triglycerides [DECARLI and LIEBER, 1967] and light and electron microscopy [RUBIN and LIEBER, 1968a]. Activities of aniline hydroxylase [GANG *et al.*, in press], pentobarbital hydroxylase [RUBIN and LIEBER, 1968b] were determined in liver homogenates, microsomal ethanol oxidation (MEOS) in liver microsomes [LIEBER and DECARLI, 1970a] and alcohol dehydrogenase (ADH) in the cytosol [BONNICHSEN and BRINK, 1955]. Blood samples were also taken for measurements of total cholesterol, total protein, albumin, bilirubin, phosphatase, glutamic oxaloacetic transaminase (SGOT), glutamic pyruvic transaminase (SGPT), creatine, urea and glucose on a SMA 12/60 Technicon Autoanalyser®.

Results

Effects of Alcohol with a High Protein Diet

Light microscopy of repeated liver biopsies revealed steatosis in the alcohol-fed animals, as illustrated in figure 1. Triglyceride measurements showed progressive fat accumulation. After three to five months there was an average sixfold increase in triglycerides (28.2 ± 5.5 mg/g in seven ethanol-fed *a* 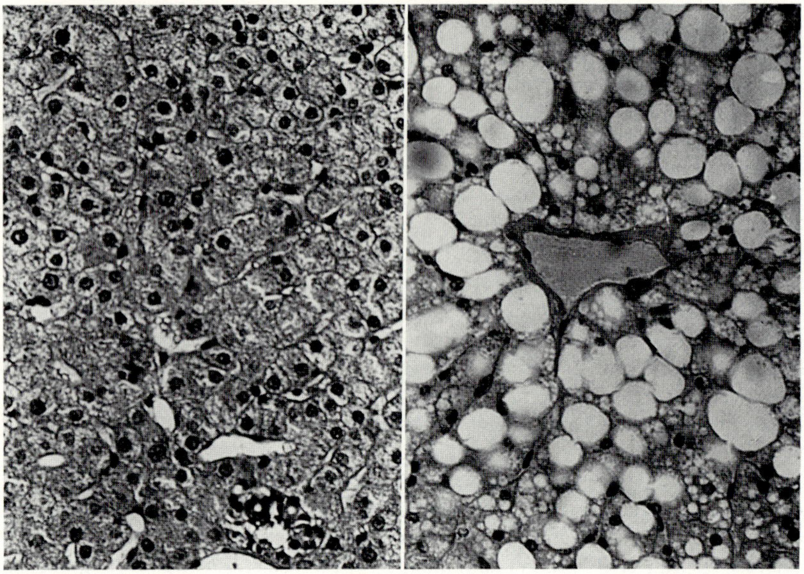 *b*

Fig. 1. Section of baboon liver shows normal hepatic architecture during *a* control period and *b* conspicuous fatty metamorphosis after 15 months of administration of ethanol with a high protein diet. HE. × 300.

animals vs. 4.6 ± 1.3 in controls; $p < 0.001$). After 15–20 months of ethanol feeding, triglycerides increased to a mean of 67.2 ± 15.5 mg/g, whereas no significant change occurred in the controls. In five baboons fed ethanol for an average of 32 months, liver triglycerides were 92.6 ± 22.8 mg/g. In the latter group, activities of aniline hydroxylase increased to 39 ± 8.2 n moles/g/min (vs. 9.3 ± 3.0 in controls; $p < 0.02$). Both pentobarbital hydroxylase and MEOS activity were 30% higher in the alcohol-fed than in the controls, but because of great variability of the results, no statistical significance was reached. ADH activity decreased slightly, but not significantly, after alcohol.

Electron microscopy (fig. 2 and 3) revealed enlarged irregular and distorted mitochondria with disoriented cristae often arranged in parallel arrays. Parallel arrays of RER were usually not seen after ethanol, while the smooth endoplasmic reticulum was proliferated and vesicular. In some cases irregular dilatation of SER was conspicuous. Occasionally cells with dilated RER were also observed. The bile canuliculi and cell borders were unchanged. Fat droplets were common in the cytoplasm.

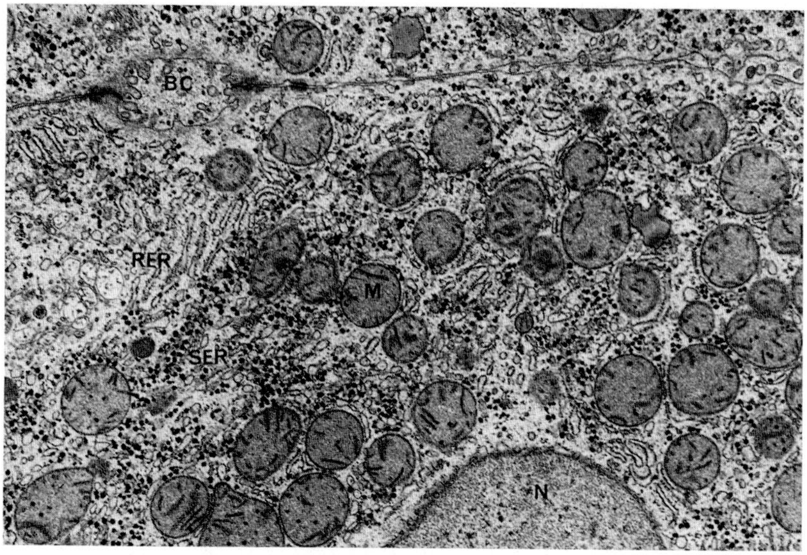

Fig. 2. Electron micrograph of a hepatocyte of a baboon fed the control high protein diet. The mitochondria (M) are of normal size. Parallel arrays of RER are noted. Small vesicles of SER in glycogen areas are present. N = nucleus; BC = bile canuliculus. × 11,000.

The only significant change noted in the blood was an increase of total cholesterol to 180 ± 11 mg/100 ml after 15–20 months of ethanol feeding (vs. 105 ± 20 in the controls; $p < 0.01$).

Effect of the Feeding of Alcohol with a Protein-Restricted Diet

The restriction of the dietary protein to 7% of total caloric intake had surprisingly little effects. Liver triglycerides of the control animals fed this protein-restricted diet for three to five months increased moderately, but not significantly, to 6.2 ± 1.3 mg/g compared to 4.6 ± 1.3 in the animals fed the high protein diet. With alcohol, steatosis developed to a degree comparable to that achieved with the high protein diet with liver triglycerides of about 60 mg/g after 15–19 months of ethanol. The enzyme and ultrastructural changes (fig. 4) were also similar. Food intake, however, was less adequate than with the high protein diet and as a consequence, some animals lost weight. In addition, alcohol intake was slightly less than in the high protein

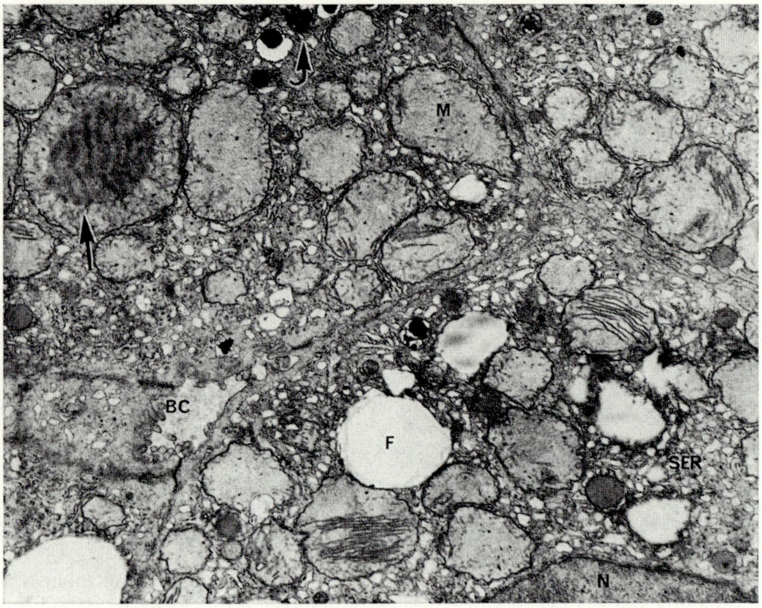

Fig. 3. Electron micrograph of the liver of a baboon fed alcohol with a high protein diet for 15 months. Mitochondria (M) are enlarged and irregular, and display disoriented parallel cristae and focally-increased matrix density (straight arrow). RER is decreased and SER proliferated and vesicular. Fat droplets are present in the cytoplasm. Occasional vesicles containing dense osmiophilic material are noted (curved arrow). BC = bile canuliculus; N = nucleus; F = fat. ×11,000.

group (33 vs. 36% of total calories). Inadequacy of protein intake reflected itself in a decrease of serum albumin from 3.37 ± 0.22 g/100 ml with the control high protein diet to 2.29 ± 0.14 ($p < 0.001$) in the control animals fed the protein-restricted diet. Alcohol had no additional effect on this parameter.

Effects of Severe Deficiency with or without Alcohol

When after 15–19 months on the protein-restricted diet, the protein intake was further reduced to 4% of total calories, a decrease in food intake resulted, with weight loss. The experiments had to be interrupted after 15 months because of various complications such as development of inanition, edema, diarrhea and infection. For that total period of time, alcohol

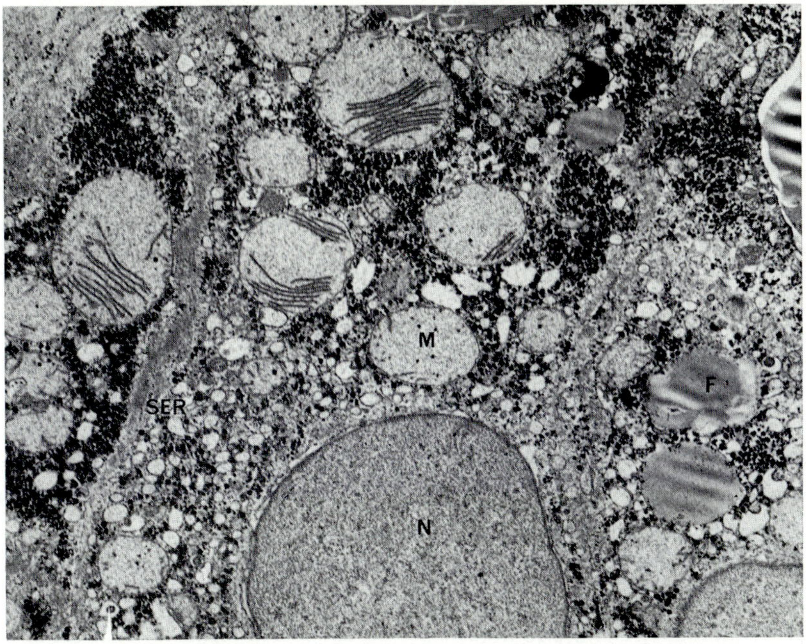

Fig. 4. Electron micrograph of the liver of a baboon fed alcohol with a protein-restricted diet for 19 months. Mitochondria (M) are enlarged and exhibit disoriented cristae, usually in parallel arrays. RER is decreased. SER is proliferated, dilated and vesicular. Fat (F) droplets are seen. N = nucleus.

intake averaged 25–30% of total calories. Lipid accumulation in the liver was variable and occurred whether or not alcohol was given. After three months of this regimen, triglycerides averaged 42.0 ± 11.6 mg/g in the six controls and 56.3 ± 12.4 in the alcohol-fed animals. After one year on this diet, the corresponding values were 104.7 ± 27.5 vs. 99.1 ± 28.2 mg/g. Under these conditions, liver enzymes and blood cholesterol still showed a trend towards an increase in the ethanol group but the changes were not statistically significant.

Discussion

The present study revealed that baboons given alcohol develop fat accumulation in the liver with striking ultrastructural changes even in the presence of an adequate diet. Similar changes had been described before after short-term ethanol administration in man [LIEBER *et al.*, 1963 and 1965; LANE and LIEBER, 1966; RUBIN and LIEBER, 1967 and 1968a; LIEBER and RUBIN, 1968] and in rats [LIEBER *et al.*, 1963 and 1965; ISERI *et al.*, 1966; RUBIN *et al.*, 1968; PORTA *et al.*, 1968]. There was considerable debate concerning the duration of these lesions in the rat. Whereas one group of investigators reported these effects to be transient [PORTA *et al.*, 1968], we found it to persist [LIEBER and DECARLI, 1970b]. The discrepancies in results is possibly due to a difference in alcohol intake. In the study in which the alcohol effect was transient, alcohol consumption was reported to decrease after four months [PORTA *et al.*, 1968]. This could have resulted in reduction in fat accumulation, since the alcohol effect upon the liver has a dose threshold [LIEBER *et al.*, 1965].

Although the fatty liver produced by alcohol in the rat resembles that of the human, there are differences in the ultrastructural lesions: In man, the endoplasmic reticulum is dilated and vesicular whereas in the rat it proliferates in the form of branching tubules. Mitochondria also show greater enlargement in man than in rats. The lesions produced in the present study in baboons resemble that of man much more than that of the rat, both by electron microscopy and also in terms of fat accumulation. The increase in triglyceride in baboons (this study) and in man [LIEBER and SPRITZ, 1966; LIEBER and RUBIN, 1968; RUBIN and LIEBER, 1968a] were comparable and more pronounced than that observed in the rat [LIEBER *et al.*, 1963 and 1965].

The present study also revealed that moderate protein restriction has no striking effects upon the liver of the baboon, an observation which is consistent with our clinical experience [RUBIN and LIEBER, 1968c]. Severe protein deficiency (4% of total calories), however, resulted in overall impairment of health which made the study of specific effects of alcohol difficult especially in view of the reduction of alcohol consumption. With this severe protein deficiency, fat accumulation occurred in the liver even without ethanol consumption, confirming similar findings previously observed in rats [KLATSKIN *et al.*, 1954; LIEBER *et al.*, 1969]. Previous studies in primates with the feeding of diets deficient in choline (or both in protein and choline) resulted in fat accumulation and the development of fibrosis [WILGRAM *et al.*, 1958; WILGRAM, 1959; HOFFBAUER and ZAKI, 1965]. In our study with the administration of ethanol and diets adequate in choline (with or without protein deficiency), no histologically visible fibrosis was produced, although ethanol feeding was associated with some increase in hepatic collagen measured chemically [FEINMAN and LIEBER, 1972]. The study is continuing to determine whether fibrosis may develop after more prolonged feeding of ethanol.

References

BONNICHSEN, R.K. and BRINK, N.G.: Liver alcohol dehydrogenase; in COLOWICK and KAPLAN Methods in enzymology, vol. 1, pp. 495–503 (Academic Press, New York 1955).

DECARLI, L.M. and LIEBER, C.S.: Fatty liver in the rat after prolonged intake of ethanol with a nutritionally adequate new liquid diet. J. Nutr. *91:* 331–336 (1967).

FEINMAN, L. and LIEBER, C.S.: Hepatic collagen metabolism. Effect of alcohol consumption in rats and baboons. Science *176:* 795 (1972).

FOY, H.; KONDI, A., and MBAYA, V.: Effect of riboflavine deficiency on bone marrow function and protein metabolism in baboons. Brit. J. Nutr. *18:* 307–318 (1964).

GANG, H.; LIEBER, C.S., and RUBIN, E.: Aniline hydroxylase microassay suitable for needle biopsy specimens. J. Pharmacol. exp. Ther. (in press).

HOFFBAUER, F.W. and ZAKI, F.G.: Choline deficiency in baboon and rat compared. Arch. Path. *79:* 364–369 (1965).

ISERI, O.A.; LIEBER, C.S., and GOTTLIEB, L.S.: The ultrastructure of fatty liver induced by prolonged ethanol ingestion. Amer. J. Path. *48:* 535–555 (1966).

KLATSKIN, G.; KREHL, W.A., and CONN, H.O.: The effect of alcohol on the choline requirement. I. Changes in the rat's liver following prolonged ingestion of alcohol. J. exp. Med. *100:* 605–614 (1954).

LANE, B.P. and LIEBER, C.S.: Ultrastructural alterations in human hepatocytes following ingestion of ethanol with adequate diets. Amer. J. Path. *49:* 593–603 (1966).

LIEBER, C.S. and DECARLI, L.M.: Hepatic microsomal ethanol oxidizing system *in vitro*. Characteristics and adaptive properties *in vivo*. J. biol. Chem. *245:* 2505–2512 (1970a).

LIEBER, C.S. and DECARLI, L.M.: Quantitative relationship between the amount of dietary fat and the severity of the alcoholic fatty liver. Amer. J. clin. Nutr. *23:* 474–478 (1970b).

LIEBER, C.S. and RUBIN, E.: Alcoholic fatty liver in man on a high protein and low fat diet. Amer. J. Med. *44:* 200–207 (1968).

LIEBER, C.S. and SPRITZ, N.: Effects of prolonged ethanol intake in man. Role of dietary, adipose and endogenously synthesized fatty acids in the pathogenesis of the alcoholic fatty liver. J. clin. Invest. *45:* 1400–1411 (1966).

LIEBER, C.S.; JONES, D.P., and DECARLI, L.M.: Effects of prolonged ethanol intake. Production of fatty liver despite adequate diets. J. clin. Invest. *44:* 1009–1021 (1965).

LIEBER, C.S.; SPRITZ, N., and DECARLI, L.M.: Fatty liver produced by dietary deficiencies. Its pathogenesis and potentiation by ethanol. J. Lipid Res. *10:* 283–287 (1969).

LIEBER, C.S.; JONES, D.P.; MENDELSON, J., and DECARLI, L.M.: Fatty liver, hyperlipemia and hyperuricemia produced by prolonged alcohol consumption, despite adequate dietary intake. Trans. Ass. amer. Physicians *76:* 289–300 (1963).

PORTA, E.A.; KOCH, O.R.; GOMEZ-DUMM, C.L.A., and HARTROFT, W.C.: Effects of dietary protein on the liver of rats in experimental chronic alcoholism. J. Nutr. *94:* 437–446 (1968).

RUBIN, E. and LIEBER, C.S.: Early fine structural changes in the human liver induced by alcohol. Gastroenterology *52:* 1–13 (1967).

RUBIN, E. and LIEBER, C.S.: Alcohol-induced hepatic injury in non-alcoholic volunteers. New Engl. J. Med. *278:* 869–876 (1968a).

RUBIN, E. and LIEBER, C.S.: Hepatic microsomal enzymes in man and rat. Induction and inhibition by ethanol. Science *162:* 690–691 (1968b).

RUBIN, E. and LIEBER, C.S.: Malnutrition and liver disease – an overemphasized relationship. Amer. J. Med. *45:* 1–6 (1968c).

RUBIN, E.; HUTTERER, F., and LIEBER, C.S.: Ethanol increases hepatic smooth endoplasmic reticulum and drug-metabolizing enzymes. Science *159:* 1469–1470 (1968).

WILGRAM, G.F.: Experimental Laennec type of cirrhosis in monkeys. Ann. intern. Med. *51:* 1134–1158 (1959).

WILGRAM, G.F.; LUCAS, C.C., and BEST, C.H.: Kwashiorkor-type of fatty liver in primates. J. exp. Med. *108:* 361–370 (1958).

Author's address: Dr. CHARLES S. LIEBER, Section of Liver Disease and Nutrition, VA Hospital, 130 West Kingsbridge Road, *Bronx, NY 10468* (USA)

Medical Primatology 1972. Proc. 3rd Conf. exp. Med. Surg. Primates, Lyon 1972, part III, pp. 279–285 (Karger, Basel 1972)

Usefulness of Primates for Studying Drug Metabolism[1]

C. C. Smith, W. W. Weigel, Geraldine F. Wolfe and S. Mattingly

Departments of Environmental Health and Laboratory Animal Medicine, University of Cincinnati College of Medicine, Cincinnati, O.

Over the past several years our unit has been studying the metabolic fate of new antimalarial compounds. These have been developed by the US Army Research Program on Malaria to treat drug-resistant *Plasmodium falciparum* malaria encountered in recent years in Southeast Asia. The compounds have been studied as radiolabeled preparations primarily in rats and rhesus monkeys. Several of the more recent compounds have also been studied metabolically in owl monkeys *(Aotus trivirgatus)* and in human volunteers.

Some of the more important compounds which have been investigated are listed below. Their structures and position of the radiolabel are shown in figure 1.

(1) WR-3090-^{14}C (2,4,7-triamino-6-*o*-tolylpteridine, TATP).

(2) WR-38,839-^{14}C (4,6-diamino-1,2-dihydro-2,2-dimethyl-1-[3′,4′-dichlorobenzyloxy]-1,3,5-triazine hydrochloride).

(3) WR-25,979-^{3}H (1-[*p*-nitrophenyl]-3-amidinourea hydrochloride [Nitroguanil]).

(4) WR-5677-^{14}C (dypnone guanylhydrazone hydrochloride).

(5) WR-5949-^{14}C (2,4-diamino-5-[3′,4′,5′-trimethoxybenzyl]-pyrimidine [Trimethoprim]).

(6) WR-9792-^{14}C (4-fluoro-4′-trifluoromethylbenzophenone guanylhydrazone hydrochloride).

(7) WR-30,090-^{14}C (6,8-dichloro-2-[3′,4′-dichlorophenyl]-α-[di-N-butylaminomethyl]-4-quinolinemethanol hydrochloride).

1 Supported in part by US Army contract DADA 17-67-C-7065. Contribution No. 1062 from the US Army Research Program on Malaria.

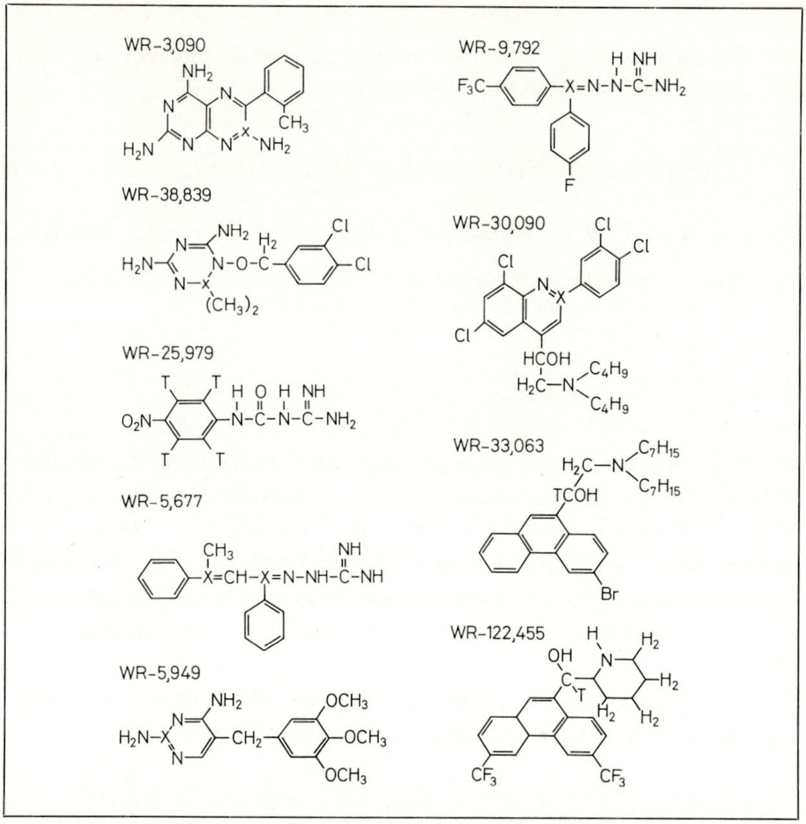

Fig. 1. Chemical structure and position of radiolabel of new experimental antimalarial drugs. X = ^{14}C; T = ^{3}H.

(8) WR-33,063-^{3}H (6-bromo-α-[di-N-heptylaminomethyl]-9-phenanthrenemethanol hydrochloride).

(9) WR-122,455-^{3}H (α-[2-piperidyl]-3,6-bis[trifluoromethyl]-9-phenanthrenemethanol hydrochloride).

The first compound, WR-3090, was almost completely absorbed and was rapidly and almost completely excreted by monkeys in the urine primarily as unchanged drug [1]. On the other hand, rats excreted the compound (as ^{14}C) about equally in urine and feces and the urine contained several metabolites.

WR-38,839 is an active folic acid antagonist which was well absorbed and rather rapidly excreted [1]. About equal amounts of radioactivity were recovered in urine and feces in monkeys whereas in the rat, fecal excretion accounted for better than 90% of the dose.

Nitroguanil (WR-25,979) is an interesting compound. It appeared to be hypotensive in monkeys in single doses of 25 mg/kg and was fairly rapidly excreted [1]. Total recovery of ^{3}H declined rapidly with time especially in rats. In this species only about 50% of the ^{3}H label could be accounted for after 24 h in the urine, feces and total animal tissues. Similar recovery data were obtained in rhesus monkeys. It was postulated that the ^{3}H on the ring was metabolized extensively to HTO, part of which escaped collection.

WR-5677 (Dypnone guanylhydrazone) was interesting because urinary excretion in rats accounted for only 4% of the dose whereas monkeys excreted 16–17% via this pathway [2]. The blood level curves in monkeys indicated probable conversion to metabolite(s); this interpretation was corroborated by TLC studies of the urine. One interesting metabolic possibility would be cyclization to the asymetrical triazine shown below.

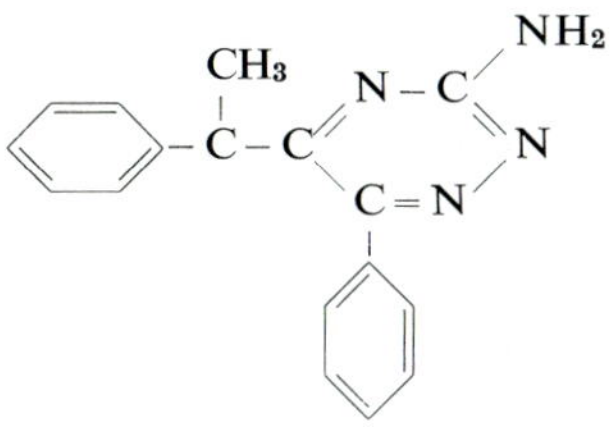

Thus, the compound is known to be metabolized but the metabolic products have not yet been identified.

Trimethoprim (WR-5949) is a compound that has been employed in treating drug-resistant malaria in Viet-Nam usually in combination with a long-acting sulfonamide. Such combinations are also used to treat certain bacterial infections. The compound (as ^{14}C) is excreted rather rapidly in both rats and monkeys [2]. Excretion occurs primarily via the urine. Using TLC we obtained evidence in both species of several urinary metabolites.

WR-9792, a guanylhydrazone, presented an unusual metabolic pattern. In monkeys it is tightly bound to organs and tissues especially the liver and lung [2]. For periods as long as 12 days after a single oral dose of 5 mg/kg almost 30% was recovered in the animal's organs and tissues. There was evidence of extensive tissue binding also in the rat.

WR-30,090 was the first of a series of quinoline or phenanthrene methanols that we have studied [3]. In monkeys and in rats this compound appeared to be poorly absorbed. Although 10% of the label was recovered in the tissues, average excretion in urine accounted for only 0.2% of the dose. There were two monkeys in which 2.5% was excreted in the urine, a finding which suggests that there may be considerable individual variation in excretion patterns.

WR-122,455 exhibited an unusual metabolic pattern. Peak concentrations of radioactivity in tissues of owl monkeys occurred as late as four days after a single oral dose of 35 mg/kg and radioactivity could be detected more than 30 days after dosing [2]. In the same species biliary excretion was prominent and there was extensive binding of the compound and/or its metabolites in tissues such as liver, lung and spleen.

For the three compounds WR-38,839, WR-5677 and WR-33,063, which have been studied also in human volunteers, the metabolic patterns in humans appear to follow the patterns obtained in rhesus monkeys [2–5]. However, insufficient data on identification of metabolites are available as yet to permit rigorous comparison of the metabolic pathways.

In the second portion of the paper we will discuss our experiments with rhesus monkeys in which we have introduced biliary cannulae. All the monkeys in table I were prepared using the following operative procedure. Through a single incision in the common duct one tube of PE-160 polyethylene was inserted into the gall bladder and a second PE-160 tube was threaded into the duodenum. The opposite ends of these tubes were exteriorized and connected by a sleeve of PE-200. Bile was collected for timed periods usually 5, 10 or 20 min by disconnecting the sleeve. Aliquots from these bile samples were assayed for total ^{14}C or ^{3}H by the standard procedures used in this laboratory [6]. The animals were maintained throughout the experiments in primate chairs.

WR-38,839-^{14}C was administered to monkeys 1–3 as indicated in table I. Peak levels of the drug (as ^{14}C) occurred in the bile 4–6 h after dosing. Biliary excretion over a three- to five-day period accounted for 6–14% of the dose. The experiments had to be terminated, however, because of plugging of the cannula or its removal by the monkey.

The fourth animal was given an oral dose of WR-122,455-^{3}H. However, the experiment had to be terminated on the seventh day after dosing because the animal seriously damaged its biliary cannula. Data on this animal suggested strongly that although there was some bile flow, biliary stasis was present. The excretion pattern of WR-122,455 in this animal was so different from that we had observed in normal monkeys that no additional animals with this type of biliary cannula were investigated. We concluded that this

Table I. Data on female rhesus monkeys with recirculating biliary cannulae

Monkey No.	Drug	Dose mg/kg	Observation period, days	
			post-dose	post-surgery
1	WR-38,839-^{14}C	10	5	16
2	WR-38,839-^{14}C	10	5	15
3	WR-38,839-^{14}C	10	3	17
4	WR-122,455-^{3}H	5	7	21

procedure was accompanied by technical problems which made the maintenance of animals with intact cannulae and adequate bile flow for extended periods very difficult.

In the next experiment (No. 5, table II), we tried using only an exit tube of PE-160 tubing. The monkey's bile was replaced with bovine bile and Initol (Hill Packing Company, Topeka, Kans.) administered orally morning and night. WR-122,455 was administered on the third postoperative day and was accompanied by a striking reduction in bile flow for the first 72 h. Later there was increased bile production averaging 50–60 ml per day. Bile flow was adequate up to the 20th day when the flow stopped abruptly and the experiment was terminated. Although this animal appeared to be some improvement over the previous ones, it still excreted 14% of its dose of WR-122,455 in the urine which was considerably more than the 5–7% we had observed in normal monkeys. This finding suggested the presence of some biliary stasis causing increased metabolism to polar metabolites excreted in the urine.

Our next approach consisted of combining the restraint jacket developed

Table II. Data on female rhesus monkeys with non-recirculating biliary cannulae

Monkey No.	Drug	Dose mg/kg	Observation period, days	
			post-dose	post-surgery
5	WR-122,455-^{3}H	5	20	24
6	WR-122,455-^{3}H	5	60	87
7	WR-33,063-^{3}H	30	30	197
	HTO (2 expts)		53	
8	HTO (3 expts)		88	184

at the Washington Primate Center in Seattle and a modification of the bile cannulation procedure perfected by Dr. D. SMALL and his collaborators at Boston University [7]. Using this general approach we prepared five additional animals, three of which are reviewed briefly in this report.

Monkey No. 6, to which we also administered WR-122-455-^{3}H, appeared to excrete the compound similarly to normal noncannulated monkeys. Bile flow was adequate for 87 days, at which time flow ceased. At this time the animal showed no evidence of jaundice, and it was assumed that a shunt had developed between the cannulated bile duct and the intestine, permitting the animal to excrete its bile in a more or less normal fashion.

Monkey No. 7 was administered WR-33,063-^{3}H as indicated in table II. We planned to condition this animal for about two weeks before drug administration. However, by day 8 it was apparent that the animal was consuming abnormal amounts of water. This became so pronounced that a diagnosis of psychogenic polydipsia was made. Administration of pitressin did not affect the animal's water intake or specific gravity of the urine. The monkey's water intake was restricted to 440 ml/day during the first ten days following administration of WR-33,063, after which the animal was allowed to drink *ad libitum*. In this cannulated monkey excretion of WR-33,063 in urine and feces was quantitatively almost identical to that which we observed in normal monkeys. Because of this animal's polydipsia, she offered us an opportunity to examine the effect of abnormal water intake and urine output on the excretion of tritiated water.

We were able to show that when monkeys were maintained on a very restricted water intake (ca. 100 ml/day), we could recover only 40–45% of a dose of HTO in urine and feces over a 21-day period. Presumably, the remainder was excreted via the lungs. In contrast, we were able to recover about 80% of the HTO in urine and feces in the same period when water intake and/or urine excretion exceeded 700 ml/day.

Although the use of the special jacket and the improved operative procedure has permitted us to maintain animals with functional biliary cannulae for periods up to six months, we have encountered three fairly serious complications: (1) the unpredictable occurrence of biliary stasis; (2) polydipsia; and (3) development of edema of the lower extremities.

We have been advised recently by Dr. D. BENNETT [personal commun.] of the Dow-Corning Corporation of the development of new techniques for studying bile excretion in primates. Although we have not had personal experience with these procedures, they seem to provide methods for overcoming several of the difficulties that we have encountered when we have attempted to maintain monkeys with biliary cannulae in primate chairs for extended periods.

References

1 Smith, C.C.; Walker, H.W.; Weigel, W.W., and Wolfe, G.F.: Unpubl. observations (1969).

2 Smith, C.C.; Weigel, W.W.; Wolfe, G.F.; McOwen, J.M.; Stefanovíc, G., and North, B.: Unpubl. observations (1970).

3 Rozman, R.S.; Smith, C.C., and Ryer, F.: Metabolic fate of WR-30,090 (6,8-dichloro-2-[3′, 4′-dichlorophenyl]-α-[di-N-butylaminomethyl]-4-quinolinemethanol HCl) in monkey and rat. Unpubl. observations.

4 Smith, C.C.; Dann, R.E.; Arnold, J., and Rozman, R.: Metabolic fate of WR-33,063-^{3}H (6-bromo-α-[di-N-heptylaminomethyl]-9-phenanthrenemethanol HCl) in humans. Unpubl. observations.

5 Smith, C.C.; Weigel, W.W.; Ryer, F., and Rozman, R.: Metabolic fate of WR-33,063-^{3}H (6-bromo-α-[di-N-heptylaminomethyl]-9-phenanthrenemethanol HCl) in monkey and rat. Unpubl. observations.

6 Smith, C.C.; Weigel, W.W., and Wolfe, G.F.: Unpubl. observations (1968).

7 Strasberg, S.M.; Dorn, B.C.; Small, D.M., and Egdahl, R.H.: The effect of biliary tract pressure on bile flow, bile salt secretion, and bile salt synthesis in the primate. Surgery *70:* 140–146 (1971).

Authors' address: Dr. Carl C. Smith, PhD, Dr. Walter W. Weigel, Dr. Geraldine F. Wolfe, and Dr. Steele Mattingly, Departments of Environmental Health and Laboratory Animal Medicine, University of Cincinnati College of Medicine, *Cincinnati, OH 45219* (USA)

Medical Primatology 1972. Proc. 3rd Conf. exp. Med. Surg. Primates, Lyon 1972, part III, pp. 286–295 (Karger, Basel 1972)

Use of Primates in Teratological Investigations[1]

J. G. Wilson

Children's Hospital Research Foundation and Departments of Pediatrics and Anatomy, University of Cincinnati, Cincinnati, O.

The advantages and disadvantages of using nonhuman primates in teratological studies has recently been reviewed in some detail [Wilson, 1972] and only generalities will be discussed here. Two genera, *Papio* (baboons) and *Macaca* (several species), have been shown to be promising for use in the evaluation of human teratic risk. Although it has been estimated that the cost is not much greater for maintaining breeding colonies of these primates than for pedigreed dogs or miniature pigs, this may change because the future supply of primates is uncertain. The main issue, however, concerns whether the use of primates offers a greater degree of security in the preclinical evaluation of the safety of drugs and other chemicals than the more widely used rodents and rabbits. Because of the relatively greater cost, the limited supply of animals and the difficulty of handling these animals, primates must be reserved for special purposes.

Better tests than are now in use can be devised, but to do so requires new protocols and a new concept including, among other things, the use of different levels of evaluation in different types of test animals (table I). The first level would consist of a teratogenicity screen employing large numbers of a readily available animal, such as rat or mouse for the purpose of finding the embryotoxic range of dosage. A test substance causing no significant embryotoxicity at several multiples of the anticipated human dose would advance to the second level of testing in which a carnivore (dog, cat or ferret), *or* an ungulate (pig or sheep) would be used, depending on which showed greater similarity to man in the metabolism of the compound in question. Information on metabolism would be accumulated in the course of routine pharma-

1 Supported in large part by contracts with the US Food and Drug Administration.

Table I. A new concept in teratogenicity testing

Order of test	Purpose	Suitable species	Number of pregnant animals
1st level	find embryotoxic dose range	rat, mouse, hamster *or* rabbit	as needed 100 or more
2nd level	confirm or adjust above	a carnivore *or* an ungulate	about 36
3rd level	only if 2nd level results are equivocal	alternate to that used in 2nd level	about 36
4th level	only if use in human pregnancy needed or likely	*Macaque* or *Papio*	about 36

Tests would terminate at 2nd level in most situations.

cological studies. The higher costs and lower fecundity of this second test animal, e.g. dogs or pigs, would dictate the use of smaller numbers than in the initial screen, but this would be acceptable because the general range of effective dosage would already have been defined. The second level test would be for the purpose of confirming and revising embryotoxic dosage found at the first level.

The results of the second level test would determine whether further animal investigation was necessary. If the compound caused no adverse effects at, for example, 10 times expected human use-level and exposure during pregnancy was thought unlikely, it might be considered ready for clinical trial without further animal tests. In case there was any uncertainty about the margin of safety between the dose that causes embryotoxicity in the second level test and the therapeutic level in man, and if the compound were one likely to involve exposure of pregnant women, a third level of sub-primate tests might be justified (table I).

A fourth level involving nonhuman primates would be recommended only for either of two specific situations: (1) drugs clearly needed to control severe discomfort or disease during pregnancy (e.g. anticonvulsants, hypoglycemics) or (2) drugs that are almost certain to be taken inadvertently during the early part of undiagnosed pregnancies (e.g. contraceptives, antiemetics). Another situation might on occasion justify use of primates for embryotoxicity testing. If, after a drug or an agricultural or household chemical had been approved and in use for a time, there were scattered reports that raised some question of low level of embryotoxicity, intensive tests in pregnant primates with doses elevated well above human exposure levels could help resolve the problem.

The foregoing has implied that embryotoxicity tests in nonhuman primates do indeed provide an added measure of security. This is probably true when they are used in sequence with other subprimate tests as proposed above. It remains to be proven, however, that in absolute terms primates are more reliable predictors of human embryotoxic risk than are other mammals. Careful scrutiny of available literature [WILSON, 1972] reveals that man and other primates do not have identical teratogenic sensitivity to more than two or three types of agents, namely thalidomide, sex hormones and probably ionizing radiations. A degree of similarity in embryotoxic response could be found as regards infections and some chemical agents, but it is already clear that an exact correlation in teratogenic susceptibility does not exist. Then, preference for simian primates can be justified only if they can be shown to be more like man in embryotoxic sensitivity than other test species. Such comparison should take into account all of the following: (1) overall phylogenetic relatedness, (2) similarity of maternal metabolism of chemicals, (3) comparability of placental transfer functions, and (4) likeness in embryonic reactions to extrinsic agents.

(1) *Phylogenetic relatedness.* The phylogenetic closeness of the simian primates to man has been offered as ample justification of their use as test animals, but this is no longer acceptable as sufficient reason in itself. It would be surprising, however, if this did not impart some similarity in embryotoxic sensitivity, in view of resemblance in other ways, such as (a) in the anatomical and temporal aspects of early embryogenesis, (b) in placental structure and known aspects of placental function, and (c) in reproductive physiology generally.

(2) *Metabolic relatedness.* SMITH [1968, 1969] has reviewed the literature to compare the accuracy with which rhesus monkey and dog would predict metabolic pathways in man as regards 11 assorted drugs. It was found that monkey and dog each showed close similarity to man in five instances; but monkey showed fair similarity in four additional instances, as against two for dog; and dog showed no metabolic similarity in four cases, whereas monkey was totally unlike man in only one case. With 12 additional compounds dog was again found to metabolize like man in about half of the tests but 'in man and rhesus monkey there was close correspondence between the metabolic patterns'. When dog, monkey and man were compared as to the presence of seven enzymatic pathways, dog was found to be strikingly different from the two primates, which were almost identical. PETERS [1971] has compared

different primate species with man as regards seven toxicologic and metabolic characteristics, and concluded that the rhesus monkey reacts more like man than does squirrel monkey in a ratio of 5:2, demonstrating that among simian primates those closest to man metabolize drugs more as does man.

Table II. Effects of diphenylhydantoin as seen in 100-day rhesus monkey fetuses from dams given large doses early in pregnancy[1]

Fetus No.	Maternal treatment		Condition of fetus			
	daily dose mg/kg	gestation days treated	weight g	external	autopsy	skeleton
♂ 3a	25 i.d.	22–24	145	normal	normal	normal
– 29c	50 i.d.	19–21	aborted on day 29			
♀ 11c	25 b.i.d.	22–24	118	normal	normal	small talus
♀ 90a	5 b.i.d.	25–45	141	normal	normal	normal
♂ 13f	5 b.i.d.	25–45	129	normal	retrocaval right ureter[2]	normal
♀ 73b	5 b.i.d.	25–45	141	normal	normal	normal
♀ 71b	5 b.i.d.	25–45	136	normal	retrocaval right ureter	normal
♀ 83b	10 b.i.d.	24–44	132	normal	normal	normal
♀ 59d	10 b.i.d.	25–45	121	normal	normal	normal
♂ 29f	10 b.i.d.	23–43	152	normal	normal	normal
♂ 38d	10 b.i.d.	20–40	134	? neck webbing	normal	normal
♂ 33e	20 b.i.d.	22–42	122	normal	retrocaval right ureter	absent talus
♀ 50d	20 b.i.d.	24–44	144	normal	3 cusps on mitral valve	normal
♂ 13g	20 b.i.d.	20–40	146	normal	normal	cervical ribs
12 controls	vehicle or none	–	142 ± 12			several skeletal variations[3]

1 Data reproduced by courtesy of US Food and Drug Administration which supported this work.
2 Retrocaval right ureter has not been previously seen in rhesus monkeys.
3 Skeletal variants include one with no ossification of talus, two with extra pr. ribs, two with extra rudimentary ribs, one 'knobby' ribs.
$\pm$ = Standard deviation.

(3) *Similarity of placental transfer.* Placental structure and circulation are highly analogous in man and rhesus monkey [RAMSEY and HARRIS, 1966; PANIGEL, 1971] but little is known about the function of either type of placenta during the period of organogenesis when the respective embryos are teratogenically most vulnerable.

(4) *Reaction within the embryo.* Too little is known about the reactions within embryos of different species to make a discussion of this subject useful at this time. Nevertheless, the choice of the most appropriate species for evaluation of human teratogenic risk should take into consideration the following questions: (a) do embryos of man and of the test animal

Table III. Effects of LSD on the first 100 days of intrauterine development in rhesus monkeys[1]

Fetus	Maternal treatment		Condition of fetus			
No.	dose × repeated μg	gestation days treated	weight g	external	autopsy	skeleton
♂ 22a	75	22	131	normal	? slight hydroceph.	normal
♂ 35a	75	25	154	normal	normal	normal
♂ 2a	100	29	150	normal	normal	cervical ribs
♀ 11b	200	27	145	normal	normal	cervical ribs 'knobby' ribs
♂ 16b	200 × 3	24, 26, 28	159	normal	normal	normal
♀ 10b	200 × 3	22, 24, 26	95	retarded	normal	retarded
♀ 17d	200 × 12	20–46	151	normal	normal	normal
♀ 51a	200 × 12	19–45	136	normal	normal	normal
♀ 38a	200 × 12	22–45	131	normal	normal	normal
♂ 58c	200 × 12	21–47	159	normal	normal	normal
– 53c	200 × 3	20–25	aborted on day 25			
♀ 71a	200 × 12	23–49	141	normal	normal	normal
♀ 39c	200 × 12	21–47	129	normal	normal	normal
♂ 10g	200 × 12	20–46	159	normal	normal	normal
12 controls			142 ± 12	normal	normal	several variations[2]

1 Data reproduced by courtesy of US Food and Drug Administration which supported this work.

2 Skeletal variants include one with no ossification of talus, two with extra pairs ribs, two with extra rudimentary ribs, one with 'knobby' ribs.

have comparable capabilities to metabolize or excrete foreign chemicals; and (b): are such chemicals bound or incorporated and do they have pharmacological effects in embryos of either man or test animal?

Use of Primates in a Multilevel Test for Embryotoxicity

When comparative data are available on maternal metabolism, placental transfer, and embryonic reaction that would indicate that primates are more appropriate than other animals, primates should be used in embryotoxicity testing for the special purposes already mentioned. Because of the limitations on numbers of primates available, they should be used only after extensive studies in other mammals have been completed, and as the last step before clinical trials are begun. There are two basic schedules that have been used for teratological testing in primates. One is essentially a chronic course of treatments repeated daily or at other frequent intervals throughout most of the period of organogenesis (approximately days 20 through 45 in rhesus monkeys). Two or more dosage levels are used, with the highest at or near the maximal tolerated chronic dose for adult females, with several pregnancies

Table IV. Embryotoxicity screen using 15 pregnant monkeys

Gestation, age in days	Developmental events	Dosage		
		X	X/2	X/4
20–23	1–11 pairs of somites, neural folds and early neural tube, heart primordia appear	1	1	1
24–27	neural tube closes, brain vesicles form, branchial arches develop, heart chambers indicated, limb buds appear	1	1	1
28–31	optic cup and lens forming, pharyngeal region differentiates, heart septation begins, midgut loop herniates	1	1	1
32–35	face and sense organs form, heart septa completed, ureteric buds dividing, cartilage skeleton appears, digit rays seen	1	1	1
42–45	palate closing, skeletal ossification begins, renal glomeruli forming, external genitals developing	1	1	1
Total		5	5	5

X = maximum tolerated dose for adult female monkeys.

assigned to each dosage group. LSD and diphenylhydantoin have been studied in this way (tables II and III).

This protocol is simple in design but has the disadvantage of other chronic treatment; it entails the possibility that maternal adaptative mechanisms may cause spurious results. For example, prolonged treatment with a test drug could induce or inhibit metabolizing enzymes, or cause pathology in maternal liver or kidneys. If treatment were begun several days before the embryos reach the peak of their teratologic sensitivity, these adaptative changes could occur and cause appreciable alterations in maternal blood levels.

The second type of test protocol is designed specifically to avoid such difficulties (table IV). The duration of treatment is limited to three- or four-day periods, with several such short-duration groups dispersed throughout the period of organogenesis. Five such four-day treatment periods will cover

Table V. Sodium cyclamate embryotoxicity screen in rhesus monkeys[1] (fetuses removed by hysterotomy on days 99–101)

Maternal treatment		Condition of fetus			
gestation days treated	daily dose mg/kg	weight g	external	autopsy	skeleton
20–23	500	127	normal	normal	normal
	2,000	154	normal	normal	13 pairs ribs
24–27	500[2]	24[2]	normal	normal	immature
	500	151	normal	normal	normal
	2,000	149	normal	normal	normal
28–31	500[2]	fetus found dead at 51 days			
	500	156	normal	normal	normal
	2,000	159	normal	normal	normal
32–35	500	127	normal	normal	normal
	2,000	159	normal	4 lobes left lung	13 pairs ribs
42–45	500	125	normal	normal	normal
	2,000	119	normal	normal	retarded
12 controls		142 ± 12	normal	normal	several variations

1 Data reproduced by courtesy of the US Food and Drug Administration which supported this work.

2 Hysterotomy early because of placental separation and hemorrhage.

the more important developmental events in monkey organogenesis. Only one or two animals are used at each treatment span and dosage because this initial screen is followed by tests of additional pregnant monkeys at all treatment spans and dosages that produce embryotoxicity. Two or three dose levels are used, with the highest near the maximum tolerated level (table IV), Sodium cyclamate and cyclohexylamine have been studied by this protocol (tables V and VI).

If highest tolerated level is the starting point for dosage selection (table VII), one or more fractions of this should be tested, preferably to find a level at which definite embryotoxicity occurs. Whichever method of dose selection is used, additional pregnant animals must be tested for confirmation at the lowest level that produces embryotoxicity. When an embryotoxic level is found, a lower dose that is known or thought to be nonembryotoxic, based on the short-term test, should be given over the entire span of organogenesis in ten additional monkeys to rule out the possibility of cumulative effects, such

Table VI. Cyclohexylamine embryotoxicity screen in rhesus monkeys[1] (fetuses removed by hysterotomy on days 99–101)

Maternal treatment		Condition of fetus			
gestation days treated	daily dose mg/kg	weight g	external	autopsy	skeleton
20–23	25	122	normal	accessory spleen	normal
	50	114	normal	1 umbilical a.	normal
	75	120	normal	normal	normal
24–27	25	155	normal	normal	normal
	50	144	normal	normal	normal
	75	119	normal	normal	retarded
28–31	25	118	normal	normal	normal
	50	19[2]	normal	normal	immature
	75	137	normal	normal	normal
32–35	25	137	normal	normal	13 pair ribs
	50	132	normal	normal	11 pair ribs
	75	aborted on day 67			
42–45	25	133	normal	normal	normal
	50	145	normal	normal	normal
	75	151	normal	normal	normal

1 Data are reproduced with the consent of the US Food and Drug Administration which supported this work.
2 Hysterotomy on day 68 because of threatened abortion.

Table VII. Minimal embryotoxicity study in monkeys

a) Short-term screen

	Number of pregnant monkeys/short-term period				
Days treated	20–23	24–27	28–31	32–35	42–45
Dose X[1]	2	2	2	2	2
<X	2	2	2	2	2

1 Highest tolerated dose.

b) Chronic treatment through organogenesis

Dose: highest no-effect level.
Duration of treatment: days 20 through 45.
Number of pregnancies: 10.
5 interrupted day 100 for fetal examination.
5 to term for 3 months' postnatal study.
Control: 6 pregnant monkeys Rx chronic/vehicle.
3 interrupted day 100 for fetal examination.
3 to term for 3 months' postnatal study.

as pathology in maternal kidney or liver, that might only be seen after more prolonged treatment.

Pregnancy in five of the ten monkeys given such long-term treatment are to be interrupted for routine fetal examination by hysterotomy on day 100 of gestation, but the remainder are to go to normal delivery, weighed weekly thereafter, and observed for behavior, muscular coordination and sensory modalities for at least three months postnatally. At the end of the postnatal observation period, surviving young should be X-rayed and subjected to *post mortem* examination.

References

PANIGEL, M.: La perméabilité du placenta chez l'homme et certains primates non humains; dans TUCHMANN-DUPLESSIS Malformations congénitales des mammifères, p. 27–48 (Masson, Paris 1971).

PETERS, J. H.: Observations on utility of subhuman primates as models of man for drug studies. Proc. west. pharmacol. Soc. *14:* 72–75 (1971).

RAMSEY, E. M. and HARRIS, J. W. S.: Comparison of uteroplacental vasculature and circulation in the rhesus monkey and man. Contrib. Embryol. Carneg. Inst. *38:* 59–70 (1966).

SMITH, C. C.: Predicting drug metabolic pathways in man; in VAGTBORG Use of nonhuman primates in drug evaluation, pp. 469–479 (University of Texas Press, Austin 1968).

SMITH, C.C.: Value of nonhuman primates in predicting disposition of drugs in man. Ann. N.Y. Acad. Sci. *162:* 604–609 (1969).

WILSON, J.G.: Abnormalities of intrauterine development in non-human primates; in DICZFALUSY and STANDLEY Symp. on the Use of Non-Human Primates for Research on Problems of Human Reproduction (World Health Organization, Training Center on Human Reproduction, Karolinska Institute, Stockholm 1972).

Author's address: Dr. J.G. WILSON, Children's Hospital Research Foundation and Departments of Pediatrics and Anatomy, University of Cincinnati, Elland and Bethesda Avenues, *Cincinnati, OH 45229* (USA)

Cardiovascular Studies

Medical Primatology 1972. Proc. 3rd Conf. exp. Med. Surg. Primates, Lyon 1972, part III, pp. 298–305 (Karger, Basel 1972)

Primate Cardiology[1]

Keynote Address

Z. FEJFAR

Cardiovascular Diseases Unit, World Health Organization, Geneva

In delivering the introductory address at this Conference, I am aware of the honour which has been bestowed on me as well as my responsibility to the audience. I propose to discuss the problem from the viewpoint of a human primate physician with cardiological orientation and to outline where investigations on nonhuman primates might bring us closer to the solution of diseases which we often call 'typical human conditions'.

Although we do not know all answers to prevention of rheumatic fever and rheumatic heart disease, this disease has ceased to be in the forefront of cardiovascular problems in most affluent societies. It does not, therefore, require specific studies on apes and monkeys. Neither shall I consider the broad aspects of congenital malformations of the circulatory system, as surgical correction of most of them is now possible from infancy, and various species of mammals have and can be used for training in the relevant techniques. The emphasis needs to be on early diagnosis of the malformations during fetal life and on the advancement of knowledge of the developmental physiology, with a view to prevent malformations or to terminate the pregnancy at the earliest stage.

There may be particular cardiac diseases, for example, those caused by parasitic infestation like Chagas' heart disease, in which arrhythmias and conduction defects terminating in ventricular fibrillation are frequent. Experimental studies should clarify the pathogenesis, especially that of ventricular fibrillation in acute coronary heart disease.

There is also an urgent need to study more profoundly the immune me-

1 This paper was presented as the keynote address on cardiovascular diseases at the Third Conference on Experimental Medicine and Surgery, Lyon, June 21–23, 1972.

chanisms resulting from damage of the myocardial cell by the parasite which might be involved in the pathogenesis of chronic Chagas' heart disease. Comparative study of the American and African trypanosomiasis in different species with varying immune characteristics might be one way to approach the problem of the pathogenesis and treatment of a disease which strikes several million people in the Latin American Continent. Investigations on immune mechanisms in experimental trypanosomiasis in New World and Old World monkeys could be rewarding in this respect, and throw new light on the development of the chronic disease in man.

Arterial hypertension and ischaemic heart disease with coronary atherosclerosis as a basis are, of course, front runners in cardiovascular human pathology. The first is the commonest circulatory disease the world over, the second is a primary cause of death in affluent societies and a running-up problem among the upper social strata in the developing world. For both conditions we still lack satisfactory animal models in spite of many years of tremendous efforts. Essential hypertension is known to evolve from labile elevation of blood pressure and is characterized often at this stage by an increased cardiac output and an insufficient vasodilatation, i.e. relatively increased peripheral vascular resistance [9]. This initial phase goes over to that of fixed, permanent hypertension, where cardiac output is within normal limits, while peripheral vascular resistance rises further. Still later, the humoral phase with an elevation of renin and angiotensin formation, accelerates the vascular damage in vital organs.

While transient elevation of pressure through stimulation of certain parts of the central nervous system is well known and documented, only rarely have attempts to produce chronic hypertension in this way been successful. FOLKOW and RUBINSTEIN [10] achieved this by repeated hypothalamic stimulation in rat and there are reports on persisting elevation of blood pressure in dogs caused by experimental derangements of habitual condition reflexes [1, 6, 11, 15].

The 'salt story' of hypertension [5] also needs further testing. I wonder whether colonies of monkeys living in a relatively free way, or manipulated (isolation, exposure, high salt intake), could be of help in clarifying the pathogenesis of the beginning phase of hypertension.

The two major aspects for prevention of ischaemic heart disease are pathogenesis of the development of heart attacks (acute myocardial infarction, sudden death) and aetiology of coronary atherosclerosis.

As for the first one, there are innumerable experimental studies in which branches of coronary arteries were occluded or ligated. The baboons appear very interesting because of a rather homogeneous morphology of the coronary vascular system which is similar to man, while coronary vessels in a dog – a most commonly studied animal – differ [21]. A particular feature in the dog is a larger septal vessel originating from the proximal part of the anterior descending branch of the left coronary artery. Baboons and perhaps other monkeys may be suitable for studying pathogenesis of malignant arrhythmias, i.e. those leading, if not treated, to ventricular fibrillation.

Figure 1 shows prevalence of atherosclerotic lesions in the left coronary artery in the autopsy material related to a population in Malmö, Prague and three areas of the USSR. In the age group 35–44 years, more than 80% of males presented fibrous plaques, calcifications or complicated lesions. In females a similar frequency could be found in a 10-year-older age group. Atherosclerosis occurs, however, already in childhood.

Comparison of the natural history of atherosclerosis, with the distribution of recognized coronary risk factors during lifetime, shows that most of them appear to play a role only after the onset of atherosclerotic damage (fig. 2). The scheme illustrates findings from studies of population groups and cannot be related to individual subjects. Elevated levels of serum cholesterol

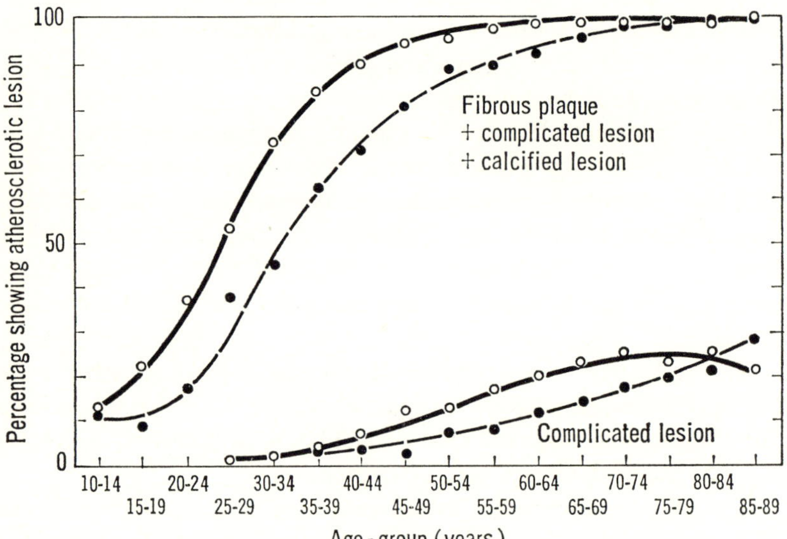

Fig. 1. Age distribution of atherosclerotic lesion in left anterior descending coronary artery among 17,455 autopsy specimens (○ men; ● women) examined in a WHO collaborative study in Czechoslovakia, Sweden and the USSR [26].

appear to be the first biochemical symptom of atherosclerosis. Overnutrition and relation of the child towards its social environment appear to be the first important environmental exposures requiring adaptation in this respect. The scheme underlines that atherosclerosis is primarily a problem of the very early phase of life, while in adulthood a combination and accumulation of several factors promote and provoke coronary accident.

Research into aetiology and pathogenesis of atherosclerosis has been mostly carried out in rabbits, pigs and birds. The question whether nonhuman primates are suitable for such studies has been answered in the affirmative way a long time ago, as can be seen, among others, in the papers from the Conference on Experimental Medicine and Surgery in Primates, 1967 [7]. I do not feel qualified enough to indicate where the pig or swine [3, 18] and where this or that species of monkeys would be preferable in studying spontaneous or experimental atherosclerosis. It seems that one needs to extend comparative studies into a number of species including nonhuman primates.

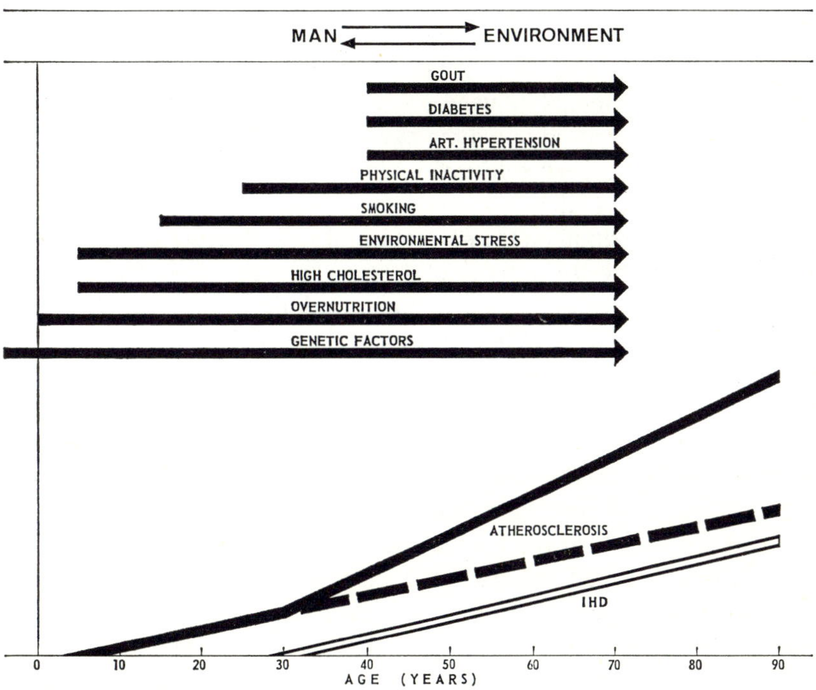

Fig. 2. Risk factors in atherosclerosis and ischaemic heart disease (IHD), by age. WHO Chronicle *25/8:* 3 [1971].

One has to take into account that atherosclerotic lesions are rather rare in wild animals, and also other characteristics including blood lipids change in captivity. There appears a clear trend in captive monkeys to elevation of blood cholesterol [23] and to more marked lesions in the aorta and in coronary vessels [16]. Splitting of the internal elastic membrane and fibroblastic proliferation in the intima of coronary vessels, are similar to changes observed in man early in life [24].

Most studies have been done in adult animals. In humans, low levels of blood cholesterol have been found at the time of birth, and already in early childhood the difference between children from affluent groups as compared to poorer ones has been demonstrated [20, 25]. Different age distribution of cholesterol has been described by BAEDER [2] in monkeys. The levels were relatively high (around 200 mg/dl) in infant monkeys and later on markedly decreased.

Studies on the quantity and quality of food in infants and children as well as parallel investigations on serum lipids and on types of lipoproteins are now beginning to appear more and more often. They need to be supplemented by research on the metabolic turnover of lipids and of other major food constituents, and on the importance of trace elements, as well as by investigations of the hormonal influences at that age. This might be a fruitful field for further investigation on young nonhuman primates.

Much less has been achieved by investigating the reaction of the child towards its first, i.e. family environment, although such studies might provide important information on the natural history of atherosclerosis. The complicated methodology has been one of the many reasons why such investigations have been only seldom made in man, and particularly in the child. As outlined by CHARVÁT *et al.* [4], reaction of the organism to mental or physical strain is rather similar and uniform. The stimulus which is perceived as dangerous or worrying is transmitted through neurohumoral mechanisms towards muscles which become ready for action (avoiding the problem by running away or facing it by the fight), and by circulatory, respiratory and metabolic preparation for this muscular function. Similar modification appears during physical activity and also when the organism is threatened by failing heart [8]. The 'civilized' human primates exposed to such a threat, even if it is only imaginative, usually suppress muscular action and the haemocirculatory and metabolic preparation remains unused. It remains to prove whether this hypothesis can explain long-term alteration in man repeatedly or continuously exposed to such worrying situations. Because of a similarity between the behaviour of monkeys and man [19], they appear uniquely suited for such research. Pioneering studies in Sukhumi [14] and investigations in other primate centres, demonstrate that one can study a number of parameters in monkeys exposed to psychic strain or to stimulation of brain centres.

Monkeys and apes seem to be particularly suitable for combined investigation of behaviour, metabolism and haemocirculation in the animals living semi-free in colonies, using telemetric methods for monitoring them within their natural groups. Follow-ups, and manipulation studies in young monkeys, be it by influencing nutrition, social life such as isolation or crowding, sedentary life, or other habits known to be the product of our civilization, would be an excellent addition to research on inbred mice [12], or birds [17] living in colonies.

Cardiology is definitely moving more and more towards clarifying the effects of the community life on the individual – ecology of our civilization – in relation to the development of hypertension, atherosclerosis and ischaemic heart disease. Research on the semi-free and on the domesticated, 'civilized' nonhuman primates might advance considerably our thinking, help to develop methodology to be used on ourselves, and contribute thus to the prevention of ischaemic heart disease, the epidemics of our civilization. One of the many problems is that individual monkeys of the same genus may respond differently to the same stimulus [22]. Little attention has been given to individual differences [27], although this is as obvious a necessity in long-term investigations as is the proper care and prevention of infections and infestations and the maintenance of optimal nutrition [13].

One should of course always take into consideration whether other animal species which are more readily available and cheaper to obtain, to breed or keep, are not equally or more suitable. From some published data it seems to me that people experienced in comparative medicine are rather cautious in promoting the use of monkeys while clinicians like myself are perhaps more on the optimistic side.

Every problem requires a particular choice of the most suitable animal, upon which the research worker himself must decide. I have, therefore, attempted to outline only some general trends in cardiovascular research in relation to the possible use of nonhuman primates.

References

1 ANOKHIN, P.K.: The physiological basis of the pathogenesis of hypertensive states. Proc. Joint WHO-Czechoslovak Cardiological Society Symposium on the Patho-

genesis of Essential Hypertension, Prague 1960, p. 199–222 (State Medical Publishing House, Prague 1961).

2 BAEDER, D.H.: A comparison of blood lipid fractions of various experimental animals, including the baboon; in The baboon in medical research, p. 301–321 (University of Texas Press, Austin 1965).

3 BIJLENGA, G.; DAHME, E.; DETWEILER, D.K.; GRESHAM, G.A.; GRUNBERG, W.; HOWARD, A.N.; KAGAN, A.R.; KAPLAN, M.M.; NIE, C.J. VAN; RUBARTH, S.; STERNBY, N.H.; STUNZI, H.; UEMURA, K., and WHITNEY, J.C.: Comparative studies of atherosclerosis in swine. Bull. Wld Hlth Org. *36:* 457–465 (1967).

4 CHARVÁT, J.; DELL, P., and FOLKOW, B.: Mental factors and cardiovascular diseases. Cardiologia *44:* 124–141 (1964).

5 DAHL, L.K.: Effects of chronic excess salt ingestion. Experimental hypertension in the rat. Correlation with human hypertension; in The epidemiology of hypertension, pp. 218–239 (Grune & Stratton, New York 1967).

6 EHRLICH, V.: General discussion of third working session. The central nervous system and essential hypertension I; in Proc. Joint WHO-Czechoslovak Cardiological Society Symposium on the Pathogenesis of Essential Hypertension, Prague 1960, pp. 163–167 (State Medical Publishing House, Prague 1961).

7 GOLDSMITH, E.I. and MOOR-JANKOWSKI, J., ed.: Experimental medicine and surgery in primates. Ann. N.Y. Acad. Sci. *162:* 80–155 (1969).

8 FEJFAR, Z. und FEJFAROVÁ, M.: Hämodynamische Veränderungen bei Kreislaufstörungen (VEB Verlag Volk und Gesundheit, Berlin 1961).

9 FEJFAR, Z. and WIDIMSKY, J.: Juvenile hypertension. Proc. Joint WHO-Czechoslovak Cardiological Society Symposium on the Pathogenesis of Essential Hypertension. Prague 1960, pp. 33–42 (State Medical Publishing House, Prague 1961).

10 FOLKOW, B. and RUBINSTEIN, E.H.: Cardiovascular effects of acute and chronic stimulation of the hypothalamic defence area in the rat. Acta physiol. scand. *68:* 48–57 (1966).

11 GOREV, N.N.: General discussion of third working session. The central nervous system and essential hypertension I. Proc. Joint WHO-Czechoslovak Cardiological Society Symposium on the Pathogenesis of Essential Hypertension, Prague 1960, pp. 167–168 (State Medical Publishing House, Prague 1961).

12 HENRY, J.P. and CASSEL, J.C.: Psychosocial factors in essential hypertension. Recent epidemiologic and animal experimental evidence. Amer. J. Epidem. *90:* 171–200 (1969).

13 KERR, G.R.: Nutritional requirements of subhuman primates. Physiol. Rev. *52:* 415–467 (1972).

14 LAPIN, B.A. and YAKOVLEVA, L.A.: Comparative pathology in monkeys (Thomas, Springfield 1963).

15 MIASNIKOW, A.L.: The significance of disturbances of higher nervous activity in the pathogenesis of hypertensive disease. Proc. Joint WHO-Czechoslovak Cardiological Society Symposium on the Pathogenesis of Essential Hypertension, Prague 1960, pp. 153–162 (State Medical Publishing House, Prague 1961).

16 MIDDLETON, C.C.; CLARKSON, T.B.; LOFLAND, H.B., and PRICHARD, R.W.: Atherosclerosis in the squirrel monkey. Arch. Path. *78:* 16 (1964).

17 RATCLIFFE, H.L.: Ecological factors associated with atherosclerosis in zoo animals; in Cerebral vascular diseases (Grune & Stratton, New York 1966).

18 Ratcliffe, H.L.; Luginbühl, H., and Pivnik, L.: Coronary, aortic and cerebral atherosclerosis in swine of 3 age-groups. Implications. Bull. Wld Hlth Org. *42:* 225–234 (1970).

19 Romer, A.S.: The vertebrate story (University of Chicago Press, Chicago 1960).

20 Scrimshaw, N.S.; Balsam, A., and Arroyave, G.: Serum cholesterol levels in school children from three socioeconomic groups. Amer. J. Nutr. *5:* 629–633 (1957).

21 Seljeskog, E.L., Hitchcock, C.R., and Groover, M.E.: Coronary artery studies in dog and Kenya baboon utilizing surgically induced myocardial infarctions; in The baboon in medical research, pp. 557–566 (University of Texas Press, Austin 1965).

22 Smith, O.A.: General discussions on influence of personality on cardiovascular disease. Proc. Int. Symp. Neural and Psychological Mechanisms in Cardiovascular Disease, Stresa 1971 (Il Ponte, Milano, 1972).

23 Strong, J.P.; Rosal, J.; Deupree, R.H., and McGill, H.C., jr.: Diet and serum cholesterol levels in baboons. Exp. molec. Path. *5:* 82–91 (1966).

24 Vlodaver, Z.; Medalie, J., and Neufeld, H.N.: Coronary arteries in immature monkeys. Preliminary report of the relationships to activity and diet. J. Atheroscler. Res. *8:* 923–933 (1968).

25 Whyte, H.M. and Yes, I.L.: Serum cholesterol levels of Australians and natives of New Guinea from birth to adulthood. Austr. Ann. Med. *7:* 336–339 (1958).

26 Work of WHO in Cardiovascular Diseases in 1971. Annual report of the Director-General. Off. Records of WHO 197, pp. 71–77 (WHO, Geneva 1972).

27 Zill, M.: Behavioral testing in laboratory animals and man. Proc. Int. Symp. Neural and Psychological Mechanisms in Cardiovascular Disease, Stresa 1971 (Il Ponte, Milano, 1972).

Author's address: Dr. Z. Fejfar, Chief Cardiovascular Diseases, World Health Organization, Avenue Appia, *CH-1211 Geneva 27* (Switzerland)

Medical Primatology 1972. Proc. 3rd Conf. exp. Med. Surg. Primates, Lyon 1972, part III, pp. 306–312 (Karger, Basel 1972)

Chimpanzee and Baboon as Biochemical Models for Human Atherosclerosis

V. BLATON, D. VANDAMME and H. PEETERS

Simon Stevin Institute for Scientific Research, Brugge

Introduction

Much of the vascular research in nonhuman primates has been concerned with the production of atherosclerosis. Many factors that are considered to aggravate the disease have been investigated. Numerous dietary experiments and intensive investigations on the role of cholesterol have been made. These studies were prompted by the hope that simians may respond to experimental induction of hypercholesterolemia and atherosclerosis with reactions more closely resembling those of man than of other experimental animals [GRESHAM *et al.,* 1965]. Although a major part of our investigations [BLATON *et al.,* 1970; PEETERS *et al.,* 1970] has been on baboons *(Papio cynocephalus)* and chimpanzees *(Pan troglodytes schweinfurthii)*, we realize the importance of gathering more comparative information on several species kept under the same conditions [PEETERS and BLATON, 1969, 1973] in order to provide a broader basis for selection of primate species for studies of experimental atherosclerosis.

The use of baboons in the atherosclerotic field seems to offer certain advantages. In the wild these animals develop diffuse fatty streaks [LINDSAY and CHAIKOFF, 1957], and some adult animals show lesions in the aorta complicated by hemorrhage into the plaque [MCGILL *et al.,* 1960]. Experimental work demonstrated that atherosclerosis [GRESHAM *et al.,* 1965; HOWARD *et al.,* 1967; STRONG and MCGILL, 1967], can be induced in baboons by a cholesterol rich diet, containing egg yolk and butter. Furthermore, MORRIS and

1 Supported by grants from the NFWGO (Belgium), grant No. 1153, Franqui Foundation and the RUCA-Zoo.

GEER [1970] and LEHNER *et al.* [1971] provided the first evidence of hereditary hyperbetalipoproteinemia in primates.

More spontaneous aortic and cerebral atherosclerosis was found in chimpanzees than in any other nonhuman primates [RATCLIFFE, 1965]. Atheromatous coronary lesions similar to those of man were described by VASTESAEGER and DELCOURT [1961] in two chimpanzees *(P. t. schweinfurthii)*. Due to their prohibitive cost little is known about the effect of raised serum cholesterol level in relation to the development and prognosis of coronary heart disease in this species. In 1942, MANNING described experimental coronary atherosclerosis and thrombosis in these animals leading to a heart attack and to the death of an eight-year-old ape.

The present long-term study on the effect of hypercholesterolemic diets in chimpanzees and baboons was undertaken to establish the genesis of atherosclerosis in nonhuman primates, to investigate the validity of its extrapolation to the human disease and to relate any plasma lipoprotein change observed to those seen in the type II hyperlipoproteinemia in man.

Material and Methods

Eighteen young baboons *(P. cynocephalus)*, three females and 15 males, 12–18 months of age, were divided in equal groups and given either a control or an atherogenic diet [GRESHAM *et al.*, 1965; BLATON *et al.*, 1970]. The body weight of the animals varied while on the diet for more than four years. The weight gain in the two groups was the same as there was no obvious difference in caloric intake. As little as 18 months after starting the dietary regime it was possible to find fatty streaks in the aorta, strikingly similar to those found in man [GRESHAM *et al.*, 1965]. It is important to emphasize that coronary and cerebral lesions were never seen during this long period of investigation. On the other hand, the control animals not been subjected to atherogenic diets also demonstrated frequent artery lesions.

Ten chimpanzees *(P. t. schweinfurthii)*, seven males and three females, two to three years of age at the beginning of the experiments, were divided into two groups, four of them were given a control diet and six of them were on an atherogenic diet [VASTESAEGER and DELCOURT, 1961; BLATON *et al.*, in press] for seven to eight years. Fatty streaks and fatty lesions were found after three years of diet. During this study one female died from myocardial infarction produced by an occluding thrombosis on stenosing lesions of the anterior descending branch of the left coronary [VASTESAEGER *et al.*, 1973]. Fasting blood was taken from the femeral artery into EDTA after tranquilization with Sernylan (Parke, Davis) as described previously [HOWARD and GRESHAM, 1966; MORTELMANS, 1969]. All methods and techniques used in separation and characterization of plasma lipoprotein fractions were described previously [BLATON *et al.*, 1966 and 1970; BLATON and PEETERS, 1971; PEETERS *et al.*, 1970].

Data obtained from baboons and chimpanzees are compared with results from normal human subjects (20–25 years of age) and from male hyperlipoproteinemic subjects (45–55 years of age) with angina pectoris or hypertensive vascular disease [HOWARD *et al.*, 1972].

Results and Discussions

Young *baboons* given the atherogenic diets developed aortic atherosclerosis similar to that seen spontaneously in old animals given a laboratory stock diet for four years. Histologically the disease resembled the early human fatty streak and consisted of intra- and extracellular lipid, fatty acids, collagen elastin and mucopolysaccharide. Despite long-term maintenance on the diet no lesions have been observed in the coronary arteries. The only major change revealed by biochemical study of the plasma was an increase in β-lipoproteins [BLATON *et al.,* 1970] accompanied by a disproportionate increase of cholesterol and phospholipids, most pronounced in β-lipoproteins. The rise in β-lipoproteins over the α-lipoproteins leads to a pattern similar to that seen in normal man. Only after a long period of high cholesterol diet was there a lipoprotein profile of the atherogenic baboon comparable to the human type II hyperlipoproteinemia. Based on detailed analysis of lipids and fatty acids in the electrochromatographic α- and β-lipoprotein, it is concluded that the pathological effect of the atherogenic diet is due not only to an increased plasma level of β-lipoproteins but also to a change in composition of lipoproteins which decreases the stability and favours the deposition of cholesterol esters in the arterial wall (table I). The chief effets of the atherogenic diet were the increase in total cholesterol, in phosphatidyl choline (table II) especially in the β-lipoproteins, an unexpected decrease of cholesterol/phospholipid in the β-lipoproteins and an increase of cholesterol oleate. The α-lipoproteins were not appreciably affected. In our experience the β-lipoproteins appear to be the main vehicle for the transport of additional exogenous cholesterol and cholesterol esters, which indicates the difference in cholesterol metabolism between normal and atherogenic diet fed animals. The triglycerides seem to take little part in this type of experimental atherosclerosis. They are neither elevated, nor did their percentage composition in α- or β-lipoproteins change, so that their very low density lipoproteins (VLDL) concentration stayed constant. There are similarities but also differences between the induced hyperlipemic state in the baboon and type II hyperlipoproteinemia in man. The most conspicuous differences, however, are the cholesterol/phospholipid decrease in the β-lipoproteins and the percentage increase of phosphatidyl-

Table I. Lipid profile of plasma and plasma lipoproteins in man, chimpanzee and baboon

Lipid mg/100 ml	Man		Chimpanzee		Baboon	
	normal n = 4[4]	type 2[1] n = 5	C[2] n = 4	A[3] n = 6	C[2] n = 3	A[3] n = 4
T. lipids						
plasma	414	870a	746	1,429a	343	549b
α-LP	152	239a	315	322	188	257
β-LP	261	631a	430	1,107a	154	292b
T. cholesterol						
plasma	151	340a	259	606a	117	203b
α-LP	43	70a	88	95	60	96
β-LP	108	269a	171	512a	57	107b
Triglycerides						
plasma	31	84a	60	65	38	32
α-LP	13	28b	19	20	13	11
β-LP	18	56a	41	45	25	21
Phospholipids						
plasma	163	284a	295	459a	122	202b
α-LP	76	105b	166	163	82	97
β-LP	87	179a	129	296a	40	105b

1 Type II, hyperbetalipoproteinemia.
2 C = Animals under control diet.
3 A = Animals under atherogenic diet.
4 n = Number of subjects.
a = $p < 0.001$; b = $p < 0.05$.

choline in the β-lipoproteins. Diet may be one of the sources of these differences [Howard *et al.*, 1972].

The protein lipid and lipoprotein patterns of *normal chimpanzees* resemble those of man. On feeding the atherogenic diet there appears a large increase of β-lipoproteins, and lipids and fatty acids in the lipoproteins are altered similarly to the changes in the human hyperlipoproteinemia. Furthermore, fasting blood from both groups of chimpanzees shows in our experiments no appreciable VLDL, so that the experimental disease can be considered as a real type II hyperbetalipoproteinemia. Most of the results in chimpanzees reported in tables I–III are very similar to those observed in human type II hyperlipoproteinemia disease. The similar results in the lipid and phospholipid distribution in plasma and in α- and β-lipoproteins indicate the close relationship between man and chimpanzee in their reaction to changes of the environment. Moreover, the biochemical determinations in the arterial wall

Table II. Cholesterol/phosphatidylcholine (C/PC) and sphingomyelin/phosphatidylcholine (S/PC) ratios in plasma and plasma lipoproteins of man, chimpanzee and baboon

Lipid ratio	Man		Chimpanzee		Baboon	
	normal n = 4[4]	type II[1] n = 5	C[2] n = 4	A[3] n = 6	C[2] n = 3	A[3] n = 4
C/PC						
plasma	1.31	1.89	1.26	1.89	1.36	1.40
α-LP	0.82	1.08	0.78	0.80	0.98	1.41
β-LP	1.73	2.42	1.90	2.60	2.11	1.45
S/PC						
plasma	0.30	0.38	0.25	0.28	0.14	0.13
α-LP	0.29	0.29	0.19	0.16	0.12	0.12
β-LP	0.28	0.44	0.30	0.37	0.17	0.12

1 Type II, hyperbetalipoproteinemia.
2 C = Animals under control diet.
3 A = Animals under atherogenic diet.
4 n = Number of subjects.

Table III. Oleic to linoleic acid (18:1/18:2) ratios in plasma, in plasmalipoproteins, in cholesterolesters (CE) and in phosphatidylcholine (PC) of man, chimpanzee and baboon

Fatty acid ratio 18:1/18:2	Man		Chimpanzee		Baboon	
	normal n = 4[4]	type II[1] n = 5	C[2] n = 4	A[3] n = 6	C[2] n = 3	A[3] n = 4
Plasma	0.64	0.75	0.62	0.89	0.68	0.85
α-LP	0.72	0.97	0.74	1.08	0.77	0.91
β-LP	0.60	0.74	0.65	0.85	0.60	0.79
CE	0.34	0.42	0.46	0.63	0.61	0.76
α-CE	0.38	0.47	0.47	0.65	0.53	0.83
β-CE	0.36	0.45	0.45	0.67	0.50	0.61
PC	0.55	0.62	0.48	0.53	0.69	0.89
α-PC	0.55	0.60	0.46	0.53	0.72	0.85
β-PC	0.61	0.60	0.53	0.55	0.62	0.81

1 Type II, hyperbetalipoproteinemia.
2 C = Animals under control diet.
3 A = Animals under atherogenic diet.
4 n = Number of subjects.

and the histological findings in one of the chimpanzees that died from a myocardial infarction showed lesions in the coronary artery which were similar in composition and structure to those found in human atherosclerosis [VASTESAEGER *et al.,* 1973].

The main differences between *baboon and chimpanzee* under atherogenic diet consist of changes in the phospholipid concentration and distribution in the β-lipoproteins and also of the more marked influence of diet on the α-lipoproteins in the baboon. These biochemical differences must result from differences in polypeptide composition of the apoproteins. Both species fulfill many of the desirable criteria for an experimental subject to elucidate the human disease. The here presented description of the natural form of atherosclerosis in nonhuman primates in the wild as well as their experimentally induced atherosclerosis clearly demonstrate their phylogenetic similarity to man.

Acknowledgements

The authors thank Dr. J. MORTELMANS (RUCA-Zoo, Antwerpen) and Dr. M. VASTESAEGER (Centre d'Etude des Maladies des Artères coronaires, Bruxelles) for their collaboration.

References

BLATON, V. and PEETERS, H.: Integrated approach to plasma lipid and lipoprotein analysis; in NELSON Blood lipids and lipoproteins, pp. 269–331 (1971).

BLATON, V.; HOWARD, A. N.; GRESHAM, G. A.; VANDAMME, D., and PEETERS, H.: Lipid changes in the plasma lipoproteins of baboons given an atherogenic diet. I. Changes in the lipids of total plasma and of alpha and beta lipoproteins. Atherosclerosis *11:* 497–507 (1970).

BLATON, V.; VANDAMME, D.; VASTESAEGER, M.; MORTELMANS, J., and PEETERS, H.: Dietary experimental type II hyperlipoproteinemia in chimpanzees (in press).

BLATON, V.; PEETERS, H.; KEERSGIETER, W. DE; DECLERCQ, B.; DEPICKERE, D., and VANDAMME, D.: Differential fatty acid composition of alpha and beta lipoproteins; in PEETERS Protides of the biological fluids, pp. 315–321 (Elsevier, Amsterdam 1966).

GRESHAM, G. and HOWARD, A. N.: Vascular lesions in primates. Ann. N.Y. Acad. Sci. *127:* 694–701 (1965).

GRESHAM, G. A.; HOWARD, A. N.; MCQUEEN, J., and BOWYER, D. E.: Atherosclerosis in primates. Brit. J. exp. Path. *66:* 94–103 (1965).

HOWARD, A. N. and GRESHAM, G. A.: The care and use of baboons in the laboratory; in London Zoological Society, Symposium No. 17 on Recent Developments in Comparative Medicine (Academic Press, New York 1966).

HOWARD, A.N.; BLATON, V.; VANDAMME, D.; LANDSCHOOT, N. VAN, and PEETERS, H.: Lipid changes in the plasma lipoproteins of baboons given an atherogenic diet. III. A comparison between lipid changes in the plasma of the baboon and chimpanzee given atherogenic diets and those in human plasma lipoproteins of type II hyperlipoproteinemia. Atherosclerosis *16:* 257–272 (1972).

HOWARD, A.N.; GRESHAM, G.A.; MALES, C.N.; LINDGREN, F.T., and KATZBERG, A.A.: Atherosclerosis in baboons. Pathological and biochemical studies; in VAGTBORG The baboon in medical research (University of Texas Press, Austin 1967).

LEHNER, N.D.M.; CLARKSON, T.B.; BULLOCK, B.C.; LOFLAND, H.B.; ST. CLAIR, R.W., and PRICHARD, R.W.: Studies on atherosclerosis of some non human primates. Medical primatology 1970. Proc. 2nd Conf. exp. Med. Surg. Primates, New York 1969, 873–885 (Karger, Basel 1971).

LINDSAY, S. and CHAIKOFF, I.L. Atherosclerosis in the baboon. Arch. Pathol. *63:* 460–471 (1957).

MCGILL, H.C.; STRONG, J.P.; HOLMAN, R.L., and WERTHESSEN, N.T.: Arterial lesions in the Kenya baboon. Circulat. Res. *8:* 670–679 (1960).

MANNING, G.W.: Coronary disease in ape. Amer. Heart J. *23:* 719–724 (1942).

MORRIS, M.D. and GEER, W.E.: Familial hyperbetalipoproteinemia (type II hyperlipoproteinemia) in the rhesus monkey; in JONES Atherosclerosis, pp. 192–196 (1970).

MORTELMANS, J.: Tranquilization and anaesthesia; in BEVERIDGE Primates in medicine, vol. 2, pp. 113–122 (Karger, Basel 1969).

PEETERS, H. and BLATON, V.: Comparison of lipid and lipoprotein patterns in primates. Acta zool. path., Antv. *48:* 221–231 (1969).

PEETERS, H. and BLATON, V.: Comparative normal values of human and nonhuman primates; in GOLDSMITH and MOOR-JANKOWSKI Medical primatology 1972, part III, pp. 336–342 (Karger, Basel 1972).

PEETERS, H.; BLATON, V.; DECLERCQ, B.; HOWARD, A.N., and GRESHAM, G.A.: Lipid changes in the plasma lipoproteins of baboons given an atherogenic diet. II. Changes in the phospholipid classes of total plasma and of alpha and beta lipoproteins. Atherosclerosis *12:* 283–290 (1970).

RATCLIFFE, H.L.: Age and environment as factors in the nature and frequency of cardiovascular lesions in mammals and birds in the Philadelphia Zoological Gardens. Ann. N.Y. Acad. Sci. *127:* 715–735 (1965).

STRONG, J.P. and MCGILL, H.C.: Diet and experimental atherosclerosis in baboons. Amer. J. Path. *50:* 669–690 (1967).

VASTESAEGER, M.M. and DELCOURT, R.: Spontaneous atherosclerosis and diet in captive animals. Nutr. Diet. *3:* 174–177 (1961).

VASTESAEGER, M.M.; VERCRUYSSE, J., and MARTIN, J.J.: Pitfalls of experimental atherosclerosis in the chimpanzee; in GOLDSMITH and MOOR-JANKOWSKI Medical primatology 1972, part III, pp. 376–381 (Karger, Basel 1972).

Authors' address: V. BLATON, D. VANDAMME and H. PEETERS, Simon Stevin Institute for Scientific Research, Jerusalemstraat 34, *B-8000 Brugge* (Belgium)

Medical Primatology 1972. Proc. 3rd Conf. exp. Med. Surg. Primates, Lyon 1972, part III, pp. 313–323 (Karger, Basel 1972)

Studies on Progression and Regression of Experimental Atherosclerosis[1]

Techniques and Application to the Rhesus Monkey

R. G. DePalma, E. M. Bellon, W. Insull, jr., W. T. Roth and Ann V. Robinson

Departments of Surgery and Radiology, Case Western Reserve University and University Hospitals of Cleveland, Ohio, and Rockefeller University, New York City, N.Y. (Dr. W. Insull, jr.)

Treatment of atherosclerosis is best evaluated in terms of its effect on arterial lesions. Effective therapy should prevent progression of atherosclerotic lesions and ideally induce their regression. However, the essential documentation of changes in lesions by direct observation *in seriatim* has, until recently, been technically difficult. We here report in detail techniques we have developed for serial observations of individual lesions during manipulation of blood lipids in the rhesus monkey *(Macaca mulatta)*.

To evaluate changes in established atherosclerotic lesions, two requirements should be met. Detection and serial observation of specific individual lesions (plaques) are essential because of variation of response among lesions in a single animal and the variable occurrence of lesions in a group of animals. Documentation of plaque encroachment into the arterial lumen is also essential since encroachment may progress to cause significant interference with blood flow. In previous reports we have applied the principle of direct serial observation of lesions to demonstrate regression of atherosclerosis in dogs [3] and to compare experimental lesions in dogs and monkeys [4].

Materials and Methods

The experimental plan aimed to develop methods for repeated observation and tissue sampling in selected portions of the arterial tree in atherosclerotic rhesus monkeys.

1 Supported by grants in aid from the Heart Association of North East Ohio and the Mead Johnson Research Center.

Male adult rhesus monkeys weighing 8–20 kg were housed in individual cages. Prior to experimental procedures the animals were held for observation for six weeks and tuberculin tested. Atherosclerosis was induced by two methods. Six animals received a ten-percent cholesterol dietary supplement after thyroid ablation as described by Younger *et al.* [13]. Prior to starting the diet, three of these animals had biliary diversion [3] to assess the preventative potential of this procedure. Nine additional animals were fed a Wissler-Roth diet [12] modified by substituting commercial Purina monkey chow containing 5% crude fat for fat-free chow. Feeding of atherogenic diets was continued for 9 to 30 months. Serum cholesterol, triglycerides and plasma lipoproteins were measured by routine clinical methods [4]. These lipids and body weight were determined at regular intervals throughout the study. To avoid injury to the femoral artery, blood for lipid analysis was obtained only from the cephalic vein under phencyclidine sedation. To induce regression of raised lesions after their development had been documented, one animal was returned to normal feeding of Purina monkey chow for 14 months, a second underwent internal biliary diversion followed by normal diet for nine months and a third animal was placed on 4–8 g of cholestyramine daily for 12 months while continuing the Wissler-Roth regimen. After various intervals during progression or regression of lesions, animals were examined to appraise their atherosclerosis by the following techniques.

Procedures to document the presence, progression or regression of atherosclerotic lesions and to provide tissue for comprehensive pathological examination were devised. We attempted to develop procedures that would satisfy the following requirements: (1) the procedure could be repeated, i.e., did not necessitate sacrifice of animal; (2) the procedure did not provoke formation of atherosclerotic lesions nor destroy lesions under observation. No one technique could satisfy all these criteria. However, combinations of the sequential application of surgical exposure of the femoral arteries, angiography, aortotomy, surgical exposure of the superior mesenteric artery and finally comprehensive autopsy examination closely approached these ideals, providing maximum information. The initial procedure was exposure and visual examination of the femoral arteries and concurrent angiography performed under phencyclidine 2 mg/kg sedation and 1% xylocaine local anesthesia. After the exposed femoral artery was observed for lesions, arteriography was performed via the common femoral artery to visualize the coronary arteries, arch vessels, and the entire aorta as far as the level of the third lumbar vertebra. This included the visceral arteries along with the origins of the celiac axis and superior mesenteric artery; in smaller animals the iliac and femoral arteries were also visualized on the 14 × 14 inch film format. A 5F Gensini catheter was inserted into the common femoral artery using the Seldinger technique [9]. With the catheter tip in the ascending aorta, 1.5 ml/kg of 76% Renografin was injected at 800 lb/in^2 pressure. Films were made in the lateral projection using a Schonander rapid film changer at a rate of 3/sec. A 2-mm focal spot tube was employed which was estimated to resolve two line pairs/mm in a water phantom corresponding to a 15-kg animal. All animals were angiographed twice using one femoral artery on each occasion.

Surgical exposure made possible direct observation and photography of the external appearance of arteries, palpation of lesions, and, with aortotomy, inspection of the intimal surface of the infrarenal abdominal aorta. The common femoral artery and short segments of its deep and superficial branches were mobilized by blunt dissection preserving the adventitial connective tissue layer. During mobilization, the artery was kept moist and trauma kept to a minimum. The mobilized artery was observed for yellow lesions visible through its thin wall. Their appearance was recorded by color photography and their size measured directly using ophthalmic calipers. More bulky lesions, when present, could also be detected by palpation as soft bead-like masses. For histological examination, 0.5-cm segments of the superficial or common femoral arteries were excised, preserving the continuity of blood flow to the deep femoral artery from the remaining vessel. The risk of thrombosis was minimized by oversewing the stumps of the severed vessels with 5/0 or 6/0 polypropylene suture. The puncture sites in the common femoral arteries used for introduction of the Gensini catheters were also closed transversely with 6/0 interrupted polypropylene suture, maintaining blood flow to the extremity in all except the smallest animals.

The intraabdominal arteries were exposed under fluothane general anesthesia administered through an endotracheal tube. To assay the practicality of serial direct observations of the intima of the aorta, incisions 2.0–2.5 cm in length were made into the anterior wall of the infrarenal portion of the abdominal aorta. To avoid trauma to surrounding periaortic tissue which might enhance plaque formation or prevent plaque regression, the aorta was not mobilized. A blood-free field for photography was obtained by occluding the aorta with two heavy silk snares placed 3 mm proximal and distal to the aortotomy. The use of arterial clamps was avoided since it has been demonstrated that these may cause lesion-provoking injury [3]. Prior to aortotomy, regional heparinization was attained by injecting 5 ml of normal saline containing 500 units of heparin just above the aortotomy site. Bleeding from the lumbar vessels was controlled without dissection by fine bulldog clamps placed 0.5–1 cm from the orifices of visible lumbar segmental arteries. After completing observation and photography, the aorta was repaired with a continuous suture of 5/0 mersilene. When angiography demonstrated lesions in the celiac axis and superior mesenteric artery, the superior mesenteric artery was exposed at its origin from the aorta by division of small inferior pancreatic veins, and upward retraction of the pancreas and duodenum. Its external surface was inspected, photographed, and palpated.

Tissues obtained from the femoral arteries were examined for the presence of small lesions by stereomicroscopy at 10- to 20-power magnification. Sheets of fresh intima obtained from the aorta, and femoral and coronary arteries at surgery and necropsy were examined for anisotropic cholesterol-rich inclusions by polarizing microscopy at a 400-power magnification [5]. Tissue specimens were fixed for light and electron microscopy. In order to correlate and confirm the findings of repeated angiography, surgical exploration and biopsy, all animals were sacrificed and autopsied immediately after the last in a series of procedures. At autopsy the aorta, major arteries and coronary vessels were inspected, photographed and representative tissue specimens obtained for histological examination.

Results

The animals with thyroid ablation and receiving the ten-percent cholesterol dietary supplement developed hypercholesterolemia ranging from 240 to 1,000 mg/100 ml (control values 80–120 mg/100 ml) which varied from animal to animal, and with time in individual animals. Prior biliary diversion prevented significant hypercholesterolemia and atherosclerosis. The animals receiving the modified Wissler-Roth diet also exhibited variability of response with hypercholesterolemia ranging from 250 to 950 mg/100 ml, and fluctuating with time for individual animals. Plasma triglyceride concentration did not increase; lipoprotein electrophoresis showed increased concentrations of lipoprotein with β-lipoprotein mobility. Grossly visible yellow fatty streak lesions developed in all animals, except those with prior biliary diversion. On stereomicroscopy these had the appearance of typical fatty streak lesions, slightly elevated yellow areas covered with a delicate transparent intima. Examination of thin sheets of fresh intima and lesions by polarizing microscopy showed clusters of micron-sized anisotropic spherical bodies with the formée-cross image characteristic of cholesterol-ester-rich inclusions of atherosclerotic tissues [5]. Three animals with hypercholesterolemia in excess of 600 mg/100 ml consistently developed raised and more intense plaques after 12–14 months of feeding and were used for regression studies. Body weight tended to remain constant in animals developing the more intense raised lesions; animals with less severe atherosclerosis tended to gain 5–30% in weight during atherogenic feeding. Body weight increased 3–25% in three animals on regression regimens. Each of the regression regimens produced significant sustained reduction in serum cholesterol concentration (fig. 1).

Three sites in the arterial tree proved to be convenient for serial surgical

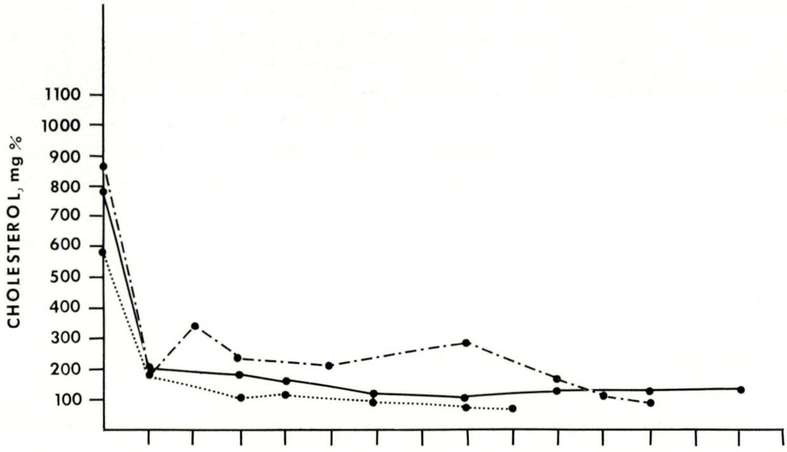

Fig. 1. Course of serum cholesterol concentration in three monkeys during plaque regression. – = Normal feeding; ···· = biliary diversion and normal feeding; –·– = cholestyramine and atherogenic diet.

and/or radiographic observation of raised plaques. These sites also commonly had fatty streaks in the less hypercholesterolemic animals. These were the common femoral arteries at their points of division into the superficial and deep branches, the aorta at the origins of the celiac axis and superior mesenteric arteries, and the posterior wall of the abdominal aorta below the origins of the renal arteries.

Raised plaques in the femoral arteries appeared externally as yellow ovoid nodules 2–4 mm in size, the larger of which also caused a visible bulge in the wall of the vessel. On transillumination and palpation these appeared to encroach on the arterial lumen (fig. 2). Generally the occurrence of lesions was found to be symmetrical for both femoral arteries. Segments of either the common or the superficial femoral arteries could be excised for later comparison with the contralateral vessel after further progression or regression of lesions. These excisions were possible without gangrene of the extremity provided circulation to the deep femoral artery was maintained. Repeated mobilization of the femoral arteries could be done three times and was not technically difficult, but resulted in mild to moderate perivascular fibrosis with thickening of the wall and loss of the normal translucency. Externally visible lesions of the femoral artery regressed in an animal in which serum cholesterol concentration was reduced from a range of 700–850 mg/100 ml to a range of 160–300 mg/100 ml by the addition of 4–8 g of cholestyramine to the atherogenic regimen for 14 months. Histological examination of the lesion site after regression showed a residual lesion of microscopic dimensions.

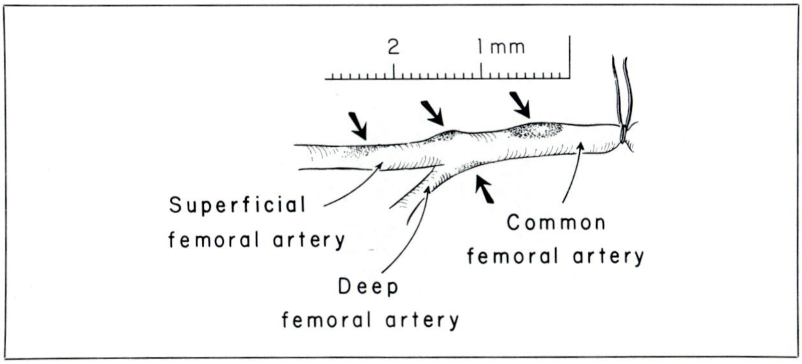

Fig. 2. Appearance of the common femoral artery and its branches with plaques visible at sites indicated by arrows.

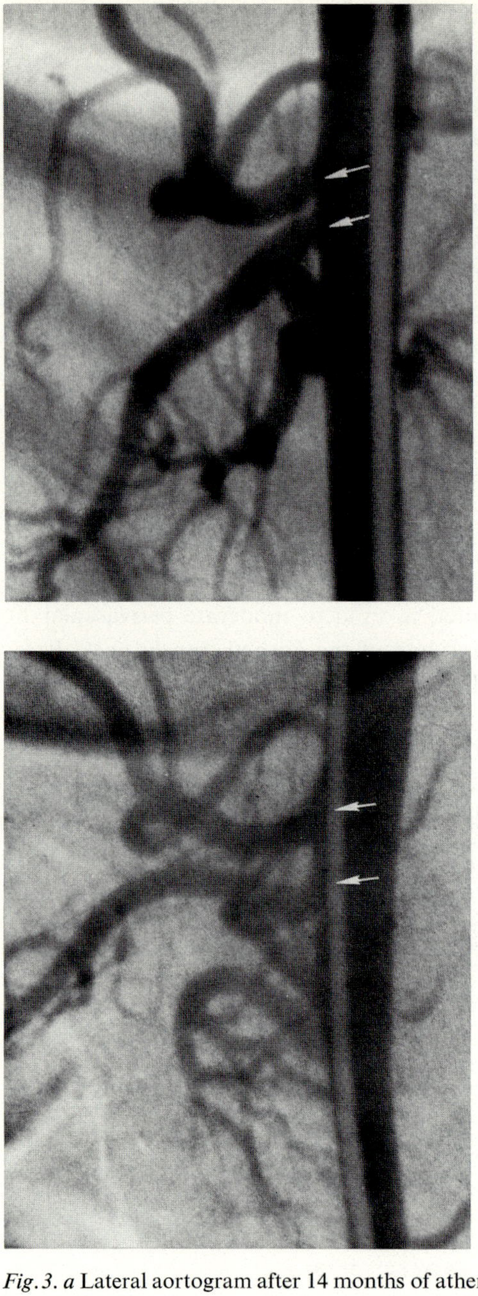

a

b

Fig. 3. a Lateral aortogram after 14 months of atherogenic feeding. Note stenoses due to plaques at origines of celiac axis and superior mesenteric arteries. *b* Lateral aortogram nine months after internal biliary diversion and normal feeding. No stenoses present. From DePalma *et al.* [4].

Plaques at the origins of the superior mesenteric artery and celiac axis appeared as stenoses on lateral aortography. In one animal nine months after reduction of serum cholesterol by internal biliary diversion, regression of these stenoses was demonstrable by serial angiography (fig. 3). In the superior mesenteric artery the lesion before treatment was circumferential when observed at laparotomy (fig. 4). Repeated exposure of this area was not practical because scarring made exposure technically difficult. In an untreated atherosclerotic animal the aortic lesions at the origins of the superior mesenteric artery and celiac axis appeared raised (fig. 5, necropsy). Histologically these lesions appeared as fibrous plaques which were moderately cellular with numerous spindle-shaped cells separated by a loose matrix which in the lesion's periphery contained fat. The retrogressed lesions in this area appeared microscopically much smaller and to have less fat content. To date there is insufficient material to establish the histologic nature of the process of regression.

The technique of aortotomy permitted visualization of plaques elevated 0.5–1 mm on the posterior wall of the aorta (fig. 6). This method of inspection did not interfere with subsequent regression of these plaques in an animal re-

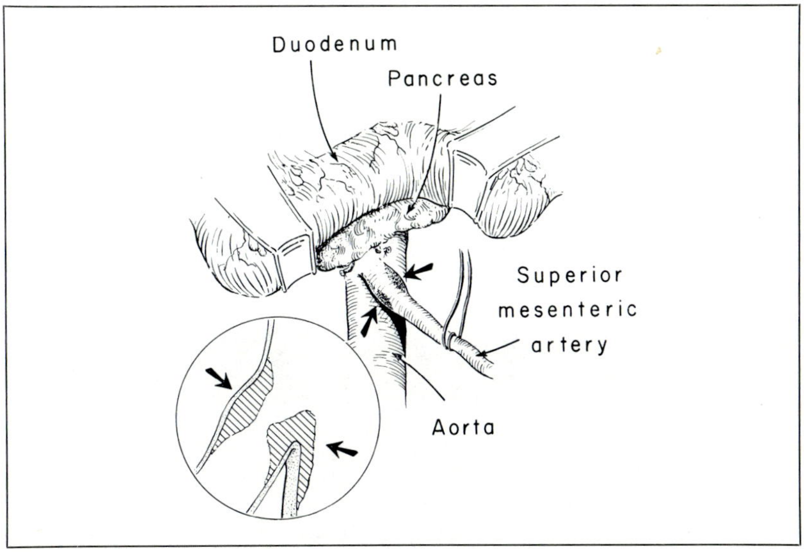

Fig. 4. Appearance of the superior mesenteric artery at surgery with plaque at sites indicated by arrows. Exposure was accomplished by division of small inferior pancreatic veins and upward retraction of pancreas and duodenum.

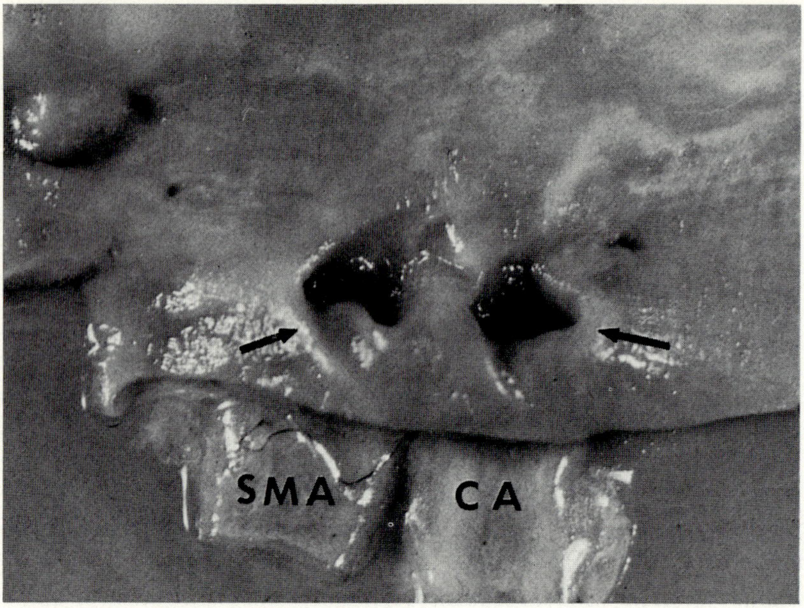

Fig.5. Necropsy appearance of raised plaques in the aorta at the origins of the celiac axis (CA) and superior mesenteric arteries (SMA) in an untreated atherosclerotic animal. The angiographic appearance of stenosis was similar to figure 3a. In the natural state the gross examination showed yellow elevated atheromatous plaques at areas indicated by arrows.

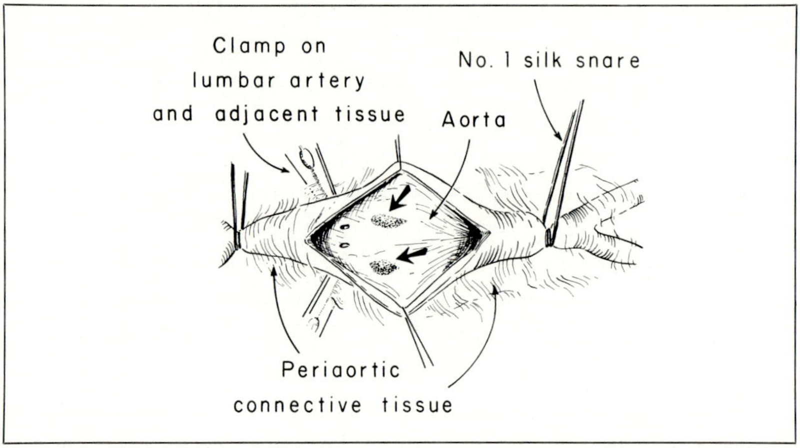

Fig.6. Appearance of aorta with intimal plaques at sites indicated by arrows. Note orifices of lumbar arteries and intact periaortic connective tissue layer.

turned to normal feeding for a 12-month period. Aortotomy was most satisfactory in animals weighing more than 10 kg.

While lateral aortography appeared to be a sensitive method for detecting changes at the origins of the visceral arteries, this technique proved to be relatively insensitive in detecting the minimally-raised lesions on the posterior wall of the abdominal aorta which could be seen at aortotomy or autopsy. Though coronary lesions were not seen by angiography in any animal, all animals demonstrated grossly visible yellow fatty streak lesions in the coronary arteries at autopsy. In untreated hypercholesterolemic animals with cholesterol in excess of 600 mg/100 ml, minimally-raised and more advanced lesions were usually present in the coronary arteries at autopsy.

Discussion

The present investigation has shown that the rhesus monkey is suitable for serial studies of arteries during progression and regression of early and intermediate experimental atherosclerotic lesions. Three different regions which frequently develop lesions are accessible for study; the femoral arteries, abdominal aorta, and origins of the major visceral arteries. Different but complementary methods of assessing lesions can be applied. Angiography and direct gross observation with recording by color photography, palpation and measurement of lesions are simple and nondestructive methods. In selected instances, i.e. in the femoral arteries, serial tissue samples for histologic examination are easily obtained. In these vessels, three specimens on separate occasions, two biopsies and one at final examination should be readily obtainable. Also, these arteries potentially can be used as entry sites for angiography four times at preselected intervals. The complementary techniques of angiography, gross *in vivo* pathology and histology can be correlated here and at other sites such as in the abdominal aorta. This approach enables study of lesion variation in different portions of the arterial system and variation among different animals. Thus, plaque changes occurring during progression and regression of the experimental disease can be described in detail.

There is a great need for an understanding of the development of atherosclerosis in man. While it is the leading cause of death in westernized countries, its pathogenesis is poorly understood and there is disagreement over methods of prevention and treatment. For these reasons, an adequate subhuman primate model for study of atherosclerosis would be most desirable.

The rhesus monkey is a highly attractive candidate for these studies on the basis of our own observations and broad experience reported in the literature. Spontaneous atherosclerosis in this species is rare or absent [2]. Mature animals are of sufficient size and are suitable for repeated surgical and angiographic procedures. Experimental atherosclerosis has been produced in females [10] as well as in males with dietary manipulation and concomitant production of hyperlipidemia. Pathologic characteristics of lesions have been described [10, 11] and complications such as gangrene of an extremity and myocardial infarction have been reported [10]. Armstrong and co-workers [1] describe uncomplicated lesions causing stenosis of coronary arteries after 17 months of feeding producing hypercholesterolemia. Wissler [11] described aortic lesions in response to feeding of saturated fat. It may be possible selectively to breed susceptible animals and evaluate genetic effects [6]. Regression of uncomplicated coronary atheromas by dietary manipulation resulting in lowered serum cholesterol concentration has recently been reported by Armstrong and co-workers [1].

The disadvantages of the rhesus monkey relate mainly to the length of time required to produce advanced lesions, difficulty in handling because of its aggressive nature and the procurement of an adequate number of animals for study [8].

The techniques described in the present report make possible a number of additional studies such as the investigation of other areas of clinical interest in the arterial tree including coronary arteries, extracranial cerebral arteries and distal peripheral arteries. Direct serial lesion observation is also applicable to other atherosclerotic primates in whom lesion distribution and type may differ from that occurring in rhesus. The clinical sensitivity of angiographic observations for minimal atherosclerotic lesions will be enhanced by exact comparison with direct morphologic findings. Thus we may be able to define a minimally detectable lesion in order to observe the earliest clinical stages of the disease. Stages in the development and induced regression (treatment) of arterial lesions can be studied in the same individual in more detail. Serial samples of tissues can be obtained for sophisticated techniques of morphology, i.e., histochemistry, electron microscopy and biochemical analysis which can be correlated with the stage of the lesion and its physiologic effects on blood flow. The relationships between blood flow, size, consistency, and composition of lesions may be more precisely defined by combining direct observation with measurement of luminal diameter and blood flow using ultrasonic techniques now available [7]. These future studies promise a greater understanding of atherosclerosis.

Acknowledgements

The authors wish to thank Dr. S. KOLETSKY for his assistance in interpreting the pathologic material.

References

1 ARMSTRONG, M.L.; WARNER, E.D., and CONNOR, W.E.: Regression of coronary atheromatosis in rhesus monkeys. Circulat. Res. *27:* 59–67 (1970).

2 COX, G.E.; TAYLOR, C.B.; COX, L.G., and COUNTS, M.A.: Atherosclerosis in rhesus monkeys. I. Hypercholesterolemia induced by dietary fat and cholesterol. Arch. Path. *66:* 32–52 (1958).

3 DEPALMA, R.G.; HUBAY, C.A.; INSULL, W., jr.; ROBINSON, A.V., and HARTMAN, P.H.: Progression and regression of experimental atherosclerosis. Surg. Gynec. Obstet. *131:* 633–647 (1970).

4 DEPALMA, R.G.; INSULL, W., jr.; BELLON, E.M.; ROTH, T.W., and ROBINSON, A.V.: Animal models for the study of progression and regression of atherosclerosis. Surgery *72:* 268–278 (1972).

5 LANG, P.D. and INSULL, W., jr.: Lipid droplets in atherosclerotic fatty streaks of human aorta. J. clin. Invest. *49:* 1479–1488 (1970).

6 MORRIS, M.D. and GREER, W.E.: Familial hyper Beta-lipoproteinemia (type II hyperlipoproteinemia) in the rhesus monkey; in JONES Atherosclerosis. Proc. 2nd Int. Symp., pp. 192–196 (Springer, New York 1970).

7 MOZERSKY, D.J.; HOKANSON, E.; BAKER, D.W.; SUMNER, D.S., and STRANDNESS, D.E.: Ultrasonic arteriography. Arch. Surg. *103:* 663–667 (1971).

8 ROTH, W.T.: The over kill. Oryx *9:* 354–356 (1968).

9 SELDINGER, S.I.: Catheter replacement of needle in percutaneous arteriography. A new technique. Acta radiol. *39:* 368–376 (1953).

10 TAYLOR, C.B.; MANALO-ESTRELLA, P., and COX, G.E.: Atherosclerosis in rhesus monkeys. Arch. Path. *76:* 239–249 (1963).

11 WISSLER, R.W.: Recent progress in studies of experimental primate atherosclerosis; in MIRAS, HOWARD and PAOLETTI Progress in biochemical pharmacology. Recent advances in atherosclerosis, vol. 4, pp. 378–392 (Karger, New York 1968).

12 WISSLER, R.W.; VESSELINOVITCH, D.; HUGHES, R., and ROTH, W.T.: Atherosclerosis and blood lipids in rhesus monkeys confined in widely varying spaces. Fed. Proc. *28:* 447 (1969).

13 YOUNGER, R.K.; SCOTT, H.W., jr.; BUTTS, W.H., and STEPHENSON, S.E., jr.: Rapid production of experimental hypercholesterolemia and atherosclerosis in the rhesus monkey. Comparison of five dietary regimens. J. surg. Res. *9:* 263–271 (1969).

Authors' addresses: Dr. RALPH G. DEPALMA, Dr. ERROL M. BELLON, Dr. WILLIAM INSULL, jr., Dr. W. TED ROTH and ANN V. ROBINSON, Department of Surgery and Radiology, Case Western Reserve University, *Cleveland, OH 44106* and Rockefeller University, *New York City, NY* (USA)

Medical Primatology 1972. Proc. 3rd Conf. exp. Med. Surg. Primates, Lyon 1972, part III, pp. 324–335 (Karger, Basel 1972)

Sterol Metabolism in the Chimpanzee[1]

G. V. MANN[2]

Vanderbilt University School of Medicine, Nutrition Division, Nashville, Tenn.

Introduction

The striking differences of sterol metabolism among species are a deterrent to useful experimental studies [KRITCHEVSKY, 1969]. Many erroneous dogma have arisen from evidence derived from irrelevant experimental models [MANN, 1966]. The Cebidae were first shown to be susceptible to atherosclerosis in 1952 [MANN *et al.*, 1952]. Subsequently xanthomatosis was produced in rhesus by dietary overloading with cholesterol [MANN and ANDRUS, 1956]. Since then many other primate species have been studied and found useful although no one has regularly produced atherosclerotic coronary occlusions with myocardial infarction in any species [LOFLAND *et al.*, 1967].

In 1958 we undertook a comparative study of cebus, rhesus and the chimpanzee, using dietary methods developed in the earlier work. The objects were to find a more human-like model of coronary disease, to evaluate the role of diet in that model and to examine the dynamics of sterol metabolism with radioisotopic methods. The present report will describe our experience with chimpanzees which were studied over a seven- to ten-year period while maintained on a purified diet. These studies of sterol dynamics are based on the premise that the metabolic lesion in human hypercholesteremia is one of catabolism. We set out to measure the rates of cholesterol catabolism through several metabolic channels, in animals exposed to various dietary and drug treatments.

1 Supported by USPHS HEW HE03926.

2 Career Investigator 4-K6-HE-8288-11.

Chimpanzees were found to be exceptionally sensitive to dietary cholesterol – ranking with the rabbit. The physiological channels of sterol clearance in the chimpanzee were similar to those of human beings. The effects on clearance of hypocholesteremic drugs were quite variable. The chimpanzee, despite cumbersome problems of availability and handling, is a useful experimental primate for study of atherogenesis.

Methods

The chimpanzees, *Pan troglodytes,* were obtained as infants from dealers. They were transferred from a variety of human foods to the experimental, purified diet described in table I as CO. This diet is nutritionally complete and has been used as the exclusive food for Cebidae for ten years. Cebidae females have matured, conceived, delivered and nursed repeatedly on this diet alone [MANN, 1968].

The chimpanzees were caged indoors in 4 × 6 × 12 feet enclosures with sleeping shelves. They were screened from human contacts after repeated difficulty with infections.

On some occasions, as the animals reached puberty, it was necessary to sedate them for handling with phencyclidine HCl (Sernylan, Parke-Davis). This is an efficient and innocuous drug for short-term sedation.

For urine collections the animals were transferred to small collection cages overnight.

Table I. Experimental diets[1] (composition as percent)

Ingredient/Diet	CO	CO Cy	CO5	CO7Cy	CO14Cy	SBO	SBO5
Casein (purified)	20	20	20	20	20	–	–
Soy protein[2]	–	–	–	–	–	20	20
Sucrose	61	60	60	60	60	61	60
Lard	15	15	15	15	15	15	15
Isoniazide[3]	0.05	0.05	0.05	0.05	0.05	0.05	0.05
Salt mix[4]	4	4	4	4	4	4	4
Vitamin mix[5]	2	2	2	2	2	2	2
Cholesterol[6]	0	0	0.05	0.07	0.14	0	0.05
L-Cystine	0	0.4	0	0.4	0.4	0	0

1 The diets were fed once daily in amounts that were consumed in 30 min, water *ad libitum.*

2 Cl Assay Protein, Dracutt Corp., Cincinnati supplies 0.6% cystine, 1.0% methionine.

3 Added as prophylaxis for tuberculosis.

4 HEGSTED *et al.:* J. biol. Chem. *138:* 459 (1941).

5 Nutrit. Biochem. Corp., Cleveland. Prepared with cholecalciferol.

6 Armour Co. Added to diet by dissolving in lard with heat.

Carbon dioxide was collected by placing the animal in a modified autoclave tank fitted with gas valves and an air pump so that vented air could be bubbled through phenethylamine and counted for radioactivity [WALLER, 1961]. Blood was easily drawn from a forearm vein. Injections, dosings and weighings were done without sedation. Nevertheless, after the age of six to eight years these animals became difficult and unpredictable.

The radiocholesterol was $^{14}C_1$ obtained commercially and purified by chromatography on a Florosil column [CARROLL, 1961]. For injection it was dissolved in absolute ethanol, a trace of Tween 20 was added and the solution was diluted with water to give a final ethanol concentration of 15%. Such a solution remains quite clear. An i.v. dose of 1 μCi/kg body weight was used. This is sufficient for two to four months of clearance study.

Blood cholesterol was measured with the Auto Analyzer [MANN, 1961]. The specific activity of plasma cholesterol was measured with the Schoenheimer-Sperry precipitation with digitonin [SCHOENHEIMER and SPERRY, 1954]. The digitonide was dissolved in methanol and one aliquot was used for cholesterol determination, another for counting with Bray's solution.

Sebum was collected from sedated animals by applying a teflon cup containing a cigarette paper to the ether-washed forehead of animals for one to three hours [STRAUSS and POCHI, 1961]. The paper was extracted with hexane and counted.

Respiratory excretion of CO_2 was measured by counting an aliquot of the phenethylamine absorber in the tank effluent. An aliquot of urine was counted in Bray's solution.

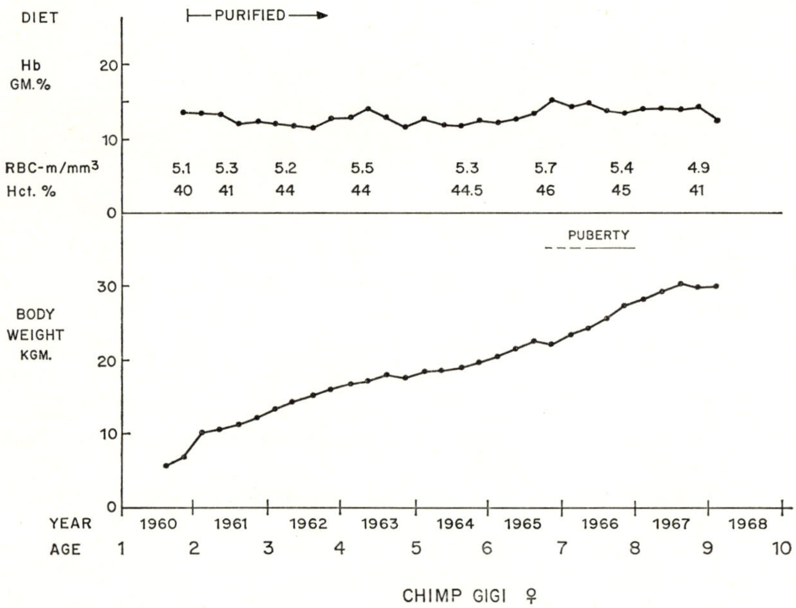

Fig. 1. Growth and blood values of a female chimpanzee, G.

Feces were collected and weighed. A 9:1 homogenate was made in ethanol with a Waring blender. Aliquots of this were taken for total nitrogen by micro-Kjeldahl and total counts in Bray's solution with quench correction. In order to avoid timed collections of feces and urine the radioactivity was expressed as counts/g N_2 in feces and counts/g creatinine in urine.

Cholesterol catabolism can be usefully quantitated as a rate of clearance of plasma cholesterol. If the level and specific activity of plasma cholesterol is known, this can be considered a metabolic pool from which cholesterol or its metabolic products are transferred to feces, urine, respiratory, CO_2, sebum and also to more secluded pools, say central nervous system or even blood vessels. Although these secluded pools cannot be measured by the noninvasive methods used here they can be estimated by a calculation balancing the biological decay of the plasma pool against the sum of the measured channels. The clearance through any particular excretory channel becomes, e.g.:

$$Cl_{total} = \frac{\text{cpm/unit time-all channels}}{\text{cpm/mg plasma cholesterol}};$$

and, e.g.:

$$Cl_{fecal} = \frac{\text{cpm/24-hour feces}}{\text{cpm/mg plasma cholesterol}}.$$

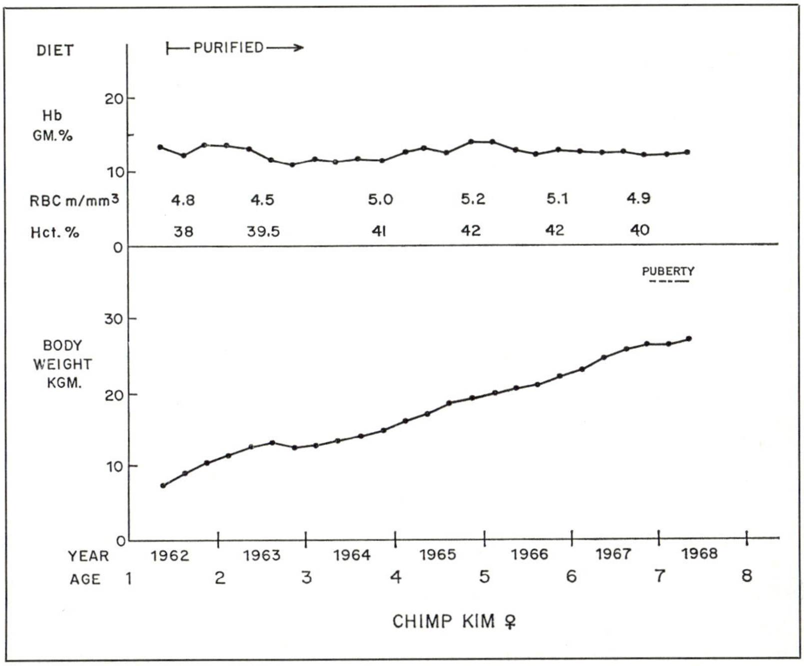

Fig. 2. Growth and blood values of a female chimpanzee, K.

This clearance reflects the milligrams of plasma cholesterol which were necessary to supply the amount of radioactivity recovered in a unit of time (or its metabolic equivalent). The method assumes that only a small amount of the steroid ring carrying the label is degraded for excretion and this is measured in the respiratory CO_2. The metabolic products of radiocholesterol found in feces and sebum are assumed to be soluble in fat solvents.

After some stormy transitional weeks these animals took the purified diet (CO) well and thrived on it. Their growth rates are shown in figures 1–3. All the observations suggest that this is a nutritionally complete diet. Toward the end of the observation the animals displayed normal pubescent changes. The blood chemistries remained within the limits described for this species [HODSON *et al.*, 1968].

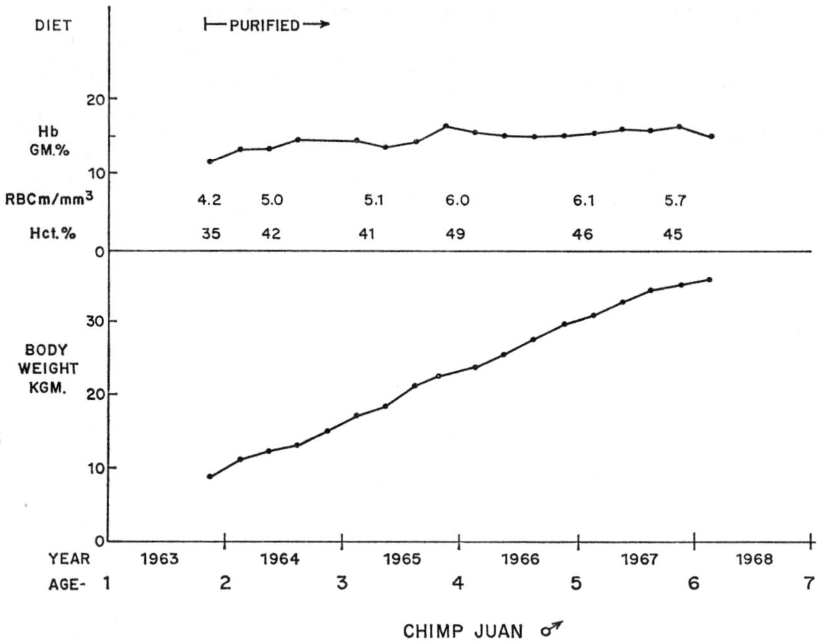

Fig. 3. Growth and blood values of a male chimpanzee, J.

Results

The chimpanzees studied were uniformly sensitive to dietary cholesterol (fig. 4). When cholesterol was added to the diet they promptly became hyper-cholesteremic. By reducing the level of dietary cholesterol it was shown that 150 mg/day would approximately double the level of serum cholesterol found in animals fed cholesterol-free diets (table II).

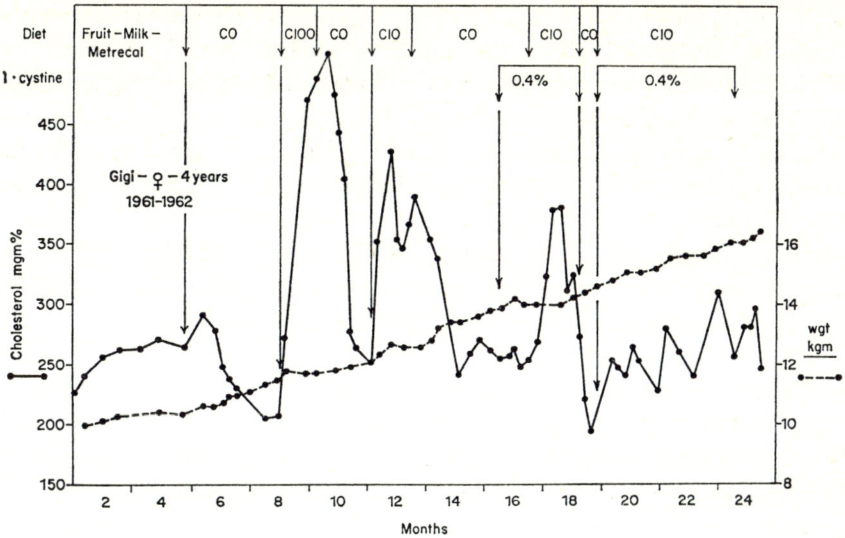

Fig. 4. Cholesteremic responses of chimp G. to several dietary mixtures. (Refer to table I). L-Cystine was added from the 16th to 24th months as indicated with one short interruption.

Table II. Comparison of species for sensitivity to dietary cholesterol (amount of dietary cholesterol necessary to increase serum level 2–3 ×)

Species	Average weight	Energy exchange	Dietary cholesterol	
	kg	kcal/kg/day	mg/day	mg/kcal/kg/day
Rabbit[1]	4	100	240	2.4
Chimpanzee[2]	40	40	150	3.7
Cebus	2	80	400	5.0
Rhesus[2]	5	90	500	5.5
Dog[3]	8	75	1,000	13
Human[4]	70	40	700	18

1 Rabbits show great individual variation [see e.g. FILLIOS and MANN: Circulat. Res. *4:* 406 (1956)].
2 Both chimpanzees and rhesus were immature.
3 Adult dogs, caged.
4 The human normal level is assumed to be 120 mg% as found in the Masai [see e.g. MANN *et al.:* J. Atheroscler. Res. *4:* 289 (1964)].

The human intake is US average, but the exposure to achieve doubling is 20–30 years.

The i.v. injection of a priming dose of 1 μCi of ring labelled radiocholesterol with subsequent determination of the specific activity (SA) of the serum cholesterol allows the construction of a biological decay curve (fig. 5 and 6). The decline in SA of serum cholesterol following injection can be resolved into two or more exponential components which are presumed to reflect the existence of hypothetical body pools with different accessibilities and turnover rates [GOODMAN and NOBLE, 1968; WHYTE *et al.*, 1969]. The initial phase of decline, reflecting mixing in pool A, can be used to measure pool size by extrapolation to time zero. The second phase of the decline of SA, corrected for A, reflects the size and turnover of a more secluded pool B.

The dimensions of certain parameters of these pools in relation to diet and serum level of cholesterol are shown in table III. There are several practical difficulties with this approach which is more titillating to computer handlers than to biochemists. The procedure requires assumptions of steady state and thus several weeks and multiple measurements of SA are necessary. The derived parameters are very sensitive to measurement errors depending as they do on the slopes of the SA with time. In practice the parameters are not very reproducible and are not useful indices of sterol dynamics.

Table III shows that low cystine diets made with soy protein tend to produce hypercholesteremia. Cholesterol added to casein diets, which are more sufficient in sulfur amino acids, also increases cholesteremia. The most useful dietary combination for chimpanzees was diet CO14Cy which subjects the

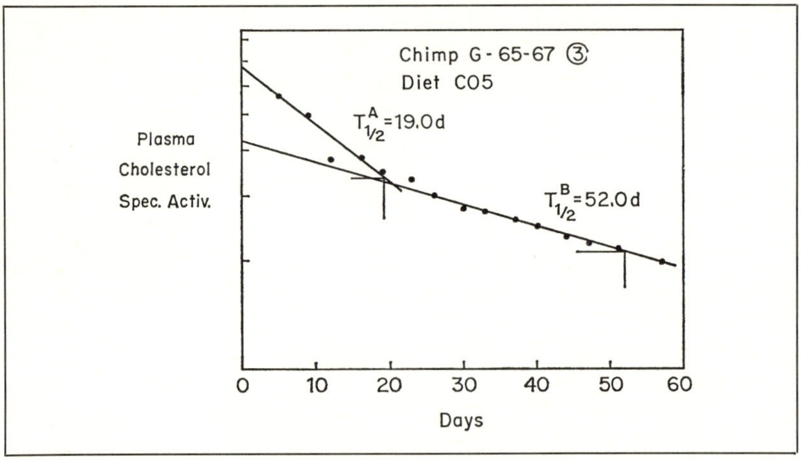

Fig. 5. The cholesterol pool in chimp G. receiving a diet without added cystine.

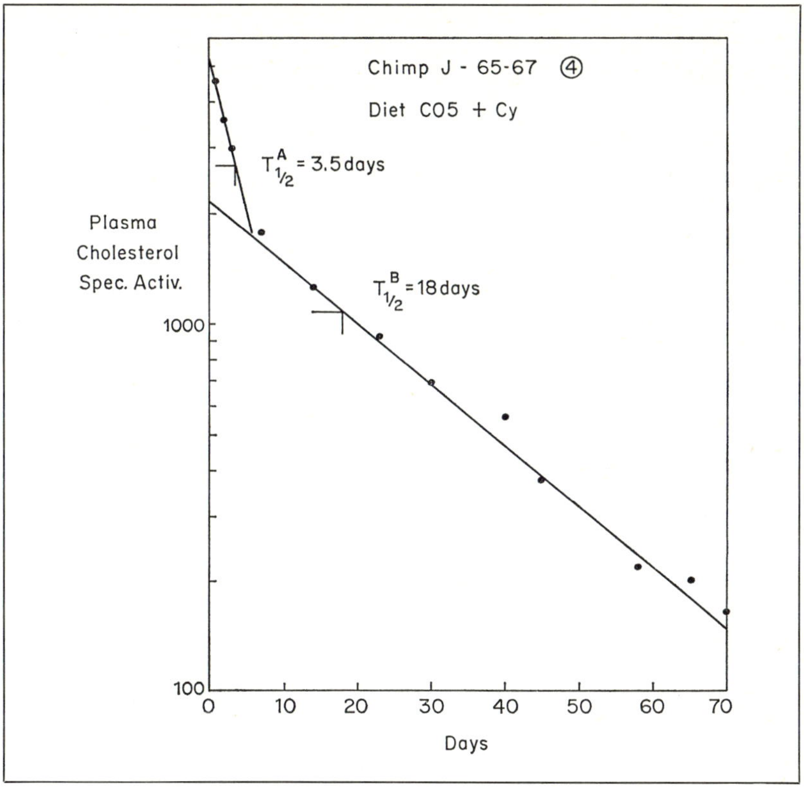

Fig. 6. Cholesterol pool kinetics in chimp J. receiving a diet with added L-cystine.

animal to a small sterol load but with added cystine keeps the cholesteremia at about double the level found on cholesterol-free diets. It is of passing interest that cholesterol level in serum and the size of pool A were reciprocally related.

Seeking a more sensitive index of sterol dynamics the clearance method was developed. This is based upon measurement of the amount of plasma cholesterol radioactivity which appears in the several physiological channels over a measured time – or its physiological equivalent. The main channels are compared in table IV for chimpanzees and man. It is apparent that the fecal channel is the main one in both species. A balance sheet which assumes a steady state suggests that the decline of activity in pool B is not entirely accounted for by the activity appearing in a unit time in the sum of all the four

Table III. Effect of diet on sterol dynamics in chimpanzees

Diet	TC mg %	Pool A mg/kg body weight	$T^1/_2$ B days
CoCy	182	2.49	58.0
CO	190	–	–
CO5	327	0.70	42.0
CO7Cy	268	1.40	71.2
Co14Cy	266	0.419	78.0
SBO	319	1.60	32.3
SBO5	336	0.78	25.2

Table IV. Comparison of rates of channel clearance of sterols in chimpanzees and man. (Adult man on an average USA diet. Chimpanzee on diet CO5) (as % of total in four channels)

Channel	Man	Chimpanzee		
		♀G	♀K	♂J
Feces	75	77	64	64
Sebum[1]	18	18	33	34
Urine	7	4	3	2
Resp. CO_2[2]	0.2	0.7	0.2	0.4

1 The sebum channel was estimated by collecting on the forehead, estimating the total surface area from height and weight and assuming the seborrheic areas are ⅓ of the total surface area.

2 The CO_2 was collected with the chimpanzees in a sedated condition. Preliminary evidence suggests that the rate of radio-CO_2 excretion is influenced by physical activity and metabolic rate.

channels measured. The unmeasured channel is probably deposition in more secluded pools, e.g. brain and vascular lesions. Nevertheless the influence of treatments for hypercholesteremia can be evaluated directly by measuring their effects on the excretion in four channels.

The effects on clearance of several drugs which are known to influence serum cholesterol in man are compared in table V. It appears that thyroid hormone, while significantly lowering the serum cholesterol, does not increase excretion of cholesterol through the main excretory channel, nor does estrogen. They are presumed to increase tissue deposition. Cholestyramine, as expected, increased the intestinal excretion, as did dietary corn oil.

Table V. Effect of drug treatments on cholesteremia and fecal sterol clearance in chimpanzees (diet CO14Cy)

Treatment	Trials	Plasma cholesterol	Sterol clearance		
			sebum mg/day	CO_2 mg/day	fecal sterol clearance mg/g N ± SEM
None	9	364	280	6	837 ± 33
Cholestyramine[1] (14 days)	9	304	202	4	1,347 ± 33 *
Thyroid hormone[2] (6 days)	9	329	356	12	761 ± 18
Estrogens[3] (14 days)	3	274	299	11	765 ± 23
Corn oil[4] (14 days)	6	302	312	19	1,107 ± 30 **

* $t = 5.86$ $p < 0.001$ cholestyramine vs. no R_x.
** $t = 4.29$ $p < 0.001$ corn oil vs. no R_x.
$t = 2.47$ $p < 0.05$ corn oil vs. cholestyramine.

1 Cholestyramine (Merck). A basic anionic exchange resin which binds bile anions. Fed to supply 10–15 g/animal/day.
2 Cytomel (Smith, Kline and French Lab.). Triiodo-thyronine, 25–150 mg/kg body weight/day for three trials of six days each.
3 Premarin (Ayerst). A blend of equine pregnancy estrogens, fed to supply 0.2–0.4 mg/animal/day for 14 days.
4 Diet CO14Cy changed to contain 15% corn oil (Mazola) in place of 15% lard for 14 days.

Discussion

The chimpanzee is the most sensitive to dietary cholesterol of any primate studied. This sample of three is too small to make generalizations about genetic variability although these three individuals behaved quite alike. The purified diet is the logical and simple way to manage such trials. All evidence indicates this is a complete diet for the animals. There is no evidence that isoniazide disturbs these animals metabolically.

The clearance technique offers a feasible method for evaluating the mechanism of hypercholesteremia and the mechanism of action of sterol active drugs. The fecal channel is the predominant route of sterol excretion. Sebum may be an underrated channel and deserves more study. The hypocholesteremic effects of thyroid hormone and estrogens seem not attributable to increased excretion. They may cause increased deposition in tissues. This may account for the noxious effects of treatment encountered with either thyroid hormone or conjugated estrogens in human subjects [Coronary Drug Project, 1972].

The vessels of these chimpanzees were not examined. ANDRUS *et al.* [1968] have described atheromatous lesions in adult chimpanzees which were treated with dietary regimens to produce hypercholesteremia during the last year of their lives. Hypercholesteremia was readily produced and correlated well with vascular lesions. The lesions were quite like those seen in all the other primates including the human. The chimpanzee may be the most prone of all the primates to atherosclerosis.

References

ANDRUS, S.B.; PORTMAN, O.W., and RIOPELLE, A.J.: Comparative studies of spontaneous and experimental atherosclerosis in primates. II. Lesions in chimpanzees including myocardial infarction and cerebral aneurysms; in PAOLETTI Progr. Biochem. Pharmacol., vol. 4, p. 393 (Karger, Basel 1968).

CARROLL, K.K.: Separation of lipid classes by chromatography on Florosil. J. Lipid. Res. *2:* 135 (1961).

Coronary Drug Project Research Group: Findings leading to further modifications of its protocol with respect to dextrothyroxine. J. amer. med. Ass. *220:* 996 (1972).

GOODMAN, D.S. and NOBLE, R.P.: Turnover of plasma cholesterol in man. J. clin. Invest. *47:* 231 (1968).

HODSON, H.H., jr.; WISECUP, W.G.; FAULKNER, M.F., and FELTS, P.E.: Baseline blood values of the chimpanzee. II. The relationship of age and sex and serum chemistry values. Folia primat. *8:* 77 (1968).

KRITCHEVSKY, D.: Experimental atherosclerosis in primates and other species. Ann. N.Y. Acad. Sci. *162:* 80 (1969).

LOFLAND, H.B.; ST. CLAIR, R.W.; MACNINTCH, J.E., and PRICHARD, R.W.: Atherosclerosis in New World primates. Arch. Path. *83:* 211 (1967).

MANN, G.V.: A method for measurement of cholesterol in blood serum. Clin. Chem. *7:* 275 (1961).

MANN, G.V.: Cystine deficiency and cholesterol metabolism in primates. Circulat. Res. *18:* 205 (1966).

MANN, G.V.: Blood changes in experimental primates fed purified diets. Pyridoxine and riboflavin deficiency. Vitam. Hormones *26:* 465 (1968).

MANN, G.V. and ANDRUS, S.B.: Xanthomatosis and atherosclerosis produced by diet in adult rhesus monkeys. J. Lab. exp. Med. *48:* 533 (1956).

MANN, G.V.; ANDRUS, S.B.; MCNALLY, A., and STARE, F.J.: Experimental atherosclerosis in cebus monkeys. J. exp. Med. *98:* 195 (1952).

SCHOENHEIMER, R. and SPERRY, W.M.: A micromethod for the determination of free and combined cholesterol. J. biol. Chem. *106:* 745 (1954).

STRAUSS, J.S. and POCHI, P.E.: The quantitative gravimetric determination of sebum production. J. invest. Derm. *36:* 293 (1961).
WALLER, F.H.: Phenethylamine for CO_2 absorption. Analyt. Biochem. *2:* 508 (1961).
WHYTE, H.M.; NESTEL, P.J., and GOODMAN, D.S.: Cholesterol distribution and turnover in obesity in man. Israel J. med. Sci. *5:* 644 (1969).

Author's address: GEORGE V. MANN, Vanderbilt University School of Medicine, Nutrition Division, *Nashville, TN* (USA)

Medical Primatology 1972. Proc. 3rd Conf. exp. Med. Surg. Primates, Lyon 1972, part III, pp. 336–342 (Karger, Basel 1972)

Comparative Lipid Values of Human and Nonhuman Primates[1]

H. PEETERS and V. BLATON

Simon Stevin Institute for Scientific Research, Brugge

Introduction

Nonhuman primates are phylogenetically, anatomically, physiologically and biochemically closely related to man. Although it is widely believed that biochemical and histological experimentation in atherosclerosis using nonhuman primates is highly relevant to human metabolism, our knowledge concerning the normal biochemistry of simian tissues and body fluids is still insufficient and more comparative work is needed.

A compendium of normal blood values for chimpanzees, baboons and marmosets was presented in the form of quantitative and descriptive tables for convenience in biochemical evaluation studies [BURNS *et al.*, 1967]. The protein and protein-bound carbohydrates in four species of nonhuman primates were considered by SU-CHEN and YU-TEH [1968]. In his review article on vascular lesions in primate animals, GRESHAM and HOWARD [1965] mentioned that these bear a general anatomical resemblance to those of man. Lipid metabolism of some resembles that of man [KRITCHEVSKY *et al.*, 1962; BLATON and PEETERS, in press] and, most important of all, many simians develop arterial lesions in the wild as well as in captivity when fed laboratory diet. Furthermore, fatty streaks induced by laboratory regimen are similar in structure and distribution to those found in *Homo sapiens*.

It is, however, of importance to establish differences as well as similarities between man and simians if results of investigations are to be properly interpreted. Much is still to be learned about the normal physiology and

1 Supported by grants from the NFWGO (Belgium), grant No. 1153, Franqui Foundation and the RUCA-Zoo.

anatomy of simians before pathological changes can be interpreted and correlated with those in man. As discussed elsewhere [PEETERS and BLATON, 1969] the relationship between lipids and fatty acids in primates is variable and needs detailed investigation.

This study is based on an integrated procedure of plasma lipid and lipoprotein analysis [BLATON and PEETERS, 1971] and is intended to compare normal values and to establish whether it is valid to extrapolate baboon and chimpanzee data to those of man.

Materials and Methods

The biochemical methods for lipoprotein, lipid and fatty acid analysis have been described earlier [PEETERS *et al.*, 1970; BLATON *et al.*, 1970]. The basic caloric component of the diet used is a freshly prepared monkey cake, supplemented with minerals and vitamins. In addition to the monkey cake, large quantities of fruit and 0.5 l of milk are being fed daily. The total intake of the control diet amounted to 10 g/kg body weight a day, which corresponds with 1.750 kcal/day. The wet control diet has a protein content of 17 g%. The lipid content of 2 g% represents 0.15% cholesterol. The chief fatty acids are palmitic (22%), oleic (31%) and linoleic (30%). Fasting blood is taken from the femoral artery of animals tranquilized with Sernylan (Parke, Davis).

The normal human values are the mean value from a group of four white males between 20 and 25 years of age. The chimpanzee belong to the species *Pan troglodytes schweinfurthii*, the baboons are *Papio cynocephalus*.

Results and Discussion

On agar electrophoresis the protein pattern of nonhuman primates is different from that of man (fig. 1), as was also shown by SU-CHEN and YU-TEH [1968] on cellulose acetate. The mobility and the percentage composition of the globulin fractions are different. A comparative study of the lipoproteins separated and interpreted according to FREDRICKSON shows a progressive decrease from baboon over the chimpanzee to man in the α/β ratio. All nonhuman primates tested by us have had more α-lipoproteins than man. Fasting blood from baboons and chimpanzees shows no appreciable very low density lipoproteins (VLDL) or prae-β-lipoproteins (fig. 2). It is to note that in our experience these low prae-β-levels are never seriously increased under atherogenic diet and neither are the triglycerides. The average plasma lipid concentration is summarized in table I and compared to human values. The chimpanzee shows total lipid values higher than man with a high cho-

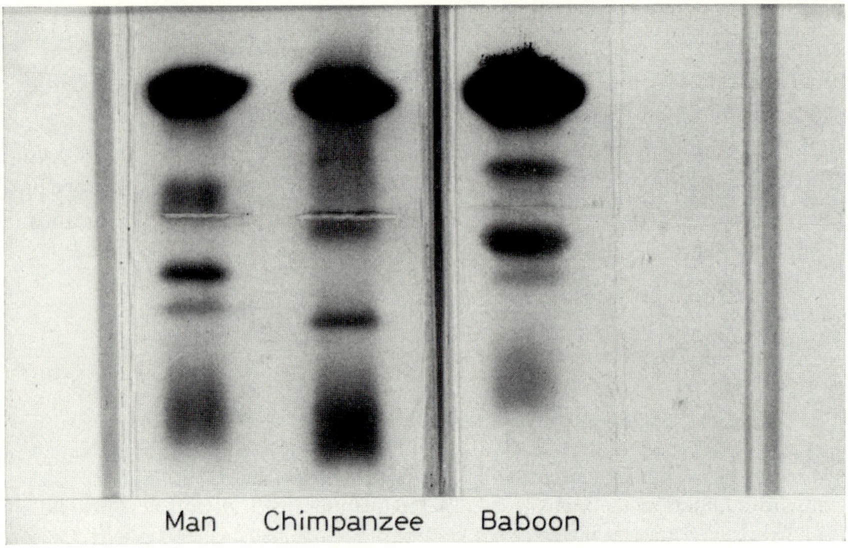

Fig. 1. Proteinogram on agar of plasma from man, chimpanzee and baboon.

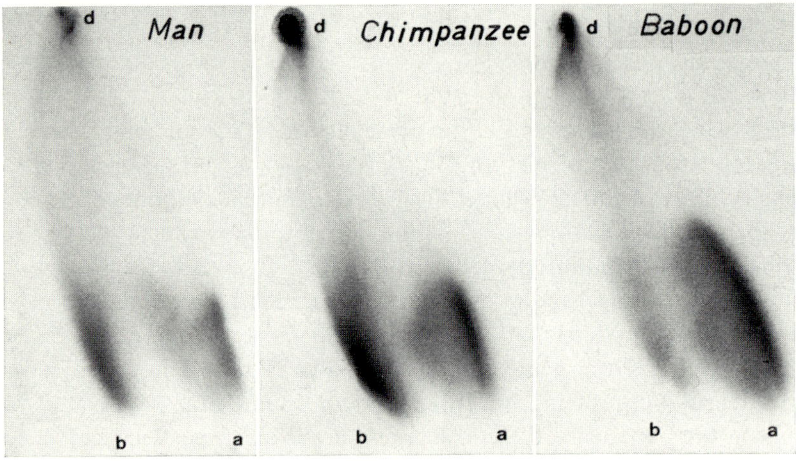

Fig. 2. Electrochromatographic lipoprotein pattern in man, chimpanzee and baboon. a = α-Lipoproteins (HDL); b = β-lipoproteins (LDL); d = startpoint, excess of dye and chylomicrons.

Table I. Lipid distribution in normal human and nonhuman primates

Subject	T.chol.	CE	F.chol.	PL	TG	C/PL	% est.chol.
Man[1]							
Plasma	151 ± 5	170 ± 9	50 ± 4	163 ± 7	31 ± 4	0.92	67
α-LP	43 ± 4	51 ± 5	12 ± 1	76 ± 3	13 ± 2	0.55	71
β-LP	108 ± 2	119 ± 4	37 ± 3	87 ± 6	18 ± 3	1.25	66
Chimpanzee[2]							
Plasma	259 ± 21	326 ± 38	65 ± 9	295 ± 18	60 ± 10	0.88	75
α-LP	88 ± 6	104 ± 14	26 ± 3	166 ± 10	19 ± 2	0.53	70
β-LP	171 ± 16	222 ± 24	39 ± 7	129 ± 10	41 ± 9	1.33	77
Baboon[2]							
Plasma	117 ± 7	162 ± 5	21 ± 4	122 ± 14	38	0.97	83
α-LP	60 ± 12	81 ± 16	12 ± 2	82 ± 19	13	0.76	81
β-LP	57 ± 5	80 ± 11	9 ± 2	40 ± 6	25	1.43	84

T.chol. = total cholesterol; CE = cholesterol ester; F.chol. = free cholesterol; PL = phospholipids; TG = triglycerides; % est.chol. = % esterified cholesterol; LP = lipoproteins.

1 Group of four normal white males between 20 and 25 years of age.
2 Average value of four individuals.

Table II. Phospholipid distribution (%) in normal human and nonhuman primates

Subject	Lyso-PC	Sph.	PC	PEt
Man[1]				
Plasma	6.8 ± 0.9	20.6 ± 1.0	68.2 ± 1.1	4.4 ± 0.7
α-LP	9.1 ± 0.8	19.1 ± 2.7	66.5 ± 0.5	5.4 ± 1.5
β-LP	7.2 ± 0.5	19.3 ± 2.6	68.6 ± 2.8	4.8 ± 0.8
Chimpanzee[2]				
Plasma	7.1	17.5	69.6	5.8
α-LP	12.5	12.8	68.2	6.5
β-LP	13.5	21.1	69.8	5.6
Baboon[3]				
Plasma	8.6 ± 2.0	9.8 ± 0.8	70.7 ± 2.7	10.9 ± 0.6
α-LP	8.1 ± 1.8	8.5 ± 1.4	73.9 ± 3.7	9.4 ± 1.3
β-LP	9.9 ± 1.1	11.4 ± 2.0	67.0 ± 2.9	11.6 ± 0.8

Lyso-PC = lysophosphatidylcholine; Sph. = sphingomyelin; PC = phosphatidylcholine; PEt = phosphatidyl ethanolamine; LP = lipoproteins.

1 Group of four normal white males between 20 and 25 years of age.
2 Average values of two determinations on pooled plasma from four individuals.
3 Average values of four individuals.

lesterol value. On the contrary, the baboon has definitely lower lipid and cholesterol levels. In both species triglyceride values are similar to man.

In the baboon and the chimpanzee, the amount of phospholipids is relatively higher than in man but the plasma cholesterol/phospholipid (C/PL) ratio is practically the same for man, chimpanzee and baboon. However, when comparing the separated lipoproteins, the C/PL ratio of the chimpanzee is more similar to that in man. The baboon shows higher ratios in α as well as in β, which may be explained as resulting differences in the phospholipid classes and in the apopolypeptide composition.

The percentage composition of the phospholipid classes is shown in table II. The chimpanzee values are very similar to those of man. In the baboon, the main difference is found in the ratio of phosphatidylcholine to sphingomyelin and phosphatidylethanolanine, both in β- and in α-lipoproteins.

The major fatty acids in plasma and in plasma lipoprotein of the three species are shown in table III. Again the chimpanzee values correspond best to those in man, whereas the baboon has more saturated fatty acids. The

Table III. Distribution of the major fatty acids in normal human and nonhuman primates

Subject	16:0[1]	16:1	18:0	18:1	18:2	20:4
Man[2]						
Plasma	21.3	3.4	7.5	23.7	37.0	7.1
α-LP	26.0	3.7	10.6	22.1	30.7	6.9
β-LP	22.2	3.9	6.3	22.9	38.5	6.2
Chimpanzee[3]						
Plasma	24.4	2.4	8.7	20.3	33.4	10.8
α-LP	26.1	2.9	10.9	20.8	28.4	10.9
β-LP	21.9	2.8	8.3	22.0	35.0	10.0
Baboon[4]						
Plasma	24.2	2.9	15.7	19.4	28.5	9.3
α-LP	25.5	2.7	17.3	19.4	25.1	10.0
β-LP	22.0	2.2	12.8	20.3	34.0	8.7

1 Major fatty acids are described by two quantities: the number of carbon atoms and the number of double bonds (e.g. 16:0).
2 Group of four normal white males between 20 and 25 years of age.
3 Average value of four individuals.
4 Average value of two plasma pools of four animals taken at an interval of six months.

striking fact shown in this table is the higher saturation percentage of α- over β-lipoproteins in all species [BLATON and PEETERS, 1969]. The arachidonic acid in α- and β-lipoproteins is higher in simians than in man.

The normal values presented here for man, chimpanzee and baboon document the differences in the lipoprotein patterns, in the plasma lipid ratios, in the plasma fatty acid composition and in the relative phospholipid composition. These differences become clearer after electrochromatographic lipoprotein separation into α- and β-fractions. The results indicate that for extrapolation from simian towards human pathology more information is required about normal biochemical values of nonhuman primates.

Acknowledgements

The authors thank Dr. J. MORTELMANS and Dr. J. VERCRUYSSE (RUCA-Zoo, Antwerpen) and Dr. M. VASTESAEGER, Centre d'Etude des Maladies des Artères coronaires, Bruxelles, for their collaboration.

References

BLATON, V. and PEETERS, H.: Lipid and fatty acid modifications in plasma lipoproteins of baboons under atherogenic diet. Acta zool. path., Antv. *48:* 233–242 (1969).

BLATON, V.; HOWARD, A.N.; GRESHAM, G.A.; VANDAMME, D., and PEETERS, H.: Lipid changes in the plasma lipoproteins of baboons given an atherogenic diet. I. Changes in the lipids of total plasma and of alpha and beta lipoproteins. Atherosclerosis *11:* 497–507 (1970).

BLATON, V. and PEETERS, H.: Integrated approach to plasma lipid and lipoprotein analysis; in NELSON Blood lipids and lipoproteins, pp. 269–331 (1971).

BLATON, V. and PEETERS, H.: Chimpanzee and baboon as biochemical models for human atherosclerosis; in GOLDSMITH and MOOR-JANKOWSKI Medical primatology 1972, part III, pp. 306–312 (Karger, Basel 1972).

BURNS, K.F.; FERGUSON, F.G., and HAMPTON, S.H.: Compendium of normal blood values for baboons, chimpanzees and marmosets. Amer. J. clin. Path. *48:* 484–494 (1967).

GRESHAM, G.A. and HOWARD, A.N.: Vascular lesions in primates. Ann. N.Y. Acad. Sci. *127:* 694–701 (1965).

KRITCHEVSKY, D.; SHAPIRO, I.L., and WERTHESSEN, N.T.: Biosynthesis of cholesterol in the baboon. Biochim. biophys. Acta *65:* 556–557 (1962).

PEETERS, H. and BLATON, V.: Comparison of lipid and lipoprotein patterns in primates. Acta zool. path., Antv. *48:* 221–231 (1969).

PEETERS, H.; BLATON, V.; DECLERCQ, B.; HOWARD, A.N., and GRESHAM, G.A.: Lipid changes in the plasma lipoproteins of baboons given an atherogenic diet. II. Changes in the phospholipid classes of total plasma and of alpha and beta lipoproteins. Atherosclerosis *12:* 283–290 (1970).

SU-CHEN, LI and YU-TEH, LI.: The protein and protein-bound carbohydrates in four species of non-human primates' sera. Proc. Soc. exp. Biol. Med. *127:* 1014–1017 (1968).

Authors' address: H. PEETERS and V. BLATON, Simon Stevin Institute for Scientific Research, Jerusalemstraat 34, *B-8000 Brugge* (Belgium)

Medical Primatology 1972. Proc. 3rd Conf. exp. Med. Surg. Primates, Lyon 1972, part III, pp. 343–349 (Karger, Basel 1972)

Spontaneous and Experimental Arterial Lesions in the Malaysian Long-Tailed Monkey

K. PRATHAP and K. S. LAU

Department of Pathology, Faculty of Medicine, University of Malaya, Kuala Lumpur

Introduction

Although there is now an extensive literature on arterial lesions in a wide variety of subhuman primates [1, 5, 6, 10], published information on atherosclerosis in the *Macaca fascicularis* is scanty [3].

M. fascicularis, is a long-tailed monkey commonly found in WestMalaysia. It lives within sight and sound of almost every village, in rubber estates, mangrove swamps and on the outskirts of most towns. Being a mixed feeder, this monkey is easily cared for in captivity and is well suited to experiments involving dietary manipulation. During the last five years we have studied spontaneous and experimentally-induced arterial lesions in this monkey. This report summarizes our findings.

Spontaneous Aortic Intimal Lesions

Autopsies were performed on 73 freshly-captured wild, adult, male monkeys to determine the extent of spontaneous arterial lesions. Aortas were fixed in 4% gluteraldehyde, stained with Sudan IV, and surface areas of intimal lesions quantitated by planimetry. Frozen and paraffin sections from all aortas were studied by light microscopy. A few selected lesions were studied by electron microscopy.

Fatty streaks were present in 66 aortas (90%). From zero to ten percent of the intimal surface was affected, with a mean of two percent. The morphology of the fatty streaks, including light microscopic and ultrastructural characteristics, was similar to that in other subhuman primates [8] and in man. The aortic valve region, the ductus scar region and a triangular area distal to the intercostal ostia were the characteristic common sites affected. Fibrous plaques were rare, with only six lesions in four aortas. All plaques were located at sites where fatty streaks normally occurred and were surrounded by a rim of sudanophilia. Complicated lesions were not seen in any of the aortas. Plasma cholesterol levels ranged from 70 to 210 mg/100 ml with a mean of 134. This corresponds to normal levels for Malaysians during the first and second decades of their life [4].

Diffuse areas of intimal roughening, seen with the naked eye in the abdominal aorta, consisted of two types of lesions when viewed under the dissecting microscope. The first of these, seen in 28 aortas (38%), consisted of closely-arranged linear intimal bands along the long axis of the aorta and forming a characteristic 'rick-rack' pattern (fig. 1). The second type of lesion

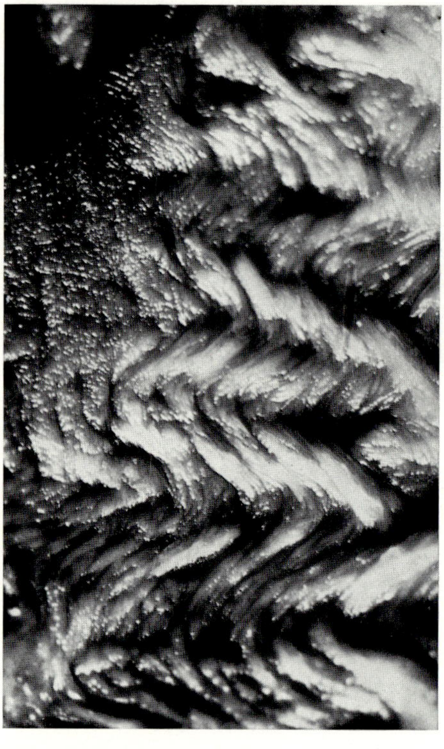

Fig. 1. 'Rick-rack' lesion seen in the abdominal aorta under the dissecting microscope. ×25.

consisted of similar intimal bands but with a wavy appearance. These lesions were not associated with intimal thickening on histological examination and are thought to be artefact caused by contraction of the muscular media.

Diet-Induced Atherosclerosis

Sixteen adult male *M. fascicularis* monkeys were divided into two equal groups and fed either a control diet or a high fat cholesterol-enriched experimental diet (containing zero to 15% total cholesterol) for periods ranging from two to four years. Within one to three months of commencing the experimental diet, the monkeys showed an elevation of their average plasma cholesterol level. This elevation was maintained within the range of 300–450 mg/100 ml throughout the experiment (fig. 2). Cholesterol levels of the control group remained unelevated. Both groups showed a gradual but steady increase in the average body weights.

All animals that were fed the experimental diet developed massive fatty

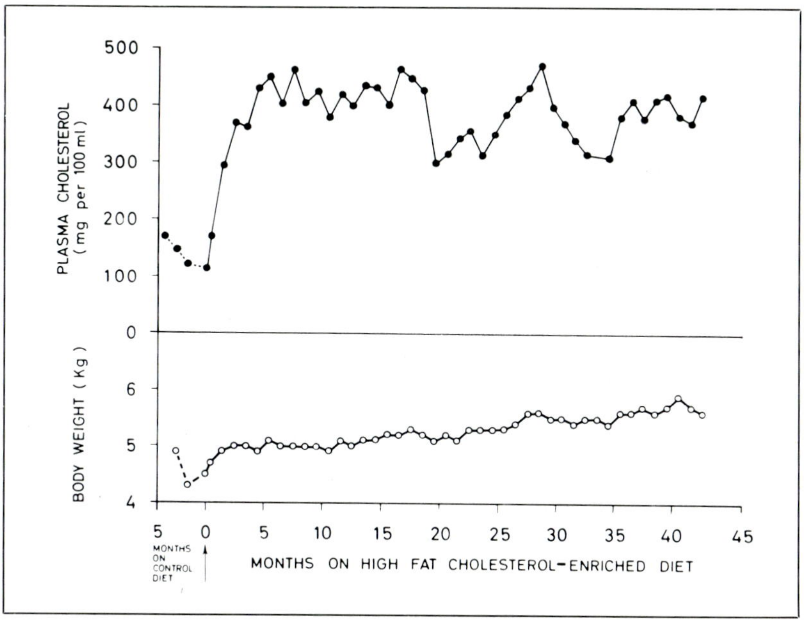

Fig. 2. Plasma cholesterol levels and body weights of monkeys fed the experimental diet. Each point represents the average of six to eight monkeys.

streaking of the aorta (fig. 3). Twenty-one to 78 % of the intimal surface was affected with a mean of 56 %. The distribution and morphology of the fatty streaks were similar to that in man. Fibrous plaques were present in aortas of all monkeys on the experimental diet. They were more common in the abdominal aorta than in the thoracic segment and were related to the ostia of arteries arising from the aorta. A variable amount of lipid was present in

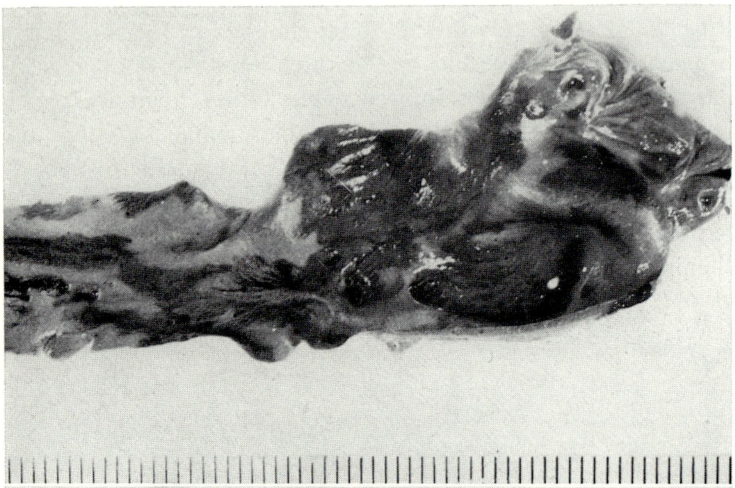

3

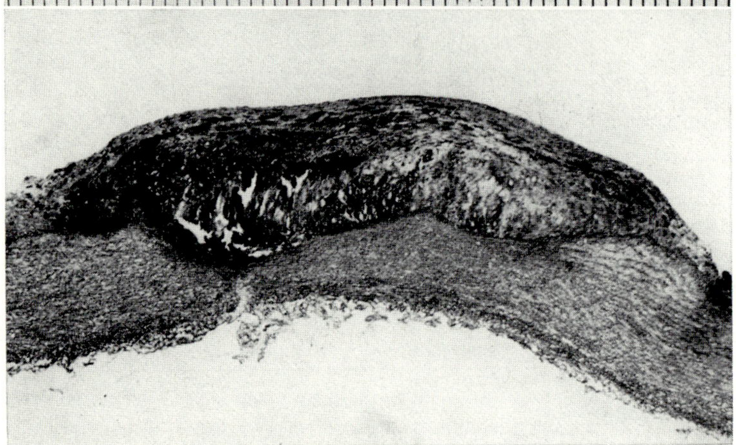

4

Fig. 3. Diet-induced fatty streaking of the aortic arch and upper thoracic aorta. Gross Sudan IV. × 1.5.

Fig. 4. Lipid-rich fibrous plaque in thoracic aorta. Oil red O. × 30.

every plaque. There were some 'soft' atherosclerotic plaques, as described in man by MONTGOMERY [7], which consisted of a lipid-rich, necrotic, juxtamedial zone covered by a fibrous cap (fig. 4). There was no grossly detectable thrombosis, hemorrhage or ulceration. Atherosclerotic lesions were also present in coronary, carotid, subclavian, iliac and femoral arteries.

Control monkeys showed only minimal fatty streaking with a mean involvement of the aortic intimal surface of two percent. Three small fibrous plaques were present in one aorta. No atherosclerotic lesions were grossly visible in any of the branches of the aorta in control monkeys.

The Fate of Mural Systemic Arterial Thrombi in Normocholesterolemic and Hypercholesterolemic Monkeys

A total of 50 monkeys were used for the study of healing arterial thrombi. Twelve monkeys were fed a high fat, cholesterol-enriched experimental diet, which resulted in a sustained elevation of their average serum cholesterol levels in the range of 300–450 mg/100 ml. The cholesterol levels of the remaining 38 monkeys that were fed a low fat diet, remained unelevated.

Sixty-six mural thrombi in the normocholesterolemic monkeys and 33 mural thrombi in the hypercholesterolemic monkeys were produced in femoral and carotid arteries by the intraluminal insertion of a catgut suture. The morphology of the resultant thrombi was studied at various intervals ranging from one hour to three years. The early natural history of the thrombi in normocholesterolemic animals was similar to that previously described in systemic arteries of pigs [2, 11]. By ten weeks the suture material had been completely removed and the thrombi were replaced by relatively avascular, lipid-free fibromuscular intimal thickenings [9]. There was no further change during the two-year period of observation (fig. 5).

In hypercholesterolemic monkeys, a small amount of lipid appeared in the thrombi during the phase of organization. Once organization was complete, however, there was no further accumulation of lipid within the thrombi. Indeed, two- and three-year-old intimal plaques contained less lipid than during the phase of organization, despite moderate hypercholesterolemia which caused the development of lipid-rich intimal plaques elsewhere in the arterial system. Foam cell aggregates developed on the luminal surface of a few healed thrombi. No evidence of hemorrhage, ulceration, central necrosis or fatty gruel was seen in any of the plaques even after three years of observation.

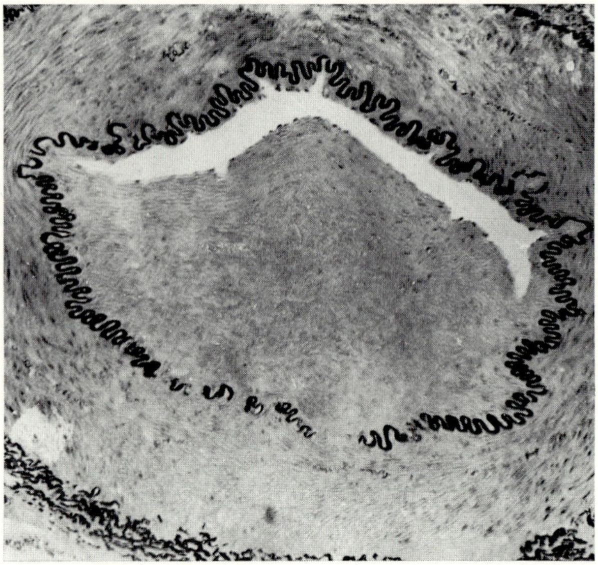

Fig. 5. Two-year-old thrombus in normocholesterolemic monkey. Elastic van Gieson. × 130.

Conclusions

(1) Fatty streaking of the aorta occurs spontaneously in 90% of free-ranging adult male *M. fascicularis*. This, together with its omnivorous nature, easy care in captivity and ready availability in Malaysia, favor this animal as a suitable model for the experimental study of atherosclerosis.

(2) Hypercholesterolemia can be readily induced in the *M. fascicularis,* as in other primate species, by feeding a high fat, cholesterol-rich diet. Persistent hypercholesterolemia regularly produces extensive atherosclerosis of the aorta and its main branches. Lesions produced include, in addition to fatty streaks, 'soft' atherosclerotic plaques.

(3) The healing of experimentally-induced mural systemic arterial thrombi in normocholesterolemic monkeys results in relatively stable, hard, fibromuscular plaques lacking the fatty gruel that is typically seen in 'soft' atherosclerotic plaques [7]. The lipid content of the plaques is slightly increased if the blood cholesterol level is raised during the phase of organisation. Nevertheless, the 'soft' lipid-rich atheromatous plaque cannot be explained on the basis of organization of mural systemic arterial thrombi even in the presence of persistent hypercholesterolemia.

References

1 GRESHAM, G.A. and HOWARD, A.N.: Vascular lesions in primates. Ann.N.Y.Acad. Sci. *127:* 696–701 (1965).

2 JORGENSEN, L.; ROWSELL, H.C.; HOVIG, T., and MUSTARD, J.F.: Resolution and organization of platelet-rich mural thrombi in carotid arteries of swine. Amer.J.Path. *51:* 681–719 (1967).

3 KRAMSCH, D.M. and HOLLANDER, W.: Occlusive atherosclerotic disease of the coronary arteries in monkey *(Macaca irus)* induced by diet. Exp. molec. Path *9:* 1–22 (1968).

4 LAU, K.S.; LOPEZ, G., and GAN, D.M.: Serum cholesterol levels in Malays, Indians and Chinese in Malaya. Med.J.Malaya *16:* 184–192 (1962).

5 LEHNER, N.D.M.; CLARKSON, T.B.; BULLOCK, B.C.; LOFLAND, H.B.; ST.CLAIR, R.W., and PRICHARD, R.W.: Studies on atherosclerosis of some nonhuman primates; in GOLDSMITH and MOOR-JANKOWSKI Medical primatology 1970, pp.873–885 (Karger, Basel 1971).

6 MALINOW, M.R. and MARUFFO, C.A.: Naturally occurring atherosclerosis in howler monkeys. J.Atheroscler.Res. *6:* 368–380 (1966).

7 MONTGOMERY, G.L.: In Scientific basis of medicine annual reviews, vol. 7, p.162 (Athlone Press, London 1959).

8 PRATHAP, K.: Spontaneous arterial lesions in wild adult Malaysian long-tailed monkeys *(Macaca irus)*. J.Path. (in press).

9 PRATHAP, K.: The morphology of two-year-old healed platelet-rich thrombi in femoral arteries of normocholesterolaemic monkeys. Light and electron microscopic observations. J.Path. (in press).

10 TAYLOR, C.B.; COX, G.E.; ESTRELLA, P.M., and SOUTHWORTH, J.: Atherosclerosis in Rhesus monkeys. II. Arterial lesions associated with hypercholesterolaemia induced by dietary fat and cholesterol. Arch.Path. *74:* 16–34 (1962).

11 WOOLF, N.; BRADLEY, J.W.P.; CRAWFORD, T., and CARSTAIRS, K.C.: Experimental mural thrombi in the pig aorta. The early natural history. Brit.J.exp.Path. *49:* 257–264 (1968).

Author's address: Dr. K. PRATHAP, Department of Pathology, Faculty of Medicine, University of Malaya, *Kuala Lumpur* (Malaysia)

Medical Primatology 1972. Proc. 3rd Conf. exp. Med. Surg. Primates, Lyon 1972, part III, pp. 350–355 (Karger, Basel 1972)

Nonhominid Primates for Experimental Cardiovascular Studies? A Fallacy!

H. L. RATCLIFFE

Institut für Tierpathologie, Universität Bern, Bern

Designs for experimental study of a disease process demand knowledge of at least its morphological characteristics from the earliest recognizable stages to its more advanced forms that impair function. Lack of adequate foundations for experimental design can lead, and in fact, has led to great waste, for it promotes erroneous concepts that can interfere with prevention and therapy.

To illustrate: relatively modern textbook discussions of tuberculosis are still based at least in part upon the results of experiments in which the disease had been induced by i.v. injection of bacilli in large numbers [VORWALD, 1932; HOPPS, 1959; WALTER and ISRAEL, 1970]. These discussions ignore other fully-documented studies that demonstrate that tuberculosis is most often an airborne infection, induced by inhalation of very few organisms, in fact usually one. Airborne tuberculosis induced in an appropriate species, for example, guinea pigs, reproduces rather completely morphological characteristics of this infection in man [RATCLIFFE and MERRICK, 1957]. Tuberculosis induced by i.v. injection does not [VORWALD, 1932; WELLS, 1955].

Similarly, experiments, presumably designed to explore the pathogenesis of cardiovascular disease, have been based upon the following assumptions: (1) lipid infiltration of the arterial intima is an initial phase in this disease process, (2) intimal lipid infiltration depends upon blood lipid levels, and (3) blood lipid levels depend upon intake [ADAMS, 1964; STRAUS and ROBERTS, 1965; TAYLOR, 1965]. Accordingly, various experimental animals have been subjected to a variety of manipulations, which certainly elevate blood lipids and induce vascular lesions. However, the significance of the results of these experiments, either in terms of pathogenesis or prevention of cardiovascular disease is questionable. Therefore, I protest the extension of experiments based on these assumptions to include nonhominid primates as experimental animals. These experiments have merely repeated with monotonous regularity exposure to the same highly-unbalanced diets and ignore other environmental factors.

Now, of course, a limited experience with the ways and wiles of man leads me to expect at best a negative response to this protest, for the results of these experimental dietary manipulations now constitute a basis for recommendations to modify extensively diets for man. These recommendations ignore the results of studies of man that demonstrate that development of cardiovascular disease, especially in younger age groups, most often reflects responses to psychosocial factors [Paul *et al.*, 1963; Dreyfuss *et al.*, 1969; Wolf, 1969; Theorell and Rahe, 1971]. They also ignore observations and experiments on lower animals that support the view that psychosocial factors are major stimuli for the development of cardiovascular disease [Ratcliffe and Snyder, 1967; Ratcliffe, 1968; Ratcliffe *et al.*, 1969; Henry *et al.*, 1971].

Thus, it may be that the present comments constitute an exercise in futility. Nevertheless, a critic should be permitted to suggest a plan that excludes both dietary manipulations and nonhominid primates.

Thus, the records of the Penrose Research Laboratory of the Zoological Society of Philadelphia, which are continuous since 1901, as well as the results of experiments based upon these records, demonstrate that mammals and birds maintained on diets of high quality ordinarily develop coronary atherosclerosis at a very slow rate [Ratcliffe, 1968]. When, however, their social environment is disturbed and they are subjected to intense psychosocial stimuli, coronary atherosclerosis has developed rapidly [Ratcliffe and Snyder, 1967; Ratcliffe *et al.*, 1969; Henry *et al.*, 1971]. Omnivorous and carnivorous mammals and birds as well as ruminants and nonruminant herbivores have shared this response with representatives of the family pongidae and other nonhominids [Ratcliffe, 1968]. Obviously then, demands for studies of cardiovascular disease with nonhominid primates as experimental animals are not supported by credible evidence. Other species can serve equally well.

But 'choice of models for experimental study of disease should be guided by the following criteria: (1) susceptibility under standard (physiological) systems of husbandry, i.e. systems that support efficient growth and reproduction, (2) ready availability at reasonable costs from established breeding lines, (3) ready trainability and size adequate for all projected laboratory procedures and (4) recognition that behavioral (psychosocial) reponses to experimental situations may determine results' [Ratcliffe and Luginbühl, 1971].

These criteria are especially applicable to experimental study of cardiovascular atherosclerosis. Obviously, however, they exclude all nonhominid primates and other exotic species and limit choice to very few species. Possibly, the most suitable of these is the domestic swine.

Here, one may object that a great majority of cardiovascular lesions induced either in exotic or experimental animals, including swine, by exposure to psychosocial stimuli have developed in the intramural coronary arteries (fig. 1). Thus, one may question the significance for mankind of intramural coronary lesions when significant lesions in man have been said by some to be limited to the proximal segments of the extramural coronary arteries [TJOTTA, 1963].

But, a detailed study of 223 hearts of adults has demonstrated that atherosclerotic lesions of the intramural coronary arteries are rarely absent in adults (fig. 2 and 3). In fact, these lesions were found in all hearts of this series, and atherosclerotic stenosis of the extramural coronary arteries correlated closely with the extent and severity of intramural coronary lesions

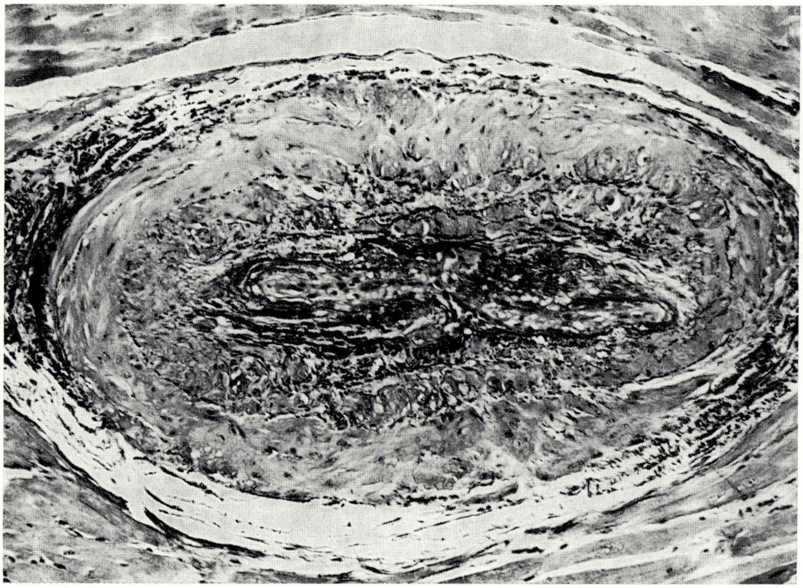

Fig. 1. Intramural coronary artery from a female swine aged 13 months. Note focal disorganization and thinning of the media, fractures and multiple replications of elastica interna, and intimal thickening by smooth muscle cells and elastic fibers which reduced lumina to a narrow slit. Formalin fixation. Weigert-Van Gieson-light green. × 170.

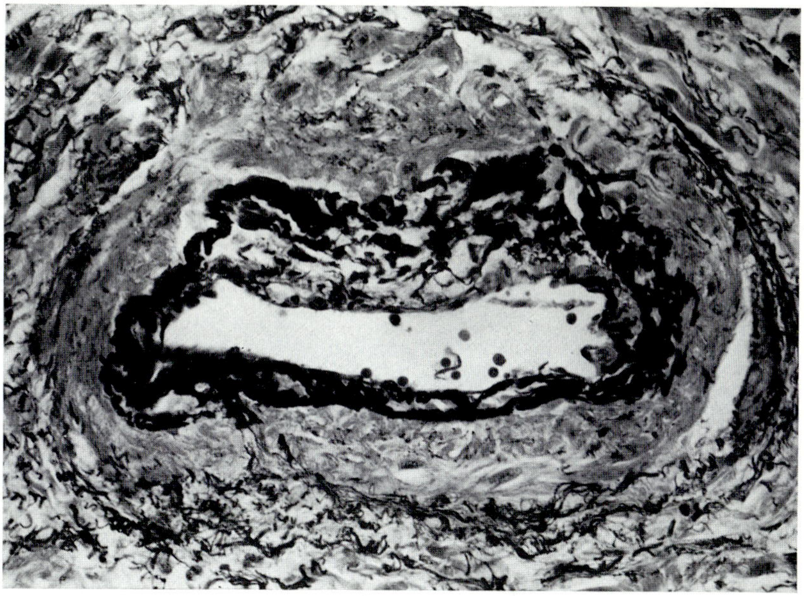

Fig. 2. Intramural coronary artery from a man, aged 68 years. Healed infarcts of myocardium, extramural arteries patent, death following resection of pancreatic carcinoma. Note focal disorganization of media and intimal thickening by dense elastic fibers among which smooth muscle cells were scattered, elastica interna not identifiable. Formalin fixation. Weigert-Van Gieson-light green. ×350.

[RATCLIFFE and REDFIELD, in press]. Further, the more advanced examples of intramural coronary atherosclerosis were commonly associated with microinfarction, whether or not macroinfarction had occurred. And in both exotic and experimental animals microinfarcts have fused to form macroscopic lesions.

Origin and progress of intra- and extramural coronary atherosclerosis have been traced to degeneration, proliferation, reorientation and migration of medial smooth muscle cells. These changes are combined with increased production of acid mucopolysaccharides, elastic and collagen fibers and fracture and replication of the elastica interna. Smooth muscle cells with their products pass through the fragmented elastica interna to accumulate under the endothelium and reduce lumina. In the deeper parts of larger lesions, especially of the extramural coronary arteries, smooth muscle cells accumulate lipid to become 'foam cells' that eventually degenerate and release their contents within the interstitium [LUGINBÜHL and JONES, 1965; RATCLIFFE *et al.*, 1970].

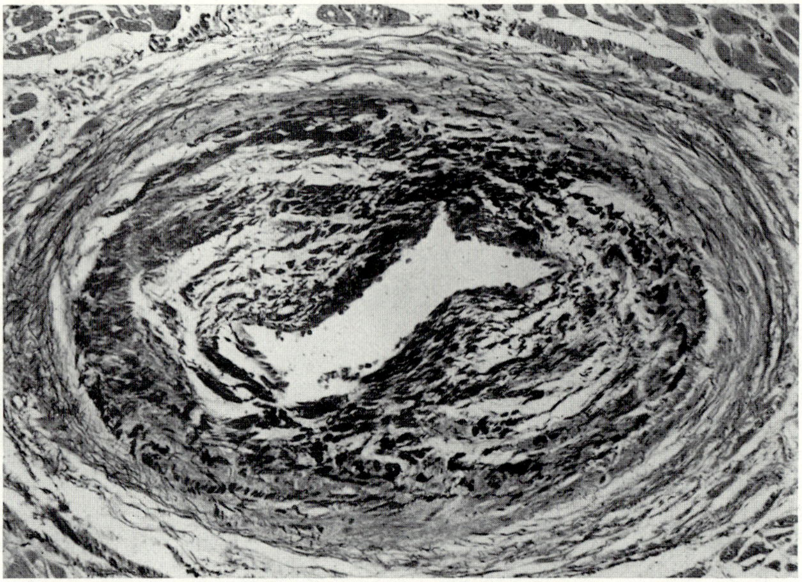

Fig. 3. Intramural coronary artery from a woman, aged 60 years. Extramural arteries patent, death attributed to myocardial weakness. Note smooth muscle cells of media largely replaced by collagen, internal elastica fragmented and partially fused with elastic fibers of lesion. Spaces in lesion occupied by mucopolysaccharide. Formalin fixation. Weigert-Van Gieson-light green. × 170.

Lesions of extramural coronary arteries have been rare in exotic animals maintained on high-quality diets [RATCLIFFE, 1968]. These lesions have been absent in swine and other experimental animals maintained on comparable diets. However, macroscopic extramural coronary lesions were found in 10 of 50 older female swine fed cooked urban garbage for eight to 14 years. This diet provided approximately 6 % protein and 12 % fat [RATCLIFFE *et al.*, 1970].

References

ADAMS, C. W. M.: Arteriosclerosis in man, other mammals and birds. Biol. Rev. *39:* 372–422 (1964).

DREYFUSS, F.; DASBERG, H., and ASSAEL, M. I.: The relationship of myocardial infarction to depressive illness. Psychother. Psychosom. *17:* 73–81 (1969).

HENRY, J. P.; ELY, D. L.; STEPHENS, P. M.; RATCLIFFE, H. L.; SANTISTEBAN, G. A., and SHAPIRO, A. P.: The role of psychosocial factors in the development of arteriosclerosis in CBA mice. Atherosclerosis *14:* 203–218 (1971).

HOPPS, H.C.: Principles of pathology, 2nd ed. (Appleton-Century-Crofts, New York 1959).

LUGINBÜHL, H. and JONES, J.E.T.: The morphology of spontaneous atherosclerotic lesions in aged swine; in ROBERTS and STRAUS Comparative atherosclerosis, pp. 3–10 (Harper & Row, New York 1965).

PAUL, O.; LEPPER, M.H.; PHELAN, W.H.; DUPERTUIS, G.W.; MACMILLAN, A.; MCKEAN H., and PARK, H.: A longitudinal study of coronary heart disease. Circulation *28:* 20–31 (1963).

RATCLIFFE, H.L.: Environment, behavior and disease; in STELLAR and SPRAGUE Progress in physiological psychology, vol. 2, pp. 161–228 (Academic Press, New York 1968).

RATCLIFFE, H.L. and LUGINBÜHL, H.: The domestic pic. A model for experimental atherosclerosis. Atherosclerosis *13:* 133–136 (1971).

RATCLIFFE, H.L. and MERRICK, J.V.: Tuberculosis induced by droplet nuclei infection. Its developmental pattern in guinea pigs and rats in relation to dietary protein. Amer. J. Path. *33:* 1121–1135 (1957).

RATCLIFFE, H.L. and REDFIELD, E.: Atherosclerotic stenosis of the extramural and intramural coronary arteries of man. Related lesions. Virchows Arch. path. Anat. (in press).

RATCLIFFE, H.L. and SNYDER, R.L.: Arteriosclerotic stenosis of the intramural coronary arteries of chickens. Further evidence of a relation to social factors. Brit. J. exp. Path. *48:* 357–365 (1967).

RATCLIFFE, H.L.; LUGINBÜHL, H., and PIVNIK, L.: Coronary aortic and cerebral atherosclerosis in swine of 3 age-groups. Implications. Bull. Wld Hlth Org. *42:* 225–234 (1970).

RATCLIFFE, H.L.; LUGINBÜHL, H.; SCHNARR, W.R., and CHACKO, K.: Coronary arteriosclerosis in swine. Evidence of a relation to behavior. J. comp. physiol. Psychol. *68:* 385–392 (1969).

STRAUS, R. and ROBERTS, J.C.: Summary of converence; in ROBERTS and STRAUS Comparative atherosclerosis, pp. 365–399 (Harper & Row, New York 1965).

TAYLOR, C.B.: Experimentally induced arteriosclerosis in nonhuman primates; in ROBERTS and STRAUS Comparative atherosclerosis, pp. 215–243 (Harper & Row, New York 1965).

THEORELL, T. and RAHE, R.H.: Psychosiocial factors and myocardial infarction. 1. An inpatient study in Sweden. J. psychosom. Res. *15:* 25–31 (1971).

TJOTTA, E.: The distribution of atheromatosis of the coronary arteries. Atherosclerosis *3:* 253–261 (1963).

VORWALD, A.J.: The early cellular reactions in the lungs of rabbits injected intravenously with human tubercle bacilli. Amer. Rev. Tuberc. *25:* 74–85 (1932).

WALTER, J.B. and ISRAEL, M.S.: General pathology (Churchill, London 1970).

WELLS, W.F.: Airborne contagion and air hygiene (Harvard University Press, Cambridge, Mass. 1955).

WOLF, S.: Psychosocial forces in myocardial infarction and sudden death; in BONDURANT Research on acute myocardial infarction, pp. 74–83 (American Heart Association Inc., New York 1969).

Author's address: Dr. H.L. RATCLIFFE, Institut für Tierpathologie, Universität, *CH-3000 Bern* (Switzerland)

Medical Primatology 1972. Proc. 3rd Conf. exp. Med. Surg. Primates, Lyon 1972, part III, pp. 356–367 (Karger, Basel 1972)

Progression and Regression of Experimental Atherosclerosis in Rhesus Monkeys[1]

H. C. Stary

Department of Pathology, Louisiana State University School of Medicine, New Orleans, La.

Introduction

We have been studying experimental atherosclerosis as induced in non-human primates by feeding diets containing cholesterol and high levels of fat. Some of the early work carried out at the Department of Pathology of Louisiana State University School of Medicine in New Orleans was in baboons, spider monkeys, and rhesus and has been previously reported [4]. In recent studies we have accepted the rhesus monkey *(Macaca mulatta)* as the most suitable experimental model to study the development of atherosclerotic lesions.

This paper is a report on two experiments in rhesus. The first deals with the progression of early aortic lesions over a period of up to 40 weeks after initiation of an experimental atherogenic diet. The purpose of this progression study was to determine the changes in serum cholesterol following the institution of the experimental diet, to correlate these changes with the extent of aortic atherosclerosis, and to investigate the nature of the developing lesions.

The second experiment deals with the regression of early aortic lesions

1 Supported by a grant-in-aid of research by the Louisiana Heart Association and by United States Public Health Service Grant HL 08974.

during periods of up to 40 weeks on commercial primate food following induction of lesions during a 12-week period on atherogenic food. A recent study indicates that large experimental lesions are not completely reversible and will, upon reduction of the serum cholesterol, be transformed into fibrous, lipid-poor plaques [3]. The intent of the present regression study was to determine whether or not small, early lesions could resorb without residual intimal thickening, to study the changes in serum cholesterol during the period following return from atherogenic to commercial primate food, and to explore the changes in the regressing lesions.

Preliminary observations on cell proliferation and ultrastructure in the developing atherosclerotic lesions of these rhesus monkeys have been reported [6, 7]. Detailed results on cell proliferation and ultrastructural changes will be published elsewhere. In this paper, the response of serum cholesterol to the dietary manipulations, and the gross observations on extent and nature of the atherosclerotic lesions in the aorta will be presented.

Methods

Experimental Design

Progression study. Fourteen male rhesus monkeys were used. Two animals (controls) received commercial primate food for eight weeks before being killed. Two animals received the atherogenic diet (see below) for four weeks, four animals for 12 weeks, and six animals for 40 weeks. One hour before being killed at the end of the experimental dietary periods, each animal received a single i.v. injection of thymidine-^{3}H to study cell proliferation in the normal aorta and in the atherosclerotic lesions.

Regression study. Eight male rhesus monkeys were used. Two animals (controls) received normal commercial primate food and were killed at the end of 52 weeks. The remaining six animals received the same experimental, atherogenic diet as that given to the animals in the progression study for 12 weeks. These six animals were selected from a group of 36 rhesus that had received the atherogenic diet for 12 weeks. The remaining animals in that group were used in a separate study [10]. The six animals selected for this study were ranked into three groups with similar mean serum cholesterols, according to mean serum cholesterol level during the induction period. After the 12-week period of lesion induction the six monkeys were returned to basal commercial primate food. Two of the animals were killed three weeks after return to the basal diet at which time the serum cholesterol levels had just returned to normal levels. This group served as lesion controls. Another two animals were killed 16 weeks following return to normal monkey food, and the last group of two animals were killed 40 weeks after reversal of the diet. Each animal in the regression study received one i.v. injection of thymidine-^{3}H eight hours, and a second injection one hour before death for studies on cell proliferation.

Animals and Experimental Diet

Male rhesus monkeys weighing 3.3–5.0 kg (mean 4.2 kg) in the 'progression study', and 5.8–7.2 kg (mean 6.4 kg) in the 'regression study' were used. The animals were obtained from Shamrock Farms, Middleton, N.Y., where they had been conditioned for six to eight weeks after importation. During this period they were dewormed, tested for tuberculosis and fed a low-fat, low-cholesterol commercial primate food. Following arrival at the laboratory the animals were maintained on baked primate food (Dietrich and Gambrills, Frederick, Md.), until the start of the experiments. The experimental atherogenic diet consisted of low-fat, low-cholesterol, baked commercial primate food supplemented with butter and beef tallow (3:1), casein, cholesterol, vitamin diet fortification mixture, and water. This diet provided 40% of the calories from carbohydrates, 20% from protein and 40% from fat. The diet contained 1 mg of cholesterol per calorie or 0.37% cholesterol by weight.

Evaluation of Aortic Lesions

Visual evaluation of atherosclerotic involvement of three aortic segments (arch, descending thoracic, and abdominal aorta) was by the method of Guzman *et al.* [5]. The grader estimated the percentage of the intimal surface area of each segment involved with any atherosclerotic lesions. He then estimated the percentage involved with fatty streaks or with fibrous plaques. Evaluations were made on two separate occasions and the mean of the two gradings was used.

Cholesterol Determination

Serum samples were obtained from all animals for determination of total serum cholesterols by the method of Abell *et al.* [1] at intervals from receival of the animals at the laboratory until they were killed. Samples were taken at one-week intervals at first, and less frequently later. Determinations were more frequent in the regression study.

Tissue Preparation

A complete autopsy was performed on each rhesus. The aorta was removed, and divided longitudinally into two equal parts. Before rinsing of the intimal surface, tissue samples were taken for electron microscopy from one lateral half. The remainder of this half of the aorta was fixed in formalin, stained with Sudan IV to determine the gross extent of lipid-containing intimal lesions, and sealed in a transparent plastic envelope by a method developed in the International Atherosclerosis Project [5]. The other lateral half of the aorta was processed for light microscopy and radioautography so that the entire vessel would be available for study. It was divided at the diaphragm, and the thoracic and the abdominal segments were each rolled into a coil which was fixed in Carnoy's solution. After embedding in paraffin, multiple sections were taken through each coil at two levels, the margin and the center of the roll. Slides were prepared for multiple stains and for radioautographic studies to be reported elsewhere.

Results

Progression Study

Most animals ate the experimental diet well. Only two of the 12 rhesus that received the experimental diet lost weight. The weight of the 14 animals in this experiment ranged from 3.3 to 5.0 kg (mean 4.2 kg) at the beginning of the experiment and from 4.2 to 5.3 kg (mean 4.6 kg) at the end (table I).

Serum cholesterol levels rose rapidly after the experimental diet was started. Maximum levels in each animal were reached after varying time periods (fig. 1). In general the steepest rise occurred within the first 15 weeks. Serum cholesterols of the three animals with the highest levels (850–1,040 mg/100 ml) leveled off after 15–30 weeks. One animal (No. 35) that had received the experimental diet for a period of 40 weeks remained resistant and the serum cholesterol did not rise above a level of 220 mg/100 ml.

Table I. Progression study. Body weights, serum total cholesterol levels (weighted mean in animals receiving the atherogenic diet for longer than four weeks), and extent of gross lesions in Sudan IV stained aortas after varying periods on the atherogenic diet

Weeks on atherogenic diet	Rhesus No.	Weight at start of experiment kg	Weight at end of experiment kg	Total serum cholesterol mg/100 ml	Percent aortic surface with lesions
0	45	4.7	4.5	130	0
(controls)	46	4.6	4.7	180	0
4	43	4.8	4.8	320	2
	44	5.0	4.9	560	9
12	27	4.0	4.7	500	11
	30	3.8	4.4	370	16
	33	3.9	4.7	760	30
	36	4.1	4.8	250	3
40	28	3.3	4.2	420	19
	29	3.8	4.6	760	69
	31	3.5	4.6	850	59
	32	4.6	4.4	680	39
	34	4.3	5.3	540	35
	35	4.1	4.4	200	2

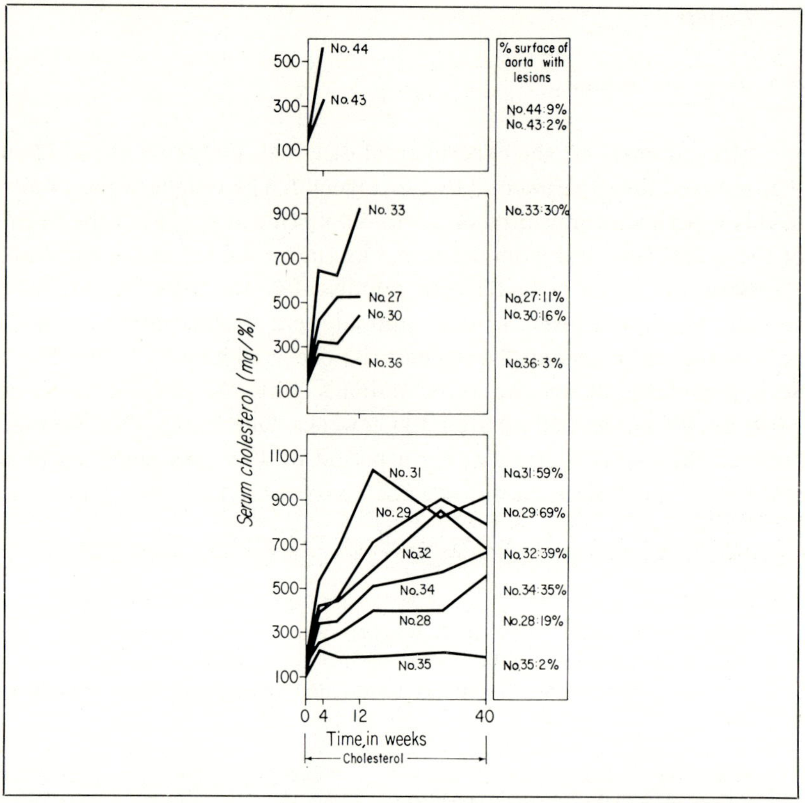

Fig. 1. Progression study. Varying susceptibility to hypercholesterolemia in rhesus receiving the atherogenic diet. The extent of gross atherosclerotic lesions in the aorta was determined after four, 12, and 40 weeks on the diet and is given in the column on the right.

Gross lesions were not seen in the aortas of the two control animals. The extent and the severity of lesions increased progressively with the duration of serum cholesterol elevation. Fatty streaks appeared as early as four weeks after start of the experimental diet (fig. 2). After 12 weeks there was marked increase in the extent and the severity of the lesions. All lesions were fatty streaks. While the six animals that had received the diet for 40 weeks still had predominantly fatty intimal streaks, the two animals with the most extensive involvement also showed early fibrous plaques in the descending thoracic aorta. No animal had complicated lesions or calcification in the aorta. The mean percentage of aortic surface involvement per group of animals increased from 5.5% at four weeks to 15% at 12 weeks, and 37% at 40 weeks. There

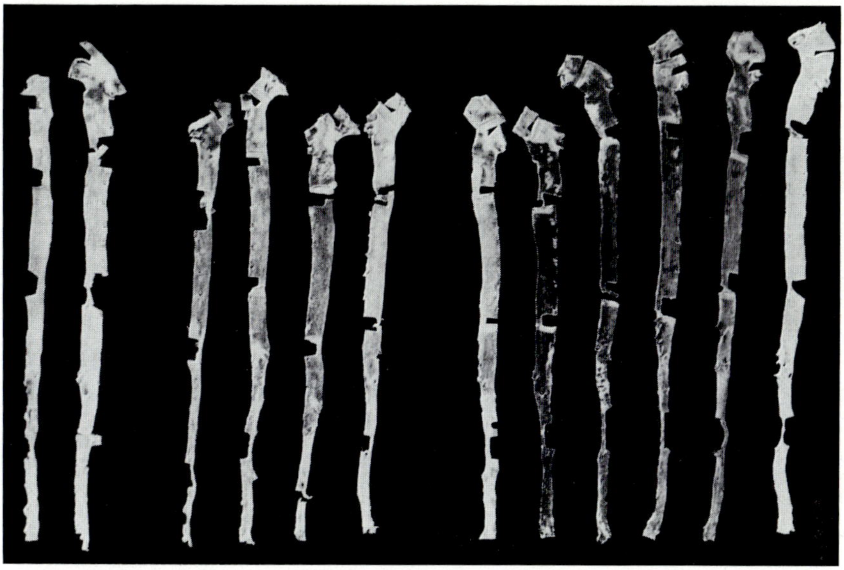

Fig. 2. Progression study. Lateral half of aortas stained with Sudan IV. Black areas in the intima represent lipid. Two aortas on the left are from rhesus that received the atherogenic diet for four weeks. The group of four aortas at left center is from animals on the diet for 12 weeks. The six aortas on the right are from animals on the diet for 40 weeks. The aorta on the extreme right is from a rhesus (No. 35) resistant to cholesterol.

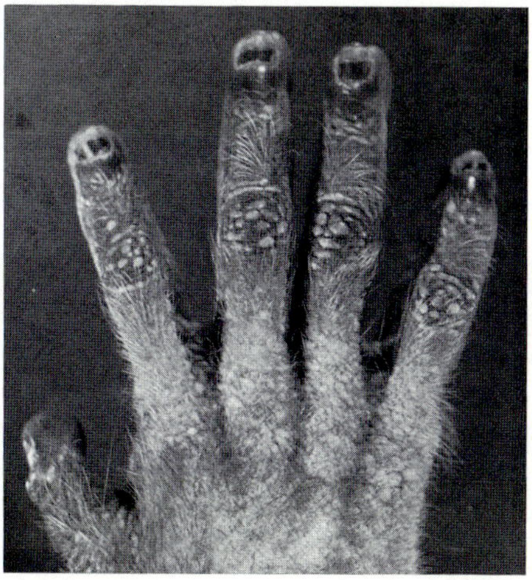

Fig. 3. Photograph of hand of rhesus No. 31 showing several groups of cutaneous xanthomata.

was a close relationship between the severity as well as the extent of intimal lesions and the degree of hypercholesterolemia (fig. 1). The two animals with early fibrous plaques (No. 29 and 31) and with the most extensive intima fatty streaks had the highest serum cholesterol levels. These two rhesus also developed cutaneous xanthomata on both hands and feet after about eight months on the diet (fig. 3).

Regression Study

The animals in the 'regression study' were older than those in the 'progression study'. The weight of the eight animals ranged from 5.8 to 7.2 kg (mean 6.4 kg) at the start of the experiment. All animals that received the

Table II. Regression study. Body weights, weighted mean total serum cholesterol levels in the 12-week period during which lesions were induced with an atherogenic diet, and extent of gross lesions in Sudan IV stained aortas after varying periods of reversal of the atherogenic diet to normal monkey food

Diet	Rhesus No.	Weight at start of experiment kg	Weight at end of experiment kg	Mean total serum cholesterol during induction period mg/100 ml	Percent aortic surface with lesions
12 weeks atherogenic,	53	6.4	6.8	290	20
3 weeks normal food	69	7.2	8.2	550	46
12 weeks atherogenic,	61	7.1	8.0	490	10
16 weeks normal food	80	6.1	8.0	380	32
12 weeks atherogenic,	57	6.4	7.8	470	8
40 weeks normal food	62	5.8	8.5	430	6
52 weeks normal food	68	6.5	8.7	110	2
(controls)	77	5.8	7.7	130	2

experimental diet gained weight during the 12-week lesion induction period. After having been returned to normal commercial primate food (regression period) the animals continued to gain weight. At the end of the experiment their weight ranged from 6.8 to 8.7 kg (mean 8.0 kg) (table II).

Serum cholesterol levels rose rapidly after beginning the experimental diet, and continued to rise during the 12-week induction period. When the animals were returned to the commercial primate food, the serum cholesterol levels fell rapidly, and normal levels were regained in one to three weeks (fig. 4). The greater part of the fall in the cholesterol level occurred within the first week following diet reversal. The variation in the speed with which serum cholesterol levels dropped from elevated levels to normal was small

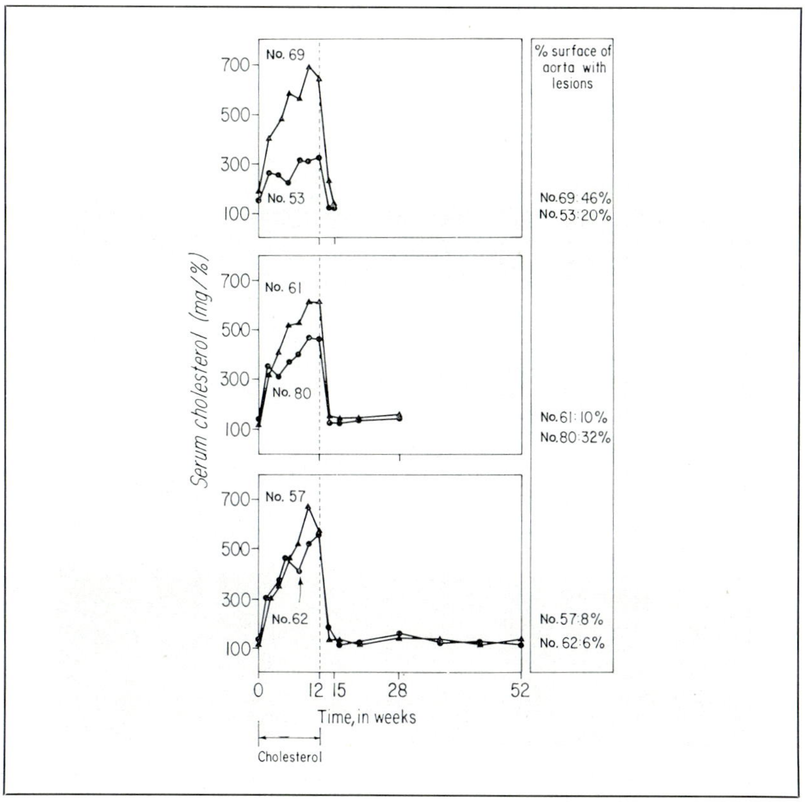

Fig. 4. Regression study. Rapid fall in serum cholesterol levels when the atherogenic diet is followed by normal primate food. The extent of gross atherosclerotic lesions was determined three, 16, and 40 weeks after diet reversal.

from animal to animal and does not appear to depend on the degree of the initial serum cholesterol elevation in this short-term experiment.

Although the animals in this regression experiment were fed the identical experimental diet as the animals in the progression study, they developed more extensive lesions in the aorta, as shown by the comparison of the group that received the experimental diet for 12 weeks in the progression study with the group that served as lesion controls in the regression study, also fed the diet for 12 weeks. The group that served as lesion controls had extensive involvement of the aortic intima with fatty streaks (mean 33 % of surface). There were no advanced lesions. After 16 weeks on the regression diet the extent of aortic involvement decreased to a mean of 21 % of intimal surface. A more striking reduction in aortic surface involvement to a mean of 7 % occurred in the two animals that received the regression diet for 40 weeks

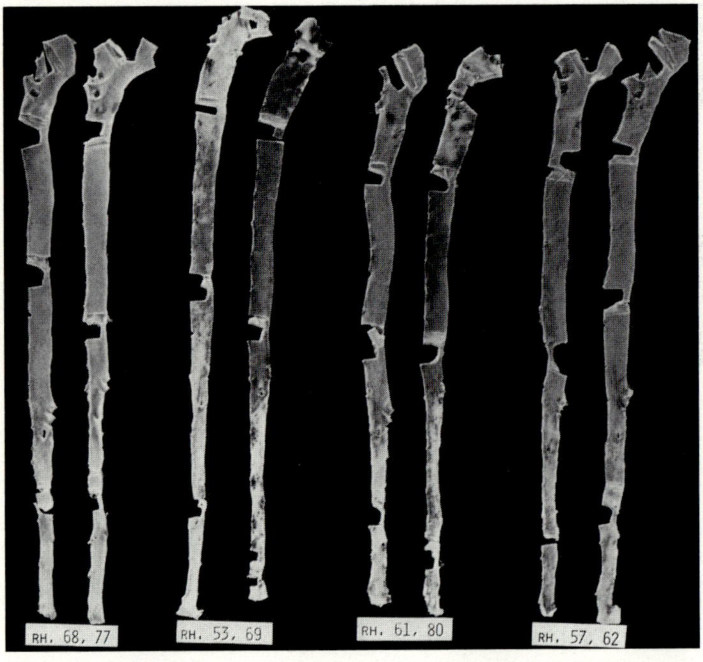

Fig. 5. Regression study. Lateral half of aortas stained with Sudan IV. Black areas in intima represent lipid. Two aortas on the left are from animals (No. 68 and 77) that received normal food. To the right are aortas from rhesus that received the atherogenic diet for 12 weeks followed by normal food for 3 (No. 53 and 69), 16 (No. 61 and 80), and 40 weeks (No. 57 and 62).

(fig. 5). While fatty streaks in the abdominal aorta showed a progressive decrease in extent and in severity, they appeared to regress at a slightly slower rate than lesions in the thoracic aorta.

Discussion

The animals showed wide individual variation in their response to the atherogenic diet. Rhesus No. 35 ate the diet for 40 weeks but remained resistant, with serum cholesterol levels close to normal for the entire period. Whether the animals were hypo- or hyperresponders to the experimental diet, the individual characteristic difference in response remained throughout the experiment. This striking variation is not as apparent in the regression study, since these animals had been preselected for more homogeneous serum cholesterol response. In general, the extent of the aortic lesions in the individual animals showed a good correlation with both the height of the serum cholesterol, and with the period of time the cholesterol remained elevated. The correlation is quite close and it appears possible to predict in the living rhesus the extent of aortic atherosclerosis from a knowledge of the degree and the duration of the serum cholesterol elevation. TAYLOR and co-workers [9] have also found a relationship between the severity of aortic lesions and the degree and period of hypercholesterolemia in rhesus, but they state that the development of lesions is not directly proportional to these factors. A similarly close correlation between serum cholesterol levels and the extent of aortic atherosclerosis was not observed in our experiments with cholesterol-fed rabbits [8]. However, in this group of rabbits the mean serum cholesterol level was 2,000 mg/100 ml. It is possible that when the serum cholesterol rise exceeds a certain level, differences in the response of the intima may become obscured. The association between serum cholesterol levels and the extent of aortic lesions might not be as close if one were to extend the duration of the study to allow development of complicated lesions. Factors other than dietary cholesterol might come into play when plaques become ulcerated or calcified. Similarly complicated lesions may not regress as readily as fatty streaks even after drastic reductions in the serum cholesterol level.

The regression study showed that early fatty streaks in the aorta can disappear when serum cholesterol is reduced to low levels. The few intimal lesions remaining after 40 weeks on the regression regimen were limited to a few areas of the aortic intima. Preliminary light and electron microscopic observations do not indicate residual lesions in areas that appear grossly uninvolved. It must be re-emphasized that the lesions studied here were early lesions, and that advanced or complicated lesions may not disappear with such facility.

In the present progression and regression studies the intimal lesions that developed during the initial 12-week period of cholesterol feeding were more severe in the older rhesus used in the regression study. This occurred even though there was no significant difference in the serum cholesterol level with manifest age. Thus the age of the animal apparently influences atherogenesis. The controls which in each experiment had received commercial primate food showed no lesions in the younger animals (No. 45 and 46). In the older control animals (No. 68 and 77) there were minimal lesions.

The aorta was not uniformly involved with lesions. The intimal lesions were consistently both more extensive and more severe in the descending segment of the thoracic aorta. This preference for location in the descending thoracic aorta did not change with the duration of hypercholesterolemia. It is possible that with even longer periods of hypercholesterolemia lesions in other segments of the aorta may begin to predominate. We have some tentative indication that the early lipid deposits in the thoracic aorta may be more active metabolically than those in the abdominal segment, since in the regression study lesions in the thoracic aorta diminished somewhat more rapidly than those in the abdominal aorta. Inasmuch as the number of animals in this regression study was small, these results must be interpreted with caution. But the tentative findings support those of ANITSCHKOW [2] who observed that in rabbits during regression of aortic lesions the lipid first disappeared from lesions located in the aortic arch and persisted longest in those located in the distal aorta.

Acknowledgements

The author is indebted to Dr. D. A. EGGEN for his advice and help with the maintenance of the rhesus monkeys.

References

1 ABELL, L. L.; LEVY, B. B.; BRODIE, B. B., and KENDALL, F. E.: A simplified method for the estimation of total cholesterol in serum and demonstration of its specificity. J. biol. Chem. *195:* 357–366 (1952).

2 Anitschkow, N.: Über die Rückbildungsvorgänge bei der experimentellen Atherosklerose. Verh.dtsch.Ges.Path. *23:* 473–478 (1928); in Zbl.allg.Path. path.Anat., suppl. ad vol.43 (1928).

3 Armstrong, M.L.; Warner, E.D., and Connor, W.E.: Regression of coronary atheromatosis in rhesus monkeys. Circulat.Res. *27:* 59–67 (1970).

4 Eggen, D.E.; Strong, J.P., and Newman III, W.P.: Experimental atherosclerosis in primates. A comparison of selected species. Ann.N.Y.Acad.Sci. *162:* 110–119 (1969).

5 Guzmán, M.A.; McMahan, C.A.; McGill, H.C., Jr.; Strong, J.P.; Tejada, C.; Restrepo, C.; Eggen, D.A.; Robertson, W.B., and Solberg, L.A.: Selected methodologic aspects of the international atherosclerosis project. Lab.Invest. *18:* 479–497 (1968).

6 Stary, H.C.: Radioautographic observations on DNA synthesis of aortic atherosclerosis in rhesus monkeys. Circulation *40:* suppl.3, p.25 (1969).

7 Stary, H.C.: Electron microscopic observations on the progression of aortic atherosclerosis in rhesus monkeys. Circulation *42:* suppl.3, p.9 (1970).

8 Stary, H.C. and McMillan, G.C.: Kinetics of cellular proliferation in experimental atherosclerosis. Arch.Path. *89:* 173–183 (1970).

9 Taylor, C.B.; Cox, G.E.; Manalo-Estrella, P., and Southworth, J.: Atherosclerosis in rhesus monkeys. Arch.Path. *74:* 28–46 (1962).

10 Tucker, C.; Strong, J.; Catsulis, C., and Eggen, D.: Regression of cholesterol-induced atherosclerotic lesions in rhesus. Circulation *44:* suppl.2, p.48 (1971).

Author's address: H.C.Stary, MD, Department of Pathology, Louisiana State University School of Medicine, 1542 Tulane Avenue, *New Orleans, LA 70112* (USA)

Medical Primatology 1972. Proc. 3rd Conf. exp. Med. Surg. Primates, Lyon 1972, part III, pp. 368–375 (Karger, Basel 1972)

Phospholipid Synthesis by the Monkey Fetus

W. A. REYNOLDS, R. M. PITKIN and L. J. FILER, Jr.

Department of Anatomy, University of Illinois, Chicago, Ill., and Departments of Obstetrics and Gynecology and Pediatrics, University of Iowa, Iowa City, Iowa

Introduction

The opportunity to sample the fetal environment came into being in the 1960's with the advent of amniocentesis. It seems likely that analysis of amniotic fluid (AF) to indicate the genetic and physiologic well-being of the fetus will reach full flowering in the 1970's. The quest for a simple, sure index of fetal maturity has not yet been resolved. Recently, GLUCK and colleagues [2] reported that lecithin (L) levels in AF rise suddenly and predictably after 35 weeks of gestation while sphingomyelin (S) levels decrease slightly at that

Table I. Experimental population and procedure

Experiment	Maternal circulation	Fetal circulation	Est. fetal age, days	Fetal weight, g
B	–	^{14}C-choline, $NaH_2P^{32}O_4$	100–110	162.5
F		^{14}C-choline, $NaH_2P^{32}O_4$	100–110	220.0
C_1	^{14}C-choline		110–120	242.3
1236	^{14}C-choline	$NaH_2P^{32}O_4$	110–120	270.0
E	–	^{14}C-choline, $NaH_2P^{32}O_4$	110–120	280.0
K	$NaH_2P^{32}O_4$	^{14}C-choline	115–125	285.0
T	–	^{14}C-choline, $NaH_2P^{32}O_4$	133[1]	295.7
C_2	–	^{14}C-choline, $NaH_2P^{32}O_4$	130–140	303.0
J	^{14}C-choline	$NaH_2P^{32}O_4$	130–140	329.0
1232	^{14}C-choline	$NaH_2P^{32}O_4$	135	335.0
L	$NaH_2P^{32}O_4$	^{14}C-choline	135	343.0
S	–	^{14}C-choline, $NaH_2P^{32}O_4$	153[1]	461.1

1 Dated pregnancy, *Macaca speciosa*.

point. Supposedly, the increase in L:S ratio is a reflection of maturation of the fetal lung, the L in AF being a derivative of lung surfactant. Currently, the L:S ratio is subject to widespread clinical trials [5, 7, 9] since it is hoped that the L:S ratio can accurately reflect fetal lung maturity and thus be used to prevent premature delivery followed by respiratory distress syndrome. However, controversy has arisen as to whether the L:S ratio represents true evidence of fetal lung maturity [2] or whether instead it is yet another index of gestational age [7]. The critical issue is the source of the L and S found in AF in late gestation.

We have embarked upon a series of experiments involving the synthesis of these two phospholipids in relation to their appearance in AF in the pregnant monkey.

Methods

Pregnant macaques (rhesus, *Macaca mulatta,* or stump-tailed, *M.speciosa*) in the last third of gestation were either purchased commercially or derived from the primate breeding colony at the University of Illinois Medical Center. Estimations of fetal age were made using data from other colonies [3, 4] as well as data compiled concerning fetal length, weight and sex with respect to species from several hundred pregnancies studied experimentally at the Illinois facility (table I) [6].

Choline chloride-1,2-^{14}C and ^{32}P-monosodium phosphate (New England Nuclear Corp., Boston, Mass. and Mallinckrodt Chemical Works, St. Louis, Mo.) were injected simultaneously into the interplacental vessels of the fetus or in some instances, one labeled compound was placed into the maternal circulation and one into the fetal circulation (table I). Choline-^{14}C and ^{32}P-phosphate levels placed into the fetal circulation ranged from 10 to 20 and 0.2 to 1.0 mCi, respectively; choline-^{14}C and ^{32}P-phosphate levels injected into maternal circulation ranged from 10 to 25 and 0.4 to 1.0 mCi, respectively. Access to the fetal circulation was gained by transilluminating the uterus in order to visualize the vasculature connecting the bipartite placenta characteristic of most macaque pregnancies, in order to insert a T-tube. Thus, the fetus is undisturbed and the amniotic sac remains intact during the sampling period. Samples of maternal venous blood, fetal blood and AF were then obtained at intervals over the next five hours. At the end of the experimental period, each fetus was delivered by cesarean section and killed. Cerebrospinal fluid (CSF) was sampled by aspiration through the cisterna magna; tracheal fluid was removed by aspiration from a tracheostomy incision. Samples of placenta, liver, trachea, brain, muscle and lung were dissected free, and weighed prior to analysis. An aliquot of each blood and AF sample was used for assaying the movement of radioactivity between the three fluid compartments: maternal blood, fetal blood and AF. Plasma and AF samples were diluted with water and Instagel (Packard Instrument Co., Downers Grove, Ill.) was added in preparation for liquid scintillation counting. All radioactivity was measured by simultaneous double-labeled counting of samples in a Packard Tri-Carb 3375 liquid scintillation counter with Absolute Activity Analyzer so that all data were derived as d.p.m. The second aliquot of each fluid sample and all tissue samples were extracted in chloroform-methanol (2:1 for fluids, 3:1 for tissues) for lipid extraction followed by chromatography on a DEAE column. The technique followed is essentially that of GLUCK and colleagues [2] with some minor modifications due to the limitations in sample size available, such as fetal blood and trachea. The isolated fractions were further purified by TLC. Each spot was identified and removed, dissolved in Aquasol (New England Nuclear Corp.) and subjected to simultaneous double-label counting.

Results and Discussion

Whether the labeled precursors were placed initially in maternal or in fetal circulation, quick access was gained to the opposite side of the placenta. For example, when ^{14}C-choline was placed in the fetal circulation (fig. 1) radioactivity appeared in the maternal circulation and AF within minutes.

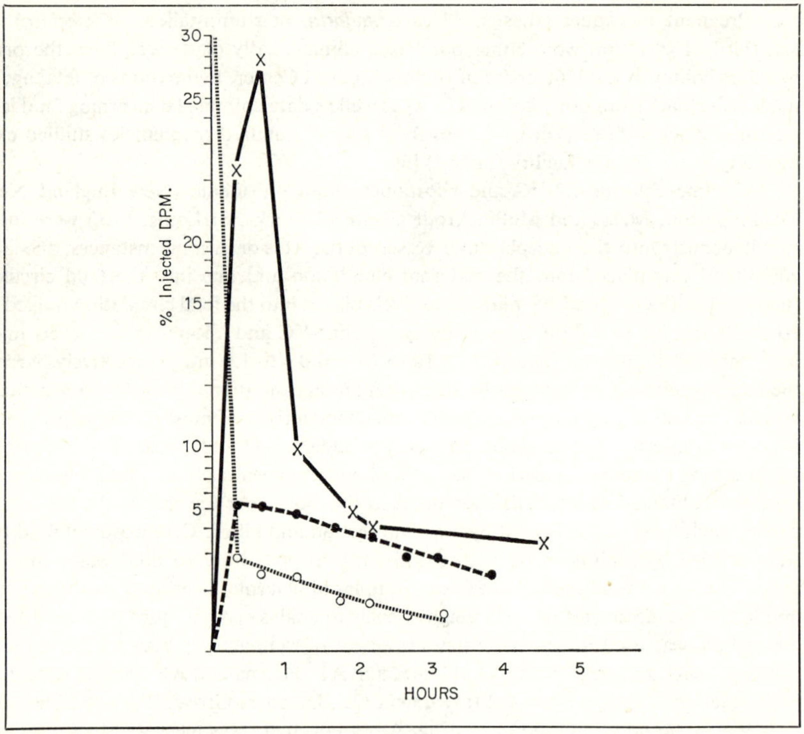

Fig. 1. Radioactivity levels following fetal administration of ^{14}C-choline. ○ = Fetal plasma; × = maternal plasma; ● = AF.

When ^{32}P-phosphate was placed in the maternal circulation (fig. 2), it quickly was found in the fetal circulation and, ultimately, in AF, but at a slower rate than for choline. It was interesting to note that, regardless of where ^{32}P-phosphate was initially administered, the fetal circulation retained a greater percentage of the injected radioactivity than did the maternal circulation. This is all the more remarkable since the maternal blood volume is some 7–10 times greater than that of the fetus.

^{14}C was incorporated into L and S in AF in a temporal sequence (fig. 3). Maximum ^{14}C-L levels were found in AF some 90 min after administration of ^{14}C-choline while peak ^{14}C-S values were observed at 3½ h postinjection. Peak levels of ^{14}C-L and ^{14}C-choline appeared in the fetal plasma in each instance about an hour before reaching maximum levels in AF (fig. 3). It was surprising to note the rapid loss of the two labeled phospholipids from AF, suggestive of a rapid rate of turnover.

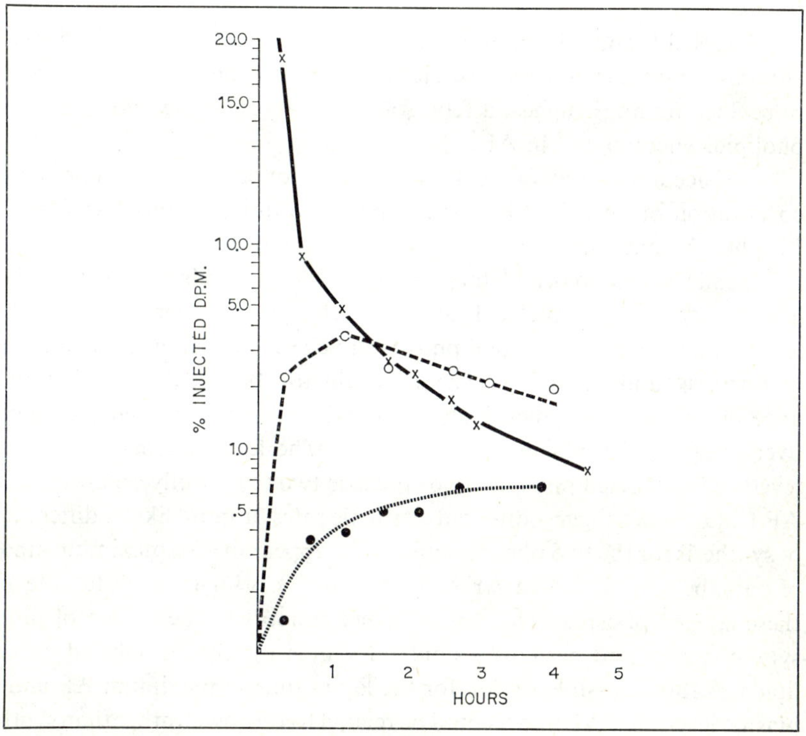

Fig. 2. Radioactivity levels following maternal administration of ^{32}P phosphate. ○ = Fetal plasma; × = maternal plasma; ● = AF.

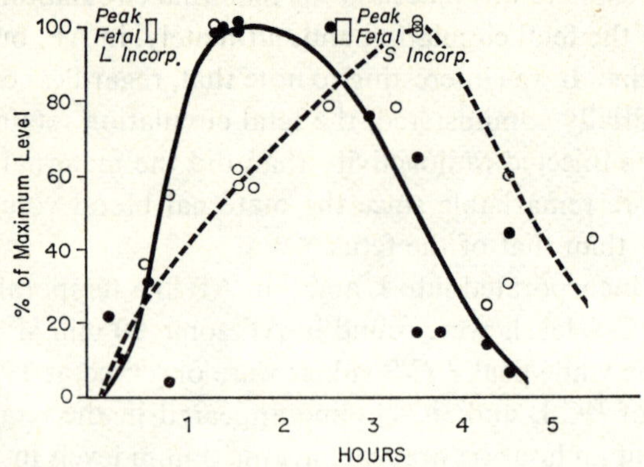

Fig. 3. AF accumulation of L (●) and S (○) after ^{14}C-choline incorporation.

Labeled L and S levels in maternal circulation were highly variable after administration and did not exhibit any peak time of ^{14}C-choline incorporation. Such findings suggest a fetal source for most of the two labeled phospholipids encountered in AF.

AF accumulations of ^{32}P-L and S were not separated in time. Peak incorporation of label in AF L and S occurred quickly, about an hour after ^{32}P-phosphate administration (fig. 4). The time of appearance of maximum AF L and S preceded peak fetal plasma ^{32}P-L and S levels by nearly two hours. The peak period of labeled L and S in fetal plasma corresponds well with maximum ^{32}P labeling of total phospholipids in fetal rabbit plasma observed by BIEZINSKI and KIMMEL [1]. These investigators believe that the slow appearance of fetal plasma labeled phospholipids reflects an inability of the fetal liver to synthesize plasma phospholipids. The fact that peak fetal plasma levels of ^{14}C-labeled phospholipids precede two temporally separate peaks of AF L and S may suggest different synthetic rates or more likely, different sites of synthesis for the two phospholipids. The appearance of maximum amounts of ^{32}P-labeled L and S in AF some two hours prior to peak fetal levels of these labeled phospholipids lends further support to the notion of different synthetic sites and perhaps a nonfetal source for the ^{32}P-labeled phospholipids. A third possible reason for the lag in time in maximum AF and fetal plasma levels of ^{32}P-L and S could be related to turnover rather than synthesis. Phospholipase C cleaves between phosphate and glycerol while phospholipase C cleaves between phosphorus and choline. Thus, it is possible that diffe-

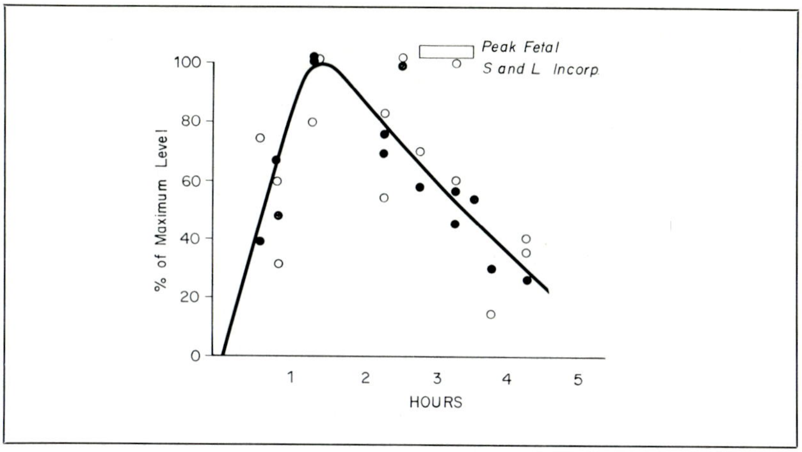

Fig. 4. AF accumulation of L (●) and S (○) after ^{32}P incorporation.

rences in enzyme activity in AF and fetal blood could account for a more rapid turnover of the ^{32}P moiety in AF than in fetal blood, shunting apparent ^{32}P maximum incorporation back to the left (fig. 4).

No obvious differences with respect to rate of incorporation of isotope were found with differences in fetal age. These experiments were acute, however, and involved pulse-labeling so that alterations in rates of phospholipid incorporation of label with increasing maturity probably could not be perceived.

Tissue levels of ^{32}P-L and S after five hours administration of the label are reflected in table II. The greatest amounts of labeled L and S were observed in the placenta, long known as an organ of extensive and rapid lipid synthesis [7].

Table II. Tissue levels of labeled L and S following ^{32}P administration

Tissue	^{32}P-L d.p.m./g	^{32}P-S d.p.m./g
Placenta	1,200–3,000	500–2,000
Liver	700–2,200	1,100–2,100
Trachea	750–1,250	700–2,000
Brain	500–1,700	400–1,600
Muscle	800–1,100	1,000–1,300
Lung	350–500	325–450
CSF	125–450	65–400

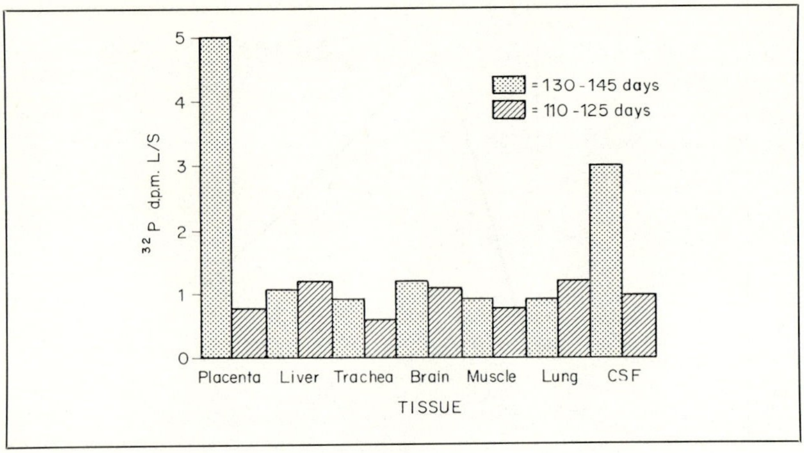

Fig. 5. ^{32}P L:S ratios in various fetal tissues.

Extensive incorporation of ^{32}P into liver L and S also occurred, similar to findings in the fetal rabbit liver [1]. The high tracheal levels and low lung levels of labeled L and S are a paradox. However, a pulse dose of label was administered some five hours prior to termination of the experiment and possibly labeled phospholipids moved from the lung into the trachea during that time.

L:S ratios in tissues following ^{32}P administration are graphed in figure 5. Only in two tissues, placenta and CSF, do the L:S ratios demonstrate a clear-cut increase as term approaches. The increasing ratio in CSF may be a phenomenon of myelination. The increasing L:S ratio in placenta supports the findings of other studies indicating an accumulation of placental phospholipids as term approaches.

Future studies will involve shorter intervals after administration of labeled precursors in order to study tissue incorporation, especially that of the respiratory tract, into phospholipids. Further, the phospholipase activity of AF in relation to L and S turnover in AF will receive close scrutiny.

References

1 BIEZINSKI, J.J. and KIMMEL, B.: Inability of fetal liver to synthesize plasma phospholipids. Proc. Soc. exp. Biol. Med. *130:* 1238 (1969).

2 GLUCK, L.; KULOVICH, M.; BORE, R.C.; BRENNER, P.H.; ANDERSON, G.G., and SPELLACY, W.W.: Diagnosis of the respiratory distress syndrome by amniocentesis. Amer. J. Obstet. Gynec. *109:* 440 (1971).

3 FUJIKURA, T. and NIEMANN, W.H.: Birth weight, gestational age and type of delivery in rhesus monkeys. Amer. J. Obstet. Gynec. *97:* 76 (1967).

4 HEUSER, C.H. and STREETER, G.L.: Development of the macaque embryo. Carnegie Contrib. Embryol. *525:* 15 (1941).

5 NELSON, G.H.: Relationship between amniotic fluid lecithin concentration and respiratory distress syndrome. Amer. J. Obstet. Gynec. *112:* 827 (1972).

6 REYNOLDS, W.A. and PITKIN, R.M.: Unpubl. obs. (1972).

7 ROUX, J.F.; NAKAMURA, J.; BROWN, E., and SWEET, A.Y.: The lecithin-sphingomyelin ratio of amniotic fluid: an index of fetal lung maturity? Pediatrics *49:* 464 (1972).

8 ROUX, J.F. and YOSHIOKA, T.: Lipid metabolism in the fetus during development. Clin. Obstet. Gynec. *1970:* 595.

9 WHITE, C.A.; MUSIALA, T.S., and WITTE, D.L.: Amniotic fluid lecithin/sphingomyelin ratio as a measure of fetal pulmonary maturity. J. Iowa St. med. Soc. *62:* 279 (1972).

Authors' address: Drs. W. ANN REYNOLDS, ROY M. PITKIN and L.J. FILER, jr., Department of Anatomy, University of Illinois at the Medical Center, *Chicago, IL* (USA)

Medical Primatology 1972. Proc. 3rd Conf. exp. Med. Surg. Primates, Lyon 1972, part III, pp. 376–381 (Karger, Basel 1972)

Pitfalls of Experimental Atherosclerosis in the Chimpanzee[1]

M. M. VASTESAEGER, J. VERCRUYSSE and J. J. MARTIN

Department of Social Cardiology, Faculty of Medicine, University of Brussels, Royal Society of Zoology and Bunge Institute, Antwerp

Introduction

Phylogeny and metabolism make pongidae closer to man than any other subhuman primates. Chimpanzees, for instance, feed naturally on an omnivorous diet comparable in most aspects to the human diet [GOODALL, 1963]. In a colony of captive chimpanzees, the mean plasma cholesterol was much higher than in any observed group of captive simians [VASTESAEGER and DELCOURT, 1966a], and the dispersion of individual values was as wide as in a western human population [DELCOURT *et al.*, 1964]. Furthermore, the first alterations of intimal sclerosis appear very early in apes as well as in humans [VASTESAEGER and DELCOURT, 1966b]. Finally, comparative studies in primates [PEETERS and BLATON, 1968] have shown that the nature and composition of plasma lipoproteins are almost identical in man and chimpanzee.

Experimental Observation

In light of the above considerations, the chimpanzee appears to be a most suitable experimental model for the study of human atherosclerosis and, in 1965, our team started experimental investigations on 16 captive chimpanzees. Eight of them were fed a 2.5-percent cholesterol high fat diet (40% of the calories being derived from fat most of which was saturated) the eight controls being kept on the usual diet of the Zoo (12% of the calories deriving from fat).

1 Supported in part by grants of the 'Fonds de la Recherche scientifique médicale' and 'Ruca-Zoo'.

After a few days on the diet, one of the animals died of haemorrhagic rectocolitis, and we had to procure a substitute for the programme. Chimpanzees for sale were not common at that time and the authors were very happy to buy from a circus a ten-year-old female, named Suzy, which had recently developed an hemiparesis of the left side after an accident but was otherwise in excellent health.

Upon introduction in the study and before being fed the experimental diet, the cholesterol levels of Suzy were fairly high (400 mg%), but still within the range of the starting values of the other experimental animals (220–420 mg%) and of the 'normal' levels in the above-mentioned colony of captive chimpanzees (120–470 mg% [DELCOURT *et al.*, 1964]).

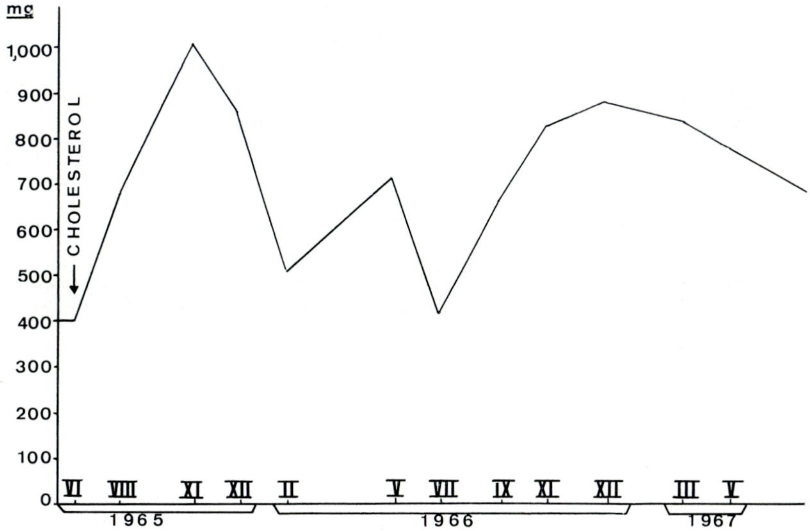

Fig. 1. Evolution of Suzy's plasma cholesterol level before and during the experiment.

In the first weeks on the diet, Suzy's blood cholesterol rose abruptly and, during the following years, it varied between 500 and 900 mg% (fig. 1).

One morning, she died unexpectedly.

Autopsy revealed that the cause of death was a large fresh infarction of the anterior wall of the left ventricle, due to an occluding thrombus on stenosing lesions of the anterior descending branch of the left coronary artery (fig. 2). Multiple stenosing atheromatous plaques were observed in the circumflex branch of the left coronary artery and in the right coronary artery. Numerous atherosclerotic plaques were also seen in the descending thoracic and in the abdominal aorta.

The macroscopic examination of the brain revealed softening in the right cerebral hemisphere: the putamen, the lateral pallidal segment, the upper part of the internal cap-

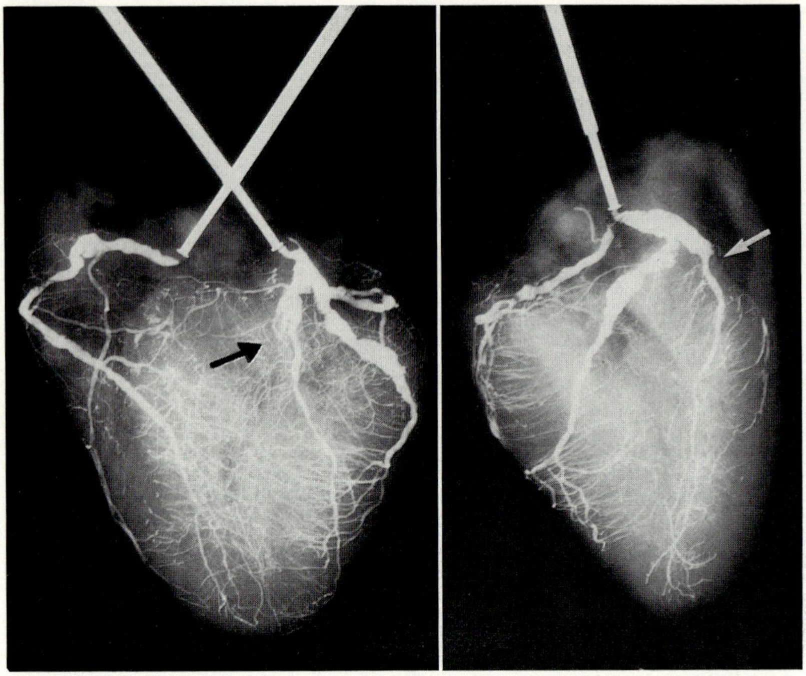

a, b

Fig. 2. Post mortem arteriography of the coronary bed of Suzy. *a* Front view. *b* Profile. → = Site of obstruction of the anterior descending branch.

sule and the juxtaventricular area of the centrum ovale were involved (fig. 3a and b). The right lateral ventricle was dilated with thalamic atrophy of the same side.

Instead of the expected traumatic lesion, the microscopic examination showed:

(a) A recanalized thrombotic occlusion of the middle cerebral artery on an atheromatous process with cholesterol crystals, calcium deposits and adventitial lymphoplasmocytic infiltration (fig. 4). The vertebral arteries also showed atheromatous lesions, whereas the smaller branches often presented fibrotic or hyaline changes.

(b) The striato-capsular necrosis was at the terminal stage of organization with cavitation surrounded by astrocytic gliosis and demyelination as in lesions of very long standing.

Fig. 3. Right cerebral hemisphere (frozen section, Spielmeyer for myelin. ×6.6). *a* Section through the lenticular nucleus (putamen + pallidum). Necrosis of the putamen, the lateral pallidal segment, the upper part of the internal capsule, the caudate nucleus and the adjacent white matter. *b* Section through the thalamus caudalis and the geniculate bodies. The necrosis is here restricted to the caudate nucleus and the surrounding white matter. Demyelination in the laterodorsal part of the thalamus.

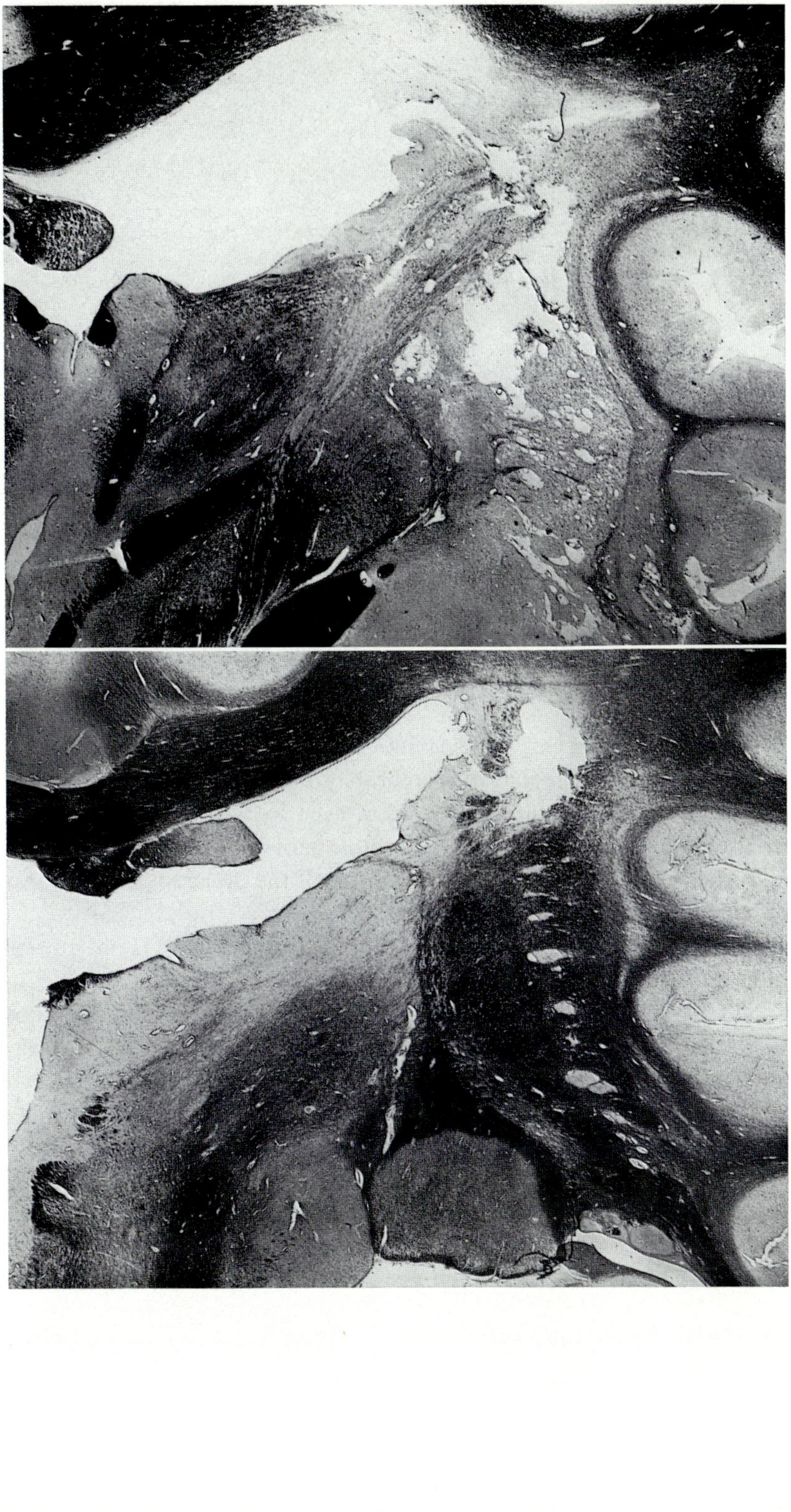

a

b

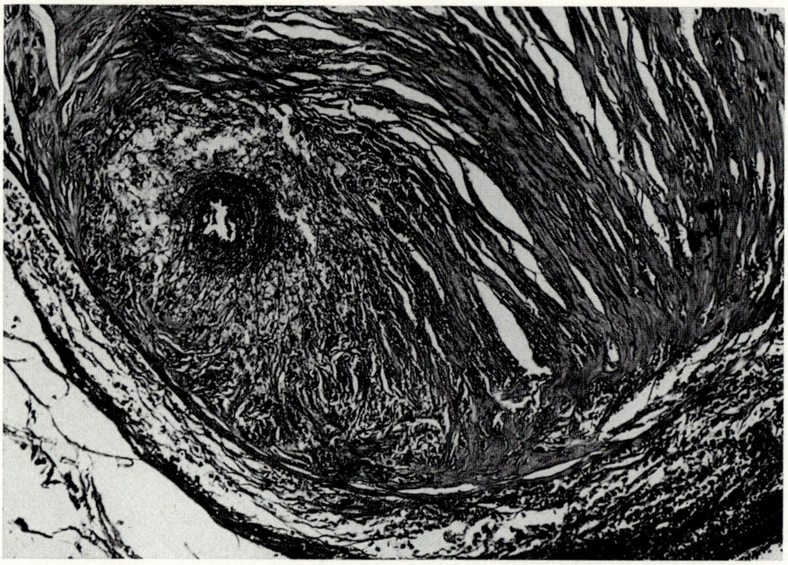

Fig. 4. Right middle cerebral artery (paraffin, HE. × 75). Severe atheromatosis with cholesterol clefts, thrombosis and recanalization, adventitial cellular infiltration.

Discussion

As hemiparesis was pre-existing before the animal was put on the diet, it is easily conceivable that the cerebral lesion developed spontaneously, i.e. before any experimental influence. So, even in the most favourable hypothesis, the diet just accelerated the evolution of spontaneous atherosclerosis, and it may well be that the natural course of the disease was little, or not at all, affected by the diet.

Early lethal myocardial infarction in the chimpanzee is not an unheard of event [MANNING, 1942] and it may well be that Suzy had essential hypercholesterolaemia. In any case, if, by chance, the initial spontaneous cerebral lesion had had no clinical expression during life, one would not have been able to detect the pre-existence of spontaneous atherosclerosis in a young adult animal, and the whole *post mortem* picture would have been erroneously attributed to the experimental intervention.

Of course, in our case, a previous angiography of the brain would have shown the pre-existing occlusion of the middle cerebral artery, but even arteriography of the cerebral or coronary bed does not enable non-stenosing plaques to be detected.

This experience places experimental atherosclerosis on the horns of a dilemma:

Either: to experiment upon species not vulnerable to spontaneous atherosclerosis and metabolically different from man; transposing the experimental data to spontaneous disease would then be very hazardous;

or: to use species vulnerable to spontaneous atherosclerosis and metabolically close to man; in such conditions of long-term experiments, sorting out the natural evolution of the spontaneous lesions from the experimental atherogenesis is a knotty, or may be, an insoluble problem.

References

DELCOURT, R.; NINANE, G.; OSTERRIETH, P. et VASTESAEGER, M.: Le métabolisme lipidique du chimpanzé. Acta cardiol. *19:* 531 (1964).

GOODALL, J.: My life among wild chimpanzees. Nat. Geogr. *124:* 272–308 (1963).

MANNING, G.W.: Coronary disease in the ape. Amer. Heart J. *23:* 719 (1942).

PEETERS, H. and BLATON, V.: Comparison of lipid and lipoprotein pattern in primates. Acta zool. Path. Antw. *48:* 221 (1968).

PEETERS, H. and BLATON, V.: Comparative biochemistry of normal human and nonhuman primates; in GOLDSMITH and MOOR-JANKOWSKI Medical primatology 1972, part III, pp. 336–342 (Karger, Basel 1972).

VASTESAEGER, M. et DELCOURT, R.: L'athérosclérose expérimentale du chimpanzé. Recherches préliminaires. Acta cardiol. *11:* 283 (1966a).

VASTESAEGER, M. and DELCOURT, R.: Some aspects of spontaneous and experimental cardiovascular disease in Old World monkeys and pongidae; in FIENNES Some recent developments in comparative medicine, pp. 179–194 (Academic Press, London 1966b).

Authors' address: Dr. MARCEL M. VASTESAEGER, Dr. J. VERCRUYSSE and Dr. J. J. MARTIN, Social Cardiology, Faculty of Medicine, University of Brussels, *Brussels* (Belgium)

Index